Typical Absences and Related Epileptic Syndromes

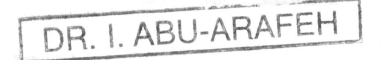
Edited by

J.S. Duncan MA DM FRCP
Senior Lecturer in Neurology
Institute of Neurology
London, UK

C.P. Panayiotopoulos MD PhD
Consultant in Clinical Neurophysiology and Epilepsy
St Thomas' Hospital
London, UK

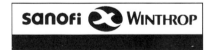

Supported by an educational grant from Sanofi Winthrop as a service to medicine

CHURCHILL COMMUNICATIONS EUROPE

CHURCHILL COMMUNICATIONS INTERNATIONAL LONDON MADRID NEW YORK AND TOKYO 1995

CHURCHILL COMMUNICATIONS EUROPE
CHURCHILL COMMUNICATIONS INTERNATIONAL

For trade and general sales a Churchill Livingstone imprint of
this publication (ISBN 0443 052697) is distributed by Churchill
Livingstone, Robert Stevenson House, 1-3 Baxter's Place, Leith
Walk, Edinburgh, EH1 3AF and by its associated companies,
branches and representatives throughout the world.

© Churchill Communications Europe Limited 1995

First published 1995

Authors' Dedication
We dedicate this book to our wives,
Liz Duncan and Thalia Panayiotopoulos,
and to our children,
Alex and Anna Duncan, Sophia and Paris Panayiotopoulos

Typeset by Saxon Graphics Ltd, Derby
Printed in Great Britain by Biddles Ltd, Guildford, Surrey

Preface

Over the last decade there have been significant advances in the understanding of the neurophysiological, anatomical and pharmacological mechanisms that underlie typical absences, at cellular, neuronal network and whole brain levels. Many new and diverse research methods have been developed and applied to this area. There has also been a dramatic increase in knowledge of the syndromes of idiopathic generalised epilepsy in which typical absences occur and the treatments that are available.

In 1993 it became apparent to us that researchers were working in several different fields, all pertaining to typical absences, and that the time was ripe to gather together the leading workers in these areas to share developments and cross-fertilise ideas. This meeting occurred over three days at a Symposium at the Royal Society of Medicine, London in June 1994, and this volume was produced out of the Symposium to draw together all aspects of current knowledge and advances in this area.

The book comprises contributions written by the Symposium participants and also includes transcripts of the discussion sessions at the end of the appropriate chapters. In some areas consensus was easily achieved. Others remain controversial, such as whether the sub-syndromes of idiopathic generalised epilepsy should be regarded as separate entities or as a neurobiological continuum. Some fields, for example the genetic basis of typical absences, still await major discoveries.

Everyone involved in this project has worked very hard to ensure that this book is available as soon as possible after the manuscripts were written. We are particularly grateful to Jenny Harry of Churchill Communications Europe for organising the publishing process so efficiently and to Sanofi Winthrop, without whose unrestricted educational grant the Symposium and this book would not have been possible.

London, 1994

John Duncan
Chrysostomos Panayiotopoulos

Contents

Contributors

Jean Aicardi
Institute of Child Health, London, UK

Eva Andermann
Montreal Neurological Institute, McGill University, Montreal, Quebec, Canada

Frederick Andermann
Montreal Neurological Institute, McGill University, Montreal, Quebec, Canada

Richard Appleton
The Roald Dahl EEG Unit, Royal Liverpool Children's NHS Trust, Alder Hey, Liverpool, UK

Gus A Baker
Dept of Neurosciences, Walton Hospital, Liverpool, UK

Samuel F Berkovic
Austin Hospital, Heidelberg, Victoria, Australia

Amedeo Bianchi
Centro Epilessia – UO Neurologia, Ospedale San Donato, Arezzo, Italy

Norman G Bowery
Dept of Pharmacology, The School of Pharmacy, London, UK

Martin J Brodie
Epilepsy Research Unit, University Dept of Medicine and Therapeutics, Western Infirmary, Glasgow, Scotland

M Bureau
Centre Saint-Paul, Marseilles, France

Zhen Cao
Dept of Medicine (Neurology), Duke University and Durham Veterans Administration Medical Centers, Durham, North Carolina, USA

David Chadwick
Dept of Neurological Science (Liverpool University), The Walton Centre for Neurology and Neurosurgery, Liverpool, UK

Astrid Chapman
Dept of Neurology, Institute of Psychiatry, London, UK

Elizabeth Chroni
Dept of Clinical Neurophysiology and Epilepsy, St Thomas' Hospital, London, UK

AML Coenen
NICI, Dept. of Psychology, University of Nijmegen, The Netherlands

Douglas A Coulter
Dept of Neurology, Medical College of Virginia, Richmond, Virginia, USA

Fritz E Dreifuss
School of Medicine, University of Virginia Health Sciences Center, Charlottesville, Virginia, USA

Bernard Duché
Dept of Neurology, University Hospital, Bordeaux, France

Connie C Duncan
Uniformed Services University of Health Sciences, Bethesda, Maryland, USA

John S Duncan
Institute of Neurology, National Hospital for Neurology and Neurosurgery, London, UK

Colin D Ferrie
Dept of Clinical Neurophysiology and Epilepsy, St Thomas' Hospital, London, UK

David R Fish
Institute of Neurology, National Hospital for Neurology and Neurosurgery, London, UK

R Mark Gardiner
University College London Medical School, The Rayne Institute, London, UK

Pierre Genton
Centre Saint-Paul, Marseilles, France

Stylianos Giannakodimos
Dept of Clinical Neurophysiology and Epilepsy, St Thomas' Hospital, London, UK

Pierre Gloor
Montreal Neurological Institute and the Dept of Neurology and Neurosurgery, McGill University, Montreal, Quebec, Canada

Lennart Gram
University Clinic of Neurology, Hvidovre Hospital, Denmark

Edouard Hirsch
Unité d'Explorations Fonctionnelles des Epilepsies, Hôpitaux Universitaires, Strasbourg, France

David A Hosford
Depts of Medicine (Neurology) and Neurobiology, Duke University and Durham Veterans Administration Medical Centers, Durham, North Carolina, USA

Italian League Against Epilepsy Collaborative Group

Ann Jacoby
Centre for Health Services Research, University of Newcastle-upon-Tyne, UK

Dieter Janz
Universitätsklinikum Rudolf Virchow, Dept of Neurology, Berlin, Germany

John Jefferys
Dept of Physiology and Biophysics, St Mary's Hospital Medical School and Imperial College of Science, Technology and Medicine, London, UK

Diane L Kraemer
Dept of Medicine (Neurology), Duke University and Durham Veterans Administration Medical Centers, Durham, North Carolina, USA

W Lason
Neuropeptide Research Dept, Institute of Pharmacology, Polish Academy of Sciences, Cracow, Poland

Tadeu Lemos
Dept of Pharmacology, The School of Pharmacy, London, UK

Miriam L Levav
Laboratory of Psychology and Psychopathology, National Institute of Mental Health, National Institutes of Health, Bethesda, Maryland, USA

Fu-hsiung Lin
Dept of Medicine (Neurology), Duke University and Durham Veterans Administration Medical Centers, Durham, North Carolina, USA

Pierre Loiseau
Dept of Neurology, University Hospital, Bordeaux, France

Richard AL Macdonell
Austin Hospital, Heidelberg, Victoria, Australia

Christian Marescaux
Unité d'Explorations Fonctionnelles des Epilepsies, Hôpitaux Universitaires, and INSERM U398, Strasbourg, France

H-J Meencke
Universitätsklinikum Rudolf Virchow, Dept of Neurology, Berlin, Germany

R Michelucci
Dept of Neurology, University of Bologna, Bellaria Hospital, Bologna, Italy

Allan F Mirsky
Laboratory of Psychology and Psychopathology, National Institute of Mental Health, National Institutes of Health, Bethesda, Maryland, USA

Jeffrey L Noebels
Dept of Neurology, Neuroscience and Molecular Genetics, Baylor College of Medicine, Houston, Texas, USA

Chrysostomos P Panayiotopoulos
Dept of Clinical Neurophysiology and Epilepsy, St Thomas' Hospital, London, UK

L Parmeggiani
Dept of Neurology, University of Bologna, Bellaria Hospital, Bologna, Italy

D Passarelli
Dept of Neurology, University of Bologna, Bellaria Hospital, Bologna, Italy

Martin Prevett
Institute of Neurology, National Hospital for Neurology and Neurosurgery, London, UK

B Przewlocka
Neuropeptide Research Dept, Institute of Pharmacology, Polish Academy of Sciences, Cracow, Poland

R Przewlocka
Neuropeptide Research Dept, Institute of Pharmacology, Polish Academy of Sciences, Cracow, Poland

David C Reutens
Austin Hospital, Heidelberg, Victoria, Australia

Edward H Reynolds
Kings College Hospital, London, UK

Douglas A Richards
Dept of Pharmacology, The School of Pharmacy, London, UK

Alan Richens
University of Wales College of Medicine, Cardiff, UK

P Riguzzi
Dept of Neurology, University of Bologna, Bellaria Hospital, Bologna, Italy

Richard O Robinson
Paediatric Neurology, Guy's Hospital, London, UK

Joseph Roger
Centre Saint-Paul, Marseilles, France

G Rubboli
Dept of Neurology, University of Bologna, Bellaria Hospital, Bologna, Italy

JWAS Sander
Institute of Neurology, National Hospital for Neurology and Neurosurgery, London, UK

Simon Shorvon
Institute of Neurology, National Hospital for Neurology and Neurosurgery, London, UK

Shelagh JM Smith
Dept of Clinical Neurophysiology, National Hospital for Neurology and Neurosurgery, London, UK

John Stephenson
Royal Hospital for Sick Children, Glasgow, UK

Gregory Stores
University of Oxford, Oxford, UK

Carlo A Tassinari
Dept of Neurology, University of Bologna, Bellaria Hospital, Bologna, Italy

ELJM van Luijtelaar
NICI, Dept. of Psychology, University of Nijmegen, The Netherlands

M Vergnes
Unité d'Explorations Fonctionnelles des Epilepsies, Hôpitaux Universitaires, Strasbourg, France

L Volpi
Dept of Neurology, University of Bologna, Bellaria Hospital, Bologna, Italy

Stephen Waltz
Universitätsklinikum Rudolf Virchow, Dept of Neurology, Berlin, Germany

Ying Wang
Dept of Medicine (Neurology), Duke University and Durham Veterans Administration Medical Centers, Durham, North Carolina, USA

Peter S Whitton
Dept of Pharmacology, The School of Pharmacy, London, UK

Arnold Wilkins
MRC Applied Psychology Unit, Cambridge, UK

John T Wilson
Dept of Medicine (Neurology), Duke University and Durham Veterans Administration Medical Centers, Durham, North Carolina, USA

Peter Wolf
Klinik für Anfallkranke Mara I, Epilepsie-Zentrum Bethel, Bielefeld, Germany

1. Historical aspects

Fritz E. Dreifuss

The definition of the absence seizure is that of the International League Against Epilepsy Classification (1981):

The hallmark of the absence attack is a sudden onset, interruption of ongoing activities, a blank stare, possibly a brief upward rotation of the eyes. If the patient is speaking, speed is slowed or interrupted; if walking, he stands transfixed; if eating the food will stop on its way to the mouth. Usually the patient will be unresponsive when spoken to. In some, attacks are aborted when the patient is spoken to. The attack lasts from a few seconds to half a minute and evaporates as rapidly as it commences.

The above describes a simple absence. In addition there may be associated mild clonic components, changes in muscle tone, either hypertonia with drooping or slumping of a body part, limbs, and there may be automatisms (gestural, oral-alimentary or quite elaborate). Mixed forms of absence frequently occur.

The first clinical description of petit mal was that of Poupart in 1705. He clearly described to the Académie Royale des Sciences simple absence occurring in a young woman (as quoted by Temkin 1945): 'At the approach of an attack the patient would sit down in the chair, her eyes open, and would remain there immobile and would not afterwards remember having fallen into this state. If she has begun to talk at the attack interruption, she takes it up again at precisely the point at which she stopped, and she believes she has talked continuously.' Tissot (1770) reported a 14-year-old girl who had had similar episodes since the age of 7 years, in which, 'One noticed a movement of the eyelids which at first seemed to be a tic, but which was soon recognized as convulsive.' Tissot distinguished between grands accès and petits accès.

Following these descriptions as epileptic seizures, there arose a terminologically induced confusion due to the introduction by Sauer (1916) and Adie (1924) of the term pyknolepsy to describe frequent small daily attacks of absence. The word pyknolepsy was derived from the tendency of the seizures to occur close to the onset of sleep, and they were frequently confused with narcolepsy or other non-epileptic absences in children (Janz, 1969). Esquirol in 1815 and Calmeil in 1824 first used respectively the terms petit mal and absence. Absence came from the use of the phrase absence d'esprit to describe the fleeing of the spirit from the eyes of the afflicted patient.

1

Hughlings Jackson in 1879 discussed the difference between complex partial seizures and absences, a distinction predicated on prolongation of alteration of consciousness and the presence or absence of automatisms. Classification of seizure types was something of a preoccupation with Jackson who, like Lennox some 60 years later, strove for a scientific classification based on anatomy, physiology and pathology. The EEG concomitant of the absence seizure was described by Gibbs, Davis & Lennox some 60 years ago. The identification of the characteristic electrographic discharge put to rest any nosological misinterpretation of absence seizures.

Adie (1924) quite clearly defined pyknolepsy as 'a disease with an explosive onset between the ages of 4 and 12 years, of very frequent, short, very slight, monotonous minor epileptiform seizures of uniform severity, which recur almost daily for weeks, months or years.' In 1935 Kinnier Wilson emphasised the identity of pyknolepsy as a variant of petit mal (Lennox & Lennox, 1960). While Berger (1933) noted rhythmic abnormal discharges in a patient with absences, it was Gibbs, Davis & Lennox (1935) who definitively identified the electroencephalographic components and stated: 'electroencephalograms from 12 patients with characteristic petit mal epilepsy show in all cases during the seizure bursts of waves great amplitude . . . at a frequency of three per second.'

Absence status epilepticus was characterised by Tucker and Forster (1950) and subsequently was described with increasing frequency as the electroencephalogram became more widely used. In absence status patients act in a stuporous, confused, dazed manner with little spontaneity and marked perseverative automatisms and these attacks might last for a matter of hours or even days (Andermann & Robb, 1972).

The introduction of split-screen video-EEG recording allowed the elaboration of clinical and EEG correlations and a definition of a repertoire of activities which are characteristically associated with absence attacks. The recording of the results of physiological experiments conducted during such events has rapidly narrowed the gap between an ideal and a utilitarian classification. Intensive observation using CCTV-EEG has shown that absence seizures may range from short interruption of activity without any concomitant movement to quite complex episodes characterised by mild clonic components ranging from the almost imperceptible to more pronounced jerking, usually synchronously with the recorded spike wave. Increase in postural tone, referred to by German neurologists as 'retropulsive petit mal', might lead to extension hypertonus. Conversely there might be decrease in postural tone, with head nodding, slumping or dropping of objects, which, if associated with myoclonic activity, has been described as 'propulsive petit mal'.

Automatisms frequently occur during absence seizures (Penry et al, 1975). These might take the form of perseveration of ongoing activity or they might be initiated during the attack in response to enteroceptive and exteroceptive stimuli (Penry & Dreifuss, 1969). Autonomic phenomena are frequent in the form of pupil dilation, colour changes, tachycardia or pilo-erection. The simple absence attack, characterised only by brief upward movement of the eyes, cessation of activity and a blank stare with interruption of consciousness, represents only about 8% of recorded attacks.

The history of behavioural evaluation during absence attacks dates back to Schwab (1939), who recorded the EEG and response to visual stimuli delivered after the onset of generalised spike wave discharges. This represented a reaction time measuring device which indicated that reaction time might run the gamut from nearly normal to significantly impaired, largely depending on the duration of the spells. Schwab also noted that sometimes the stimulus was responsible for terminating a seizure. Several studies of reaction time and response to continuous performance tests have been reported (Shimazono et al, 1953; Goldie & Green, 1961; Tizard & Margerison, 1963; Mirsky & van Buren, 1965; Goode et al, 1970). In the latter studies behaviour was evaluated at various points during the episodes. The maximal interference with reaction times appears to be within one second of the onset of the paroxysm and, though the attack may continue, responsiveness improves during the latter stages of the ongoing episode. There appear to be both sensory and motor components to disrupted behaviour. Moreover there appears to be a dichotomy between the cortical and reticular components of the absence seizure at various times during its course. Differences in spike wave morphology during different sleep stages would also suggest an increase in cortical activity during sleep and an increase in sub-cortical influences of predominantly inhibitory nature during the waking and REM sleep stages.

HISTORY OF NEUROPHYSIOLOGICAL INVESTIGATIONS

As noted earlier, Gibbs, Davis & Lennox published their seminal paper in 1935 and this was followed by further observations suggesting the generalised nature of the process. The difference between typical and atypical spike wave episodes was noted by Lennox & Davis in 1950. This represents the first EEG differentiation between the pure petit mal syndrome and the Lennox–Gastaut syndrome. Jasper & Droogleever-Fortuyn (1946) produced bilaterally synchronous spike wave EEG patterns with 3 Hz intralaminar thalamic stimulation in the cat, as had also been seen by Morison & Dempsey (1942) and was subsequently confirmed by Williams (1953). Subsequently the slow wave component was found to represent hyper-polarising inhibition.

Marcus & Watson (1966) and Bancaud et al (1974) showed that generalised spike wave discharges could also be induced by lesioning or stimulating cortical areas using bilateral lesions or mesial frontal cortex stimulation. Naquet et al (1969) showed that the photically sensitive baboon activated areas 4 and 6 from the occipital regions via cortical relays. Gloor et al (1977) produced spike wave discharges and seizures with low-frequency stimulation in animals whose cortex had been pre-treated with penicillin, and so developed the cortico-reticular theory. This represents a compromise situation between the Jacksonian concept of 'highest level seizures' and the Montreal school's 'centrencephalic seizures'. The former placed the highest level (and the origin of absence) in the 'prefrontal lobes' and the latter in an ill-defined upper brainstem organisation, the centrencephalon, whence the discharges would excite both hemispheres simultaneously (McNaughton, 1952).

In this connection it is of interest that microdysgenesis of cerebral cortical structures has been implicated as an epileptogenic mechanism in generalised epilepsies (Meencke & Janz, 1984). Mirski & Ferrendelli (1986), using pentylenetetrazol stimulation and ethosuximide suppression, suggested that the mammillo-thalamic tract, the anterior nuclei of the thalamus and the dorsal and ventral tegmental nuclei of the mesencephalon are active in mediating absence seizures. More recently a genetic absence epilepsy model has been identified in a strain of Wistar rats (Marescaux et al, 1984), and it has been found that abnormalities in calcium channels controlling thalamic neuronal excitability are involved through $GABA_B$-mediated neurotransmission in the development of spike wave discharges.

HISTORY OF GENETIC RESEARCH IN CHILDHOOD ABSENCE EPILEPSY

Tissot in 1770 recognised that the expression of epilepsy was the result of predisposing factors and precipitating factors. Lennox et al (1945), studying EEG patterns in monozygotic twins, showed that 85% had identical EEG appearances. Metrakos & Metrakos (1961) suggested an autosomal dominant mode of transmission of generalised spike and wave discharges with an age-dependent maximal penetrance regardless of the presence or absence of seizures. In the past there may have been confusion because of failure to distinguish between phenotypically similar seizure forms representing different epileptic syndromes. It is now becoming clear that pyknoleptic petit mal was a syndrome characterised by a specific type of seizure with a specific EEG pattern in the face of normal neurological development, the absence of abnormal neurological findings, the presence of normal intelligence and a strong family history of similar seizures, as well as a good response to medication and benign outcome.

Secondary or symptomatic epilepsy may present with seizures which appear identical but which occur under considerably different circumstances. Further difficulties arise when one tries to equate the inheritance of all the idiopathic generalised epilepsies which have a dominant tendency, including not only the childhood absence syndromes but also photic sensitivity-induced epilepsy, myoclonic petit mal and juvenile myoclonic epilepsy. This reinforces the need for separation of syndromic concatenations whose only claim to commonality is the presence of a generalised spike wave discharge.

OTHER FORMS OF PRIMARY GENERALISED EPILEPSIES WITH BILATERALLY SYNCHRONOUS SPIKE WAVE EEG DISCHARGES

Juvenile absence epilepsy is similar in its phenotypic characteristics of the absence seizure but has a somewhat older age of onset than pyknoleptic petit mal. Moreover it lacks the pyknoleptic characteristic and is more frequently associated with generalised tonic-clonic seizures. The response to anti-absence medication is less predictable. Some observers think that this may be a fragmentary form of juvenile myoclonic epilepsy. Historically, juvenile absence epilepsy was defined considerably later than childhood absence epilepsy, by Janz & Christian (1957).

Juvenile myoclonic epilepsy (JME)

This condition was first described by Herpin (1867) under the term 'maladie de secousse' after he had observed myoclonic jerks in his son. In 1899 Rabot noted the mild isolated upper extremity jerks, referring to this as 'impulsion'. This led Janz & Christian to speak of 'impulsive petit mal'. Janz aroused the current interest in the condition and noted the overlap between JME, juvenile absence and primary generalised tonic-clonic convulsions on waking.

JME is of historical importance because it is one of the first epileptic syndromes to be subjected to genetic linkage studies. JME is further of interest because of a tendency for sufferers to manifest photo- sensitivity, leading to an overlap in symptomatology between this condition and a number of other epileptic syndromes.

Epilepsy with photo-sensitivity

One variety of photo-sensitive epilepsy afflicts predominantly adolescent females and the manifestation is frequently absence seizures, with or without myoclonic components. Temkin (1945) ascribed the earliest reference to photo-sensitive epilepsy to Apuleius, in his book, *Apologia* in which it was stated that 'rotating a potter's wheel might provoke a fit'. Gowers (1885) described seizures in a girl going into bright sunshine. Both flickering light and pattern sensitivity became commonly recognised as the range of adequate stimuli increased to include television viewing and self-stimulation.

The history of childhood absence seizures and the pyknoleptic petit mal syndrome parallels the technological advance of the 20th century and will culminate with the identification of an abnormal gene product when the place of this syndrome is established on the human genome. At the same time the application of mathematical analysis of the spread of the spike wave discharge, which may be an age-related phenomenon, may unlock some of the secrets of epileptogenesis in the idiopathic generalised epilepsies.

REFERENCES

Adie WJ 1924 Pyknolepsy: a form of epilepsy occurring in children with a good prognosis.
Brain 47: 96–102
Andermann F, Robb JP 1972 Absence status: a reappraisal following review of 38 patients.
Epilepsia 13: 177–187
Bancaud J, Talairach P, Morel M et al 1974 'Generalized' epileptic seizures elicited by electrical
stimulation of the frontal lobe in man. Electroencephalography and Clinical
Neurophysiology 37: 275–282
Berger H 1933 Über das Elektroenkephalogramm des Menschen. Archiv für Psychiatrie 100:
301–320.
Browne TR, Penry JK, Porter RJ et al 1974 Responsiveness before, during and after spike-wave
paroxysms. Neurology 24: 659–665
Gibbs FA, Davis H, Lennox WG 1935 The electroencephalogram in epilepsy and in conditions
of impaired consciousness. Archives of Neurology and Psychiatry 34: 1133–1148
Gloor P, Quesney LF, Zumstein H 1977 Pathophysiology of generalised penicillin epilepsy in
the cat. The role of cortical and subcortical structures. II Topical application of penicillin to
the cerebral cortex and to subcortical structures. Electroencephalography and Clinical
Neurophysiology 43: 79–94
Goldie L, Green JM 1961 Spike and wave discharges and alterations of conscious awareness.
Nature 191: 200–201
Goode DJ, Penry JK, Dreifuss FE 1970 Effects of paroxysmal spike-wave on continuous visual-
motor performance. Epilepsia 11: 241–254
Gowers WR 1885 Epilepsies and other chronic convulsive diseases. Their causes, symptoms
and treatment. Wood & Co, New York
Herpin TH 1867 Des accès incomplets d'épilepsie. Baillière, Paris
Janz E 1969 Die Epilepsien. Thieme, Stuttgart
Janz D, Christian W 1957 Impulsiv-Petit mal. Journal of Neurology 176: 346–386
Jeavons PM, Harding GFA 1975 Photosensitive epilepsy. William Heinemann, London
Jasper HH, Droogleever-Fortuyn J 1946 Experimental studies on the fundamental anatomy of
petit mal epilepsy. Res Tubel Assoc Res Nerv Ihert Dis 26: 272–298
Lennox WG, Lennox M 1960 Epilepsy and related disorders. Little, Brown, Boston
Lennox WG, Gibbs FA, Gibbs EL 1945 The brain wave pattern; an hereditary trait. Evidence
of 74 'normal' pairs of twins. Journal of Heredity 36: 233–243
McNaughton FL 1952 The classification of the epilepsies. Epilepsia 1: 7–16
Marcus EM, Watson CW 1966 Bilateral synchronous spike-wave electrographic patterns in the
cat: Interactions of bilateral cortical foci in the intact, the bilateral cortical callosal and
adiencephalic preparation. Archives of Neurology 14: 601–610
Marescaux C, Micheletti G, Vergnes M, Depanlis A, Rumbach L, Warter JM 1984 A model of
chronic spontaneous petit mal-like seizures in the rat: comparison with pentylene tetrazol-
induced seizures. Epilepsia 25: 326–331
Meencke HJ, Janz D 1984 Neuropathological findings in primary generalised epilepsy: A study
of eight cases. Epilepsia 25: 8–21
Metrakos JD, Metrakos K 1961 Genetics of convulsive disorders. Part II Genetic and
electroencephalographic studies in centrencephalic epilepsy. Neurology 11: 464–483
Mirski MA, Ferendelli JA 1986 Anterior thalamic mediation of generalised pentylene tetrazol
seizures. Brain Research 399: 212–223
Mirsky AF, VanBuren JM 1965 On the nature of the 'absence' in centrencephalic epilepsy: A
study of some behavioural, electroencephalographic and autonomic factors.
Electroencephalography and Clinical Neurophysiology 18: 334–348
Morison RS, Dempsey EW 1942 A study of thalamo-cortical relations. American Journal of
Physiology 135: 281–292
Naquet R, Killam KF, Killam EK 1969 Photomyoclonic epilepsy of Papio Papio. In: Gastaut
H, Jasper HH, Bancaud J, Waltregny A (eds) The physiopathogenesis of the epilepsies. Chas
C Thomas, Springfield, Ill.
Penry JK, Porter RJ, Dreifuss FE 1975 Simultaneous recordings of absence seizures with video
tape and electroencephalography. Brain 98: 427–440
Penry JK, Dreifuss FE 1969 Automatisms associated with the absence of petit mal epilepsy.
Archives of Neurology 21: 1942–1949
Sauer H 1916 Über Gehäufte Kleine Anfälle by Kindern (pyknolepsie). Mschr Psychiatr

Neurol 40: 276–300

Schwab RS 1939 Method of measuring consciousness in attacks of petit mal epilepsy. Archives of Neurology and Psychiatry 41: 215–217

Shimazono Y, Hirai T, Okura T, Fukuda T, Yamamasu E 1953 Disturbance of consciousness in petit mal epilepsy. Epilepsia 2: 49–55

Temkin C 1945 The falling sickness. Johns Hopkins Press, Baltimore

Tissot SA 1770 Traité de l'épilepsie, faisant le tome troisième du traité des nerfs et de leurs maladies. Didot le jeune, Paris

Tizard B, Margerison JH 1963 The relationship between generalised paroxysmal EEG discharges and various test situations in two epileptic patients. Journal of Neurology, Neurosurgery and Psychiatry 26: 308–313

Tucker W, Forster FM 1950 Petit mal epilepsy occurring in status. Archives of Neurology and Psychiatry 64: 823–827

Williams D 1953 A study of thalamic and cortical rhythms in petit mal. Brain 76: 50–69

Wolf P, 1992 Juvenile absence epilepsy. In: Roger J, Bureau M, Dravet C, Dreifuss FE, Perret A, Wolf P (eds) Epileptic syndromes in infancy, childhood and adolescence. John Libbey, London

DISCUSSION

Duncan: Can we initially define typical and atypical absences?

Dreifuss: The term atypical absence is used to describe absence seizures which occur in the context of the Lennox–Gastaut syndrome, for example. The atypicality is characterised by a <3 cycles/s spike and wave on the EEG. It is usually associated with postural changes which are slower and much more pronounced that those we see in the typical absence attack and which last usually for a considerably longer period of time.

If one has in one's mind's eye the child with Lennox–Gastaut syndrome with very prolonged blinking, staring and postural tonic changes which may go on for hours, days or weeks at a time, and compare that with the blank stare of the typical absences, there is very little doubt as to which is the typical and which is the atypical absence. That is what the atypical is in reference to.

The Commission was occupied for an inordinate length of time in making these definitions. The word atypical is not used as 'not typical'. We are describing a clinical phenomenon, even leaving out the 3 cycles/s spike and wave. Atypical absence describes a condition and what it describes is the attack of absence that is seen in the context of the Lennox–Gastaut syndrome and is not just the opposite of typical. In other words, it is not just a rag-bag of a multitude of other conditions.

Panayiotopoulos: Typical absences by definition include absences with more than 2.5–3 Hz spike slow wave. Therefore, they should not be equated only with the 'classical' absences of childhood absence epilepsy, but also with 'less classical' ones like eyelid myoclonia with absences and myoclonic absence epilepsy.

Duncan: Happily we shall try to restrict ourselves to typical absences. A recurring theme over the next two days is how typical is typical and how many different kinds of typical there are.

2. Animal models of absence seizures and absence epilepsies

C. Marescaux   M. Vergnes

Absences are fundamentally different from any other kind of epileptic seizures (Berkovic et al, 1987). Human absences are concomitant with unresponsiveness to environmental stimuli and cessation of activity. They start and end abruptly and may be associated with automatisms or mild clonic components. They may occur as frequently as several hundred times per day, mainly during quiet wakefulness, inattention and in the transitions between sleep and waking; they are interrupted by attention and unexpected sensory stimulations (Jung, 1962; Guey et al, 1969). The EEG hallmark of absence seizures is the occurrence of 3 Hz bilateral and synchronous spike and wave discharges (SWD) (Loiseau, 1992; Panayiotopoulos, 1994). Another distinguishing feature of absences is the fact that they are more severe in children. Therefore, absence epilepsy is a disorder of the developing brain (Loiseau, 1992; Panayiotopoulos, 1994).

Absence seizures are pharmacologically unique. Ethosuximide and trimethadione, which are effective in absences, are ineffective in all other seizures. Reciprocally, anti-epileptic drugs which are effective in generalised convulsive and partial epilepsies (phenytoin, carbamazepine and all GABA-mimetic drugs) are known to make absences worse (Loiseau, 1992).

Absence epilepsy remains one of the most enigmatic of neurological disorders and there is no widely accepted theory of its aetiology. No structural lesion of any kind – anatomical or biochemical – has ever been identified as its substrate (Berkovic et al, 1987; Gloor & Fariello, 1988). Its cause is increasingly regarded as genetic. It seems to be provoked by an abnormal oscillatory pattern of discharges that involve a thalamo-cortical loop. These thalamo-cortical circuits may normally sustain the physiological spindles.

The study of pathophysiological mechanisms underlying absence epilepsy is dependent upon use of models. According to the degree of similarity with human diseases, three categories of animal models may be distinguished: isomorphic models with similar symptoms and occurrence; predictive models with a similar therapeutic profile; and homologous models with a similar aetiology to the considered pathology (Kornetsky, 1977). The requirements for an isomorphic and predictive model of absence seizures (Marescaux et al, 1992b) are: EEG and behavioural similarities with human absences (SWD of 5–15 s on a normal background EEG, associated with arrest of movement and reduced responsiveness); an increased occurrence of SWD by decreased arousal and a decreased occurrence of SWD by increased arousal; a pharmacological profile that reflects the results obtained in clinical practice; a potentiation of SWD by drugs inducing absence-like seizures; and an age-related developmental profile.

The experimental models discussed in this paper are pharmacologically induced or genetically determined models in rodents or cats. They meet some or all of these criteria. Rodent models are emphasised because these animals are easily obtainable and easier to work with than larger animals. When using rodent models, one must bear in mind the work of McQueen & Woodbury (1975), who demonstrated that rodents are incapable of generating 3 Hz SWD during experimental absence seizures.

PHARMACOLOGICAL MODELS IN RODENTS

The gamma-hydroxybutyrate model: an isomorphic and predictive model

Gamma-hydroxybutyrate (GHB) is a GABA metabolite which occurs naturally in mammalian brain. When given to animals, GHB produces electrographic and behavioural events which closely resemble generalised absence seizures. This phenomenon has been well described in cats, rats and monkeys (Snead, 1992). A standard dose of 300 mg/kg GHB given intraperitoneally (i.p.) reliably produces onset of bilateral SWD within 20 min of administration. The frequency of the SWD is 7–9 Hz. Associated with these hyper-synchronous EEG changes are behavioural arrest, facial myoclonus and vibrissal twitching. Similar effects are obtained with a smaller dose of the pro-drug gamma-butyrolactone (GBL).

The pharmacology of the GHB model is what one would predict for absence seizures (Snead, 1992). GHB-induced SWD are significantly decreased by anti-absence drugs such as ethosuximide, trimethadione and valproate, and enhanced by phenytoin. The GHB model is exacerbated by drugs which produce absence-like seizures in rodents and other species: pentylenetetrazol, penicillin and GABA-mimetics. The GHB model of absence seizures also has a unique developmental profile which reflects the propensity of the developing brain for the occurrence of bilaterally synchronous SWD. In rodents, the age at which animals are most sensitive to GHB is during the fourth postnatal week (Snead, 1992). Using mapping of EEG with bipolar depth recordings and lesion experiments, it has been demonstrated that the thalamus is involved in the GHB model (Vergnes & Marescaux, 1992; Snead, 1992).

In conclusion, the GHB rat model of generalised absence seizure, which meets all criteria put forward to date for experimental absences, is a useful model for the study of the mechanisms of bilaterally synchronous SWD production. GHB-induced SWD can be used to screen for anti-absence activity of potential anti-epileptic drugs.

The pentylenetetrazol model: a predictive model

Drugs effective in the treatment of absence seizures have been reported to be more potent against clonic seizures induced by pentylenetetrazol (PTZ) in a dose of 40 mg/kg or higher than against seizures produced by maximal electro-shock. A stronger relative potency against PTZ seizures has thus been used to predict efficacy against absences in drug screening programmes (Snead, 1992). In fact the electro-clinical characteristics of PTZ-induced seizures are dose-dependent. Intermediate doses (40–60 mg/kg) produce clonus restricted to the face and forelimbs responsive to anti-absence drugs; high doses ($\geq$ 80 mg/kg) produce tonic seizures unresponsive to anti-absence drugs. The idea that the clonic component of PTZ seizures are more representative of absence seizures than the tonic components finds additional support from experiments which have shown that tonic seizures occur independently of any epileptic discharge in forebrain structures, whereas clonic seizures are associated with EEG discharges emanating from the forebrain.

According to these data, the traditional model induced by high doses of PTZ appears to be predictive rather than isomorphic. However, relatively recently it was reported that low doses (10–20 mg/kg) produce bilaterally synchronous 7–9 Hz SWD associated with behavioural arrest and immobility (Marescaux et al, 1984). The low-dose-PTZ model meets the pharmacological requirement for experimental absences. SWD are aborted by anti-absence drugs and made worse by phenytoin, carbamazepine (Marescaux et al, 1984), and by GABA-ergic agonists as well as by GHB (Snead, 1992). PTZ seizures have a distinct ontogeny: spikes appear on the 12th post-natal day in rats. Moreover, thalamic mechanisms are involved in the genesis of these seizures (Snead, 1992; Vergnes & Marescaux, 1992).

EEG seizures induced by low doses of PTZ represent a useful, predictable, reproducible model of absences which can be used along with other pharmacological or genetic models in rodents to investigate basic mechanisms of SWD production, as well as to screen drugs for anti-absence activity.

The THIP model: an isomorphic but non-predictive model

Recently Fariello & Golden have proposed the use of THIP, a GABA agonist, to induce absences in rats (Fariello & Golden, 1987). THIP (5–10 mg/kg, given i.p.) results in bilaterally synchronous 4–6 Hz SWD which occur in bursts lasting 1–7 s. Behaviourally, the animals have immobility and some vibrissal twitching. This model appears to be isomorphic. However, to date there are no pharmacological data to support this hypothesis: the THIP model is not predictive as it is exacerbated by valproate (Snead, 1992). Moreover, as yet there are no data concerning ontogeny or thalamo-cortical mechanisms in the generation of THIP-induced SWD.

The feline model of penicillin-induced generalised absence epilepsy

Intramuscular injection of 300 000 IU/kg of penicillin G into a cat results in recurrent episodes of arrested activity, staring, myoclonus, facial-oral twitching and occasional progression to generalised tonic-clonic seizures. Seizure activity begins about 1 h after injection and continues for 6–8 h. The EEG shows 3–5 Hz SWD emerging from a relatively normal background. Response of feline generalised penicillin epilepsy to anti-epileptic drugs appears to parallel the clinical response in absence epilepsy: ethosuximide and valproate are effective whereas phenytoin is not (Gloor & Fariello, 1988). The feline penicillin model has been particularly useful in the study of the cellular correlates of SWD and in the study of the networks involved in the genesis of SWD.

Detailed neurophysiological studies on this model have shown that SWD reflects an abnormal oscillatory pattern of discharge involving mutually interconnected cortical and thalamic neurons. This oscillation consists of a regular alternation of brief periods of neuronal excitation characterised by action potential discharge with longer periods of neuronal silence which affect large populations of cortical and thalamic neurons in a nearly synchronous manner. Neither the cortex nor the thalamus can sustain this pattern on its own (Gloor & Fariello, 1988). SWD appear in cortex before they appear in mesial thalamus or reticular formation. Moreover, application of penicillin to wide regions of cortex, but not to thalamus, can produce SWD. Thus, experimental evidence suggests that, in feline penicillin epilepsy, SWD are caused by a state of diffuse hyper-excitability of cortical neurons affecting both hemispheres and leading secondarily to a dysfunction in thalamo-cortical projecting systems.

Pharmacological studies suggest that the ideal condition for the generation of SWD is an enhancement of both glutamate-mediated excitation and GABA-mediated inhibition. A further enhancement of GABA-ergic inhibition stabilises and prolongs SWD. Breakdown of GABA-ergic inhibition may promote the transition from non-convulsive absences to convulsive seizures (Avoli & Gloor, 1994).

THE GENETIC MODEL OF ABSENCE EPILEPSY IN RATS FROM STRASBOURG (GAERS): ROLE OF GABA$_B$ NEUROMEDIATION

EEG, behavioural and pharmacological characteristics of GAERS

We have selected a strain of Wistar rats (Genetic Absence Epilepsy Rats from Strasbourg, GAERS) in which 100% of the animals present recurrent generalised non-convulsive seizures characterised by bilateral and synchronous SWD accompanied by behavioural arrest. Spontaneous SWD (7–10 Hz 300–1000 μV, 1–75 s) start and end abruptly on a normal background EEG (Fig. 2.1). They usually occur at a mean frequency of 1.5 per

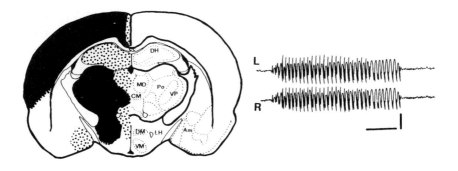

Fig. 2.1   Left panel: schematic mapping of SWD on a coronal section of a rat brain. Am, amygdala; DH, dorsal hippocampus; LH, lateral hypothalamus; DM, dorsomedial nucleus of the hypothalamus; VM, ventromedial nucleus of the hypothalamus; CM, centromedial; MD, mediodorsal; Po, posterior; VP, ventroposterior nucleus of the thalamus. Black areas, large or small SWD recorded; dots, no SWD recorded. Right panel: spontaneous bilateral cortical spike and wave discharges recorded in one GAERS. L, left; R, right. Calibration 1 s 400 μV.

min when the animals are in a state of quiet wakefulness (Vergnes & Marescaux, 1994; Marescaux et al, 1992b). During the discharges the animals have a fixed stare and are completely inert. Frequently rhythmic twitching of the vibrissae and the facial muscles is observed. Muscle tone in the neck is sometimes diminished, inducing a gradual and slight drop of the head. At the end of the SWD, a sudden extension of the head precedes the recovery of the previous position. In some instances SWD appear when the rat is moving. The movement is then suddenly interrupted and resumes as soon as the discharge stops. During SWD, animals are unresponsive to non-relevant stimuli. However, the SWD are immediately interrupted by strong and unexpected sensory stimulation (Marescaux et al, 1992b).

Drugs effective against absence seizures in humans (ethosuximide, trimethadione, valproate, benzodiazepines) suppress the SWD dose-dependently, whereas drugs specific for convulsive or focal seizures (carbamazepine, phenytoin) are ineffective. SWD are increased by epileptogenic drugs inducing absence-like seizures, such as PTZ, GHB, THIP and penicillin (Marescaux et al, 1992a; Vergnes & Marescaux, 1994).

Before 30 days of age none of the animals recorded had SWD. From 30 to 40 days, 30% developed SWD. The number of rats with SWD then increased regularly with age, reaching 100% at four months. The first SWD were rare (1 or 2/h) and short-lasting (1–3 s). The number of SWD reached a maximum (>1/min) around the age of six months. SWD could be recorded over months and they never disappeared spontaneously (Vergnes et al, 1986).

Anatomical substrate of SWD in GAERS

In order to determine which brain structures are involved in SWD, chronic and acute EEG recordings were performed with cortical and depth bipolar electrodes. The largest SWD were recorded from the fronto-parietal cortex and the postero-lateral thalamus. In some rats the beginning of the lateral thalamic SWD occasionally preceded that of the cortical SWD. Small-amplitude or delayed SWD were present in the striatum, lateral hypothalamus and ventral tegmentum (Fig. 2.1). SWD were absent or considerably reduced in the anterior and midline nuclei of the thalamus. No SWD were recorded from the limbic structures: hippocampus, septum, amygdala, cingular and piriform cortex (Vergnes & Marescaux, 1992; 1994).

The effect of various cortical and thalamic lesions on the occurrence of spontaneous SWD was also examined. Cortical ablations suppressed thalamic SWD. KCl-induced unilateral cortical spreading depression transiently suppressed SWD in the ipsilateral cortex and thalamus; SWD recovered simultaneously in both structures (Marescaux et al, 1992b; Vergnes & Marescaux, 1992). Bilateral thalamic lesions of the anterior nuclei, the ventromedial nuclei or the posterior area or lesions of the midline nuclei did not suppress cortical SWD. Large lesions of the lateral thalamus, including the specific relay and reticular nuclei, definitely suppressed ipsilateral SWD (Fig. 2.2), and PTZ, THIP or GHB failed to restore the cortical SWD (Vergnes & Marescaux, 1992; 1994). These results demonstrate that the neocortex and specific thalamic nuclei are both necessarily involved in the generation of SWD in GAERS.

In GAERS the SWD are always bilaterally synchronous, all over the cortex of both hemispheres and in the lateral part of the thalamus. In order to examine the pathways underlying bilateral synchronisation, the corpus callo-

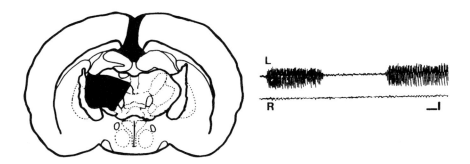

Fig. 2.2   Left panel: coronal section showing a unilateral lesion of the right lateral thalamus, with a transection of the corpus callosum. Right panel: cortical EEG recordings in the same rate. SWD are suppressed on the cortex ipsilateral to the thalamic lesion. L, left; R, right. Calibration 1 s 400 μV.

sum (CC) and the midline thalamus were sectioned. After section, 90% of SWD were asynchronous. Our results confirm that the CC is the major pathway involved in bilateralisation of spontaneous SWD in absence epilepsy in rats. Transection of the CC does not totally abolish bilateral synchronism of the SWD, suggesting that additional pathways are also involved in inter-hemispheric synchronisation of SWD. The midline thalamus is likely to fulfil this role. Full inter-hemispheric dissociation of SWD is only achieved when the midline thalamus is sectioned in addition to the CC. However, the midline thalamus plays a minor role in bilateral transfer, as destruction of this area alone does not affect occurrence of bilateral and synchronous SWD (Vergnes & Marescaux, 1994).

Genetic transmission of SWD in GAERS

In our initial colony of Wistar rats, 30% of the animals showed spontaneous SWD. Selective in-breeding produced a strain in which 100% of the rats were affected. Similarly, we selected a control strain free of SWD. These data demonstrated that SWD were genetically controlled. We analysed the mode of inheritance of SWD in GAERS by performing a classic Mendelian cross-breeding study. All offspring of parents from the control non-absence strain had a normal EEG up to 12 months. All offspring of parents from the GAERS strain showed SWD. More than 95% of the F_1 (control × GAERS) showed SWD at 12 months, demonstrating that there is a dominant transmission. Similar SWD in males and females F_1 indicate that the transmission is autosomal. Inter-individual variability for age of appearance and duration of SWD was extremely high, suggesting that the inheritance of SWD is probably not due to a single gene locus. These data are confirmed in F_2 (F_1 × F_1) and back crosses (F_1 × control) generations (Marescaux et al, 1992b; Vergnes & Marescaux, 1994).

Neurotransmitters and SWD in GAERS

Most neurotransmitters are involved in the control of SWD. GABA appears to play a prominent role. GABA-mimetics, inhibitors of seizures in many models of convulsive epilepsy, aggravate seizures in all models of generalised non-convulsive epilepsy in rodents, as well as in cats, primates or humans. The effects of GABA are mediated not only by $GABA_A$ but also by $GABA_B$ receptors which differ in terms of pharmacological profile, mechanisms of transduction, and regional distribution. In GAERS, activation of the $GABA_A$ receptors clearly increases duration of SWD, whether the drugs are administered systemically or into the specific relay nuclei of the thalamus (Marescaux et al, 1992a; 1992b).

In order to study the role of $GABA_B$ transmission in absence seizures, systemic and intra-thalamic administration were performed in GAERS using R-baclofen, an agonist, and CGP 35 348, an antagonist of $GABA_B$ receptors. Baclofen injected i.p. not only increased SWD in epileptic rats but also induced, in control rats free of spontaneous SWD, paroxysmal discharges of oscillatory activity which resemble spike and wave complexes. By contrast, i.p. or p.o. administration of CGP 35 348 efficiently suppressed the SWD. Systemic administration of the $GABA_B$ antagonist suppressed SWD aggravated by $GABA_A$ or $GABA_B$ agonists, by inhibitors of GABA re-uptake or transamination, or by GHB. CGP 35 348 also suppressed SWD induced in non-epileptic rats by GHB or pentylenetetrazol (Marescaux et al, 1992c; Vergnes et al, 1994). Similar results were obtained after intra-thalamic micro-injections of $GABA_B$ agonist and antagonists. R-baclofen injected into the specific relay nuclei or the reticular nucleus of the thalamus increased duration of SWD in GAERS and elicited rhythmic oscillations on the cortical EEG in non-epileptic control rats. By contrast, intra-thalamic injections of CGP 35 348 into the same nuclei suppressed the spontaneous SWD or the SWD aggravated by prior i.p. injection of $GABA_A$ or $GABA_B$ mimetics. Our data suggest that a dysfunction in $GABA_B$ receptor-mediated transmission is a possible mechanism involved in genetically determined SWD. The density and affinity of $GABA_B$ receptors is similar in GAERS and in control non-epileptic rats. However, the possibility of a modified transduction of $GABA_B$ receptors to the second messenger is not excluded in GAERS.

SWD in GAERS: a valid model of absence epilepsy

Similarities with human absence seizures strongly support the epileptic nature of GAERS SWD and fully agree with the requirements for an experimental model of absence seizures. GAERS spontaneous SWD can actually be considered an isomorphic and predictive model of human generalised non-convulsive absence epilepsy on the basis of EEG, behavioural and pharmacological data. Neurophysiological and genetic data suggest that these SWD and human absences are likely to be related to similar neural mechanisms. As the mechanisms involved in the thalamo-cortical dysfunction during SWD are still unknown, their analysis in GAERS may be fruitful in the investigation of the pathogenesis of generalised non-convulsive epilepsy.

REFERENCES

Avoli M, Gloor P 1994 Physiopathogenesis of feline generalized penicillin epilepsy: the role of thalamocortical mechanisms. In: Malafosse A, Genton P, Hirsch E, Marescaux C, Broglin D, Bernasconi R (eds) Idiopathic generalized epilepsies: clinical, experimental and genetic aspects. John Libbey, London (in press)
Berkovic SF, Andermann F, Andermann E, Gloor P 1987 Concepts of absence epilepsies: discrete syndrome or biological continuum? Neurology 37: 993–1000
Fariello RG, Golden GT 1987 The THIP-induced model of bilateral synchronous spike and wave in rodents. Neuropharmacology 26: 161–165

Gloor P, Fariello RG 1988 Generalized epilepsy: Some of its cellular mechanisms differ from those of focal epilepsy. Trends in Neuroscience 11: 63–68

Guey J, Bureau M, Dravet C, Roger J 1969 A study of the rhythm of petit mal absences in children in relation to prevailing situations. The use of EEG telemetry during psychological examinations, school exercises and periods of inactivity. Epilepsia 10: 441–451

Jung R 1962 Blocking of petit-mal attacks by sensory arousal and inhibition of attacks by an active change in attention during the epileptic aura. Epilepsia 3: 435–437

Kornetsky C 1977 Animal models: promises and problems. In: Hanin I, Udsin E (eds) Animal models in psychiatry and neurology. Pergamon Press, Oxford, pp1–7

Loiseau P 1992 Childhood absence-epilepsy. In: Roger J, Bureau M, Dravet Ch, Dreifuss FE, Perret A, Wolf P (eds) Epileptic syndromes in infancy, childhood and adolescence, 2nd edn. John Libbey, London, pp135–150

McQueen JK, Woodbury DM 1975 Attempts to produce spike-and-wave complexes in the electrocorticogram of the rat. Epilepsia 16: 295–299

Marescaux C, Micheletti G, Vergnes M, Depaulis A, Rumbach L, Warter JM 1984 A model of chronic spontaneous petit mal-like seizures in the rat: comparison with pentylenetetrazol-induced seizures. Epilepsia 25: 326–331

Marescaux C, Vergnes M, Depaulis A, Micheletti G, Warter JM 1992a Neurotransmission in rats' spontaneous generalized nonconvulsive epilepsy. In: Avanzini G, Engel J, Fariello R, Heinemann U (eds) Neurotransmitters in epilepsy. Epilepsy Research 8 (Suppl.) 335–343

Marescaux C, Vergnes M, Depaulis A 1992b Genetic absence epilepsy in rats from Strasbourg. A review. Journal of Neural Transmission 35 (Suppl.) 37–69

Marescaux C, Vergnes M, Bernasconi R 1992c GABAB receptor antagonists: potential new anti-absence drugs. Journal of Neural Transmission 35 (Suppl.) 179–188

Panayiotopoulos CP 1994 The clinical spectrum of typical absence seizures and absence epilepsies. In: Malafosse A, Genton P, Hirsch E, Marescaux C, Broglin D, Bernasconi R (eds) Idiopathic generalized epilepsies: clinical, experimental and genetic aspects. John Libbey, London (in press)

Snead OC III 1992 Pharmacological models of generalized absence seizures in rodents. Journal of Neural Transmission 35 (Suppl.) 7–19

Vergnes M, Marescaux C, Depaulis A, Micheletti G, Warter JM 1986 Ontogeny of spontaneous petit mal-like seizures in Wistar rats. Developmental Brain Research 30: 85–87

Vergnes M, Marescaux C 1992 Cortical and thalamic lesions in rats with genetic absence epilepsy. Journal of Neural Transmission 35 (Suppl.) 71–83

Vergnes M, Marescaux C 1994 Pathophysiological mechanisms underlying genetic absence epilepsy in rats. In: Malafosse A, Genton P, Hirsch E, Marescaux C, Broglin D, Bernasconi R (eds) Idiopathic generalized epilepsies: clinical, experimental and genetic aspects. John Libbey, London (in press)

DISCUSSION

Brodie: How does lamotrigine work in typical absences? It does not affect T-calcium channels and it clearly does not work in the GAERS model.

Duncan: If lamotrigine is inhibiting the release of glutamate, could one conceive of it working at the cortical level, interrupting the thalamo-cortical cycle?

Marescaux: One could. It would also be possible that lamotrigine acts at the thalamic level because both the thalamo-cortical and the cortico-thalamic cells are glutamatergic. The fact that lamotrigine is acting on glutamate release is not definite. I think that if lamotrigine had been synthesised 20 years ago it would be thought to act on GABA and not on glutamate. I do not feel very confident about the scientific argument. In 20 more years it will be acting on membrane potentials or something of the kind. It is a fashion effect.

Stephenson: May drugs that act on GABA$_B$ or NMDA receptors be effective in clinical practice?

Marescaux: It is quite difficult. Any time in vivo something interacts with GABA$_B$ or NMDA there is a lot of interaction with GABA$_B$ presynaptic receptors, which are located on glutamatergic cells. Any time we block GABA$_B$ receptors we also have an NMDA effect and any time we block GABA$_B$ receptors we increase aspartate and glutamate release, and we increase the risks of convulsive seizures. It is very difficult in vivo to differentiate the pre- and post-synaptic effects.

Stephenson: Does baclofen help any type of epileptic seizure?

Marescaux: It is surprisingly effective in several animal models but absolutely ineffective in humans. In humans, only a small fraction reaches the brain. Nobody knows exactly what a GABA$_B$ agonist, which crosses the blood–brain barrier very easily, can do.

Brodie: Can I ask about stiripentol? There is one study in the literature suggesting that it is effective in absence.

Marescaux: A few years ago we did a study with stiripentol and it will block absences in GAERS, but only at sedative doses. This is not very specific. Each time we put the rat into a sleepy state there are fewer absences.

Duncan: Ciba-Geigy in Basle are trialling GABA$_B$ antagonists in dementia but are not developing these drugs for absences. Are there any side-effects causing seizures in that population?

Marescaux: Nothing that I know of. I am not sure whether they will see any effect at all. Other drugs are much more potent – but not ready for use in humans.

Brodie: And 10% of those with dementia get seizures, so it is a complicated scenario.

Brodie: Does anybody know of any anti-epileptic drug that has not been mentioned that has been suggested to have anti-absence effects?

Marescaux: We have found an anti-absence effect of NMDA antagonists but with severe EEG side-effects, including the production of very strange behaviour in rats. Even in rats we can see that they are psychotic. It does not encourage the use of these drugs in humans.

In patients with Lennox–Gastaut syndrome, West's syndrome, or continuous spike-wave discharge during sleep we see a tremendous effect of corticosteroids. We are wondering if it is a classical anti-epileptic effect that we have not seen in patients with typical absences because no one has thought of using corticosteroids to treat typical absences.

We tried to use corticosteroids as chronic treatment in these rats and saw absolutely no effect on spike-wave discharges, even when they were almost dying of the effects of chronic treatment. The only thing that seemed to remain was the spike-wave discharge.

Genton: Are there any data on the effects of alcohol on generalised spikes and waves and on absence seizures on animal models or humans? Alcohol has an anti-myoclonic effect and has an effect on photo-sensitivity even in humans. Have you tried it in your rats?

Marescaux: Alcohol is a potent anti-epileptic in this model, as it is in humans. The main problems are tolerance and the short-term behavioural effects.

E Andermann: Could response to medication be helpful to us in genetic studies by: (a) further defining the phenotype and getting rid of some of the heterogeneity, and (b) using the response to medication as a guide to possible candidate genes?

Marescaux: I do not know. Initially I had the impression that resistance to valproic acid might be something very characteristic, but later gained the impression that patients were not sensitive to valproic acid for a metabolic reason. For these reasons I do not believe it will be a useful criterion.

It may be interesting to try and see if there are any differences in absences which are sensitive to valproic acid and not to ethosuximide, or absences that are sensitive to ethosuximide and not to valproic acid. But in view of the difficulties we are having with all the other criteria, I do not know if this would be pragmatic.

Brodie: The problem is if we knew how the drugs acted it would help, and, with a very few exceptions (possibly ethosuximide), we really do not know how the drugs work. We may know some mechanisms but by no means all.

Berkovic: There are anecdotal reports of monozygous twins reacting differently to anti-epileptic drugs. Lennox reported in a couple of his twins that one responded to tridione and the other did not. If we assume they are truly identical, that may not be a very smart way to go.

Marescaux: We believe there are several reasons why someone may not react to a drug. In children, for example, we are suprised by the numbers of children who are insensitive to valproic acid until we stop using the syrup and go for the classic pill. Even if they have a good blood level they do not react, but then when we go the classic pill they react. There are a lot of metabolic problems which are not understood.

3. Neurophysiological studies in animal models of absence

Douglas A. Coulter

In order to understand the cellular basis of neurophysiological circuit oscillations like the thalamo-cortical rhythms generating the spike-wave discharges (SWDs) of typical absences, we need to develop: a detailed insight into the synaptic (cellular) circuitry underlying generation of the epileptic discharges; rigorous characterisation of the intrinsic membrane (ionic) conductances activated during SWDs in the neuronal populations participating in generation of the discharge; and characterisation of the physiology and pharmacology of synaptic conductances activated during the pathological discharge.

THE THALAMO-CORTICAL CIRCUIT

The thalamus constitutes the major relay of information for sensory information to the cortex, except for olfaction. Thalamic neurons send an ordered axonal projection principally to layers III/IV and V/VI of neocortex, synapsing on both pyramidal neurons and interneurons. In turn, thalamic neurons receive a feedback projection from layer VI neurons in the same cortical area to which they project.

In addition, both the thalamo-cortical and cortico-thalamic projections send axon collaterals to the nucleus reticularis thalami (NRT), which is an entirely GABA-ergic nucleus surrounding the thalamus (Houser et al, 1980). NRT in turn provides a strong inhibitory innervation to the thalamus (Jones, 1985). Although other areas of the brain are involved in modulating and controlling thalamo-cortical rhythm generation, isolated synapses described above are capable of supporting thalamo-cortical oscillations in vitro (Coulter & Lee, 1993).

STUDIES IN ISOLATED NEURONS

Thalamic relay neurons constitute one of the few neuronal types in which single cell recordings can be directly related to behaviour: the thalamus is the primary relay for sensory information to the cortex, and thalamic neurons are not mutually interconnected. Their primary axonal targets are the neocortex and NRT, with few or no intrathalamic axonal collaterals (Jones,

1985). Hence, alterations in thalamic neuronal activity and excitability will have direct, readily interpretable consequences for both circuit properties and perception.

Characterising and comparing properties of voltage- and ligand-gated conductances on cortical and thalamic neurons provides data from which to develop a detailed model of how thalamus and cortex interact to generate rhythms. This helps define and understand cellular mechanisms of drug action involved in control of absences. Longer term, this type of framework can also help explain the nature of the pathological processes underlying this seizure disorder.

We isolated and recorded from thalamic and cortical neurons within 24 h of removal, which allowed for isolation of healthy neurons with trimmed dendritic trees, usually only leaving the primary and secondary dendrites on the cell. This acute isolation methodology facilitates high quality voltage-clamp recording and minimises potential artifactual problems.

INTRINSIC MEMBRANE CONDUCTANCES OF THALAMIC AND CORTICAL NEURONS: CHARACTERISATION AND SENSITIVITY TO ANTI-EPILEPTIC DRUGS

Thalamic neurons are endowed with an ensemble of voltage-dependent ionic conductances which are activated and inactivated by changes in membrane potential overlapping with the normal range of potentials occurring during the resting state of these cells. These conductances play a significant role in generating normal cellular behaviour in these neurons. The role of these conductances is particularly notable in the generation of the state-dependent changes in behaviour evident in thalamic neurons. In the waking state, thalamic neurons faithfully transduce information and relay it from the periphery to the cortex. As an animal falls asleep, thalamic neurons hyperpolarise (Hirsch et al, 1983), and a portion of the conductances which are inactivated at normal 'awake' membrane potentials 'de-inactivate', and alter the behaviour of thalamic neurons, and of the system as a whole.

The system becomes generally unresponsive to external input. It tends to oscillate spontaneously, generating slow sleep rhythms such as spindle waves and thalamic neurons tend to shift their action potential firing mode from a tonic, single-spike mode to a phasic, burst-firing mode (Hirsch et al, 1983). Chief among the conductances involved in these state-dependent alterations is the large, low-threshold calcium current (LTCC) in thalamic neurons, which is activated and inactivated by potentials near rest (Fig. 3.1A) and tends to trigger large bursts of action potentials riding on low-threshold calcium spikes when activated.

Three main characteristics of the LTCC stand out: the large amplitude of the current in thalamic neurons relative to other areas of the brain; the low threshold for its activation; and the voltage-dependent inactivation of the current by potentials near rest (Coulter et al, 1989b). Figure 3.1 illus-

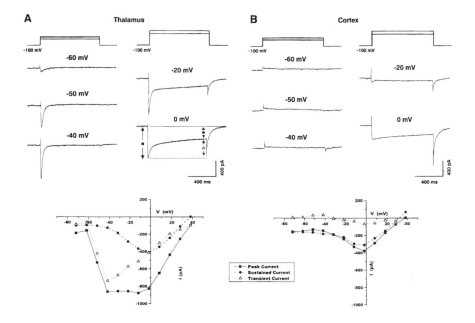

Fig. 3.1 Calcium currents in thalamus and cortex. **A** Raw traces illustrating the response of a rat thalamic (left) and cortical (right) neuron to increasing depolarising step commands from a holding potential of -100 mV, under ionic conditions designed to isolate calcium currents (Coulter et al, 1989b). Note the large, transient calcium current in the thalamic (but not the cortical) neuron, which activates at very low threshold (by –60 mV). The amplitude of the step command eliciting the current in each trace is specified above the trace. In this and all subsequent voltage-clamp traces, inward currents are downward deflections. **B** Plot of the current voltage relations for the thalamic and cortical neuron, traces from which are depicted in **A**. The peak current (squares), the sustained current (defined as the amplitude of current which does not inactivate at the end of the 1 s step; circles), and the transient current (defined as the amount of current which inactivates during the 1 s step command, or peak-sustained; triangles) are plotted against the amplitude of the step command eliciting the current. Note the large, transient current in the thalamic neuron, larger in peak amplitude than the sustained current in the same cell. Also note the lack of a transient calcium current in the cortical neuron. Both the traces and the IVs are not leak subtracted (Gibbs & Coulter, unpublished data).

trates the distinct nature of the calcium currents present in rat cortical and thalamic neurons. The thalamic neuron has a large, transient, inactivating calcium current, which activates at potentials near –70 mV. As the neuron is depolarised further, an additional, sustained calcium current begins to activate at potentials near –30 mV. The peak amplitude of the LTCC is larger than the non-inactivating, sustained calcium current. In the cortical neuron, little or no calcium current is activated until potentials near –30 mV and virtually all of this calcium current is higher-threshold and non-inactivating. The properties of the LTCC in thalamic neurons characterised in these studies demonstrate that this current is both necessary for generation of low-threshold calcium spikes and sufficient to account for the properties of this regenerative potential.

Anti-absence drugs, such as ethosuximide, dimethadione and methyl-phenyl succinimide, all blocked the LTCC in a concentration-dependent, reversible, repeatable manner (Fig. 3. 2) (Coulter et al, 1989a; 1989c;1991). Furthermore, the rising phase of the concentration-dependence of this block overlapped clinically relevant concentration ranges of these drugs, i.e. concentrations of drug achieved as free serum levels in adequately med-icated epileptic patients (Coulter et al, 1989a). Other anti-epileptic drugs, including phenytoin and carbamazepine, were ineffective in blocking LTCC in thalamic neurons. Control agents, which were ineffective clin-ically but similar in structure to ethosuximide also did not block LTCC (Coulter et al, 1989c). Valproic acid may share ethosuximide's action in blocking LTCC (Kelly et al, 1990), although this has yet to be documented in thalamic neurons. This LTCC-blocking action of ethosuximide has been demonstrated dramatically to dampen thalamic oscillations in vitro and is consistent with the efficacy of this drug against absences (Huguenard & Prince, 1994; von Krosigk et al, 1993).

FURTHER ISOLATED NEURON STUDIES

In the rhythmic state of the thalamo-cortical system, GABA-ergic inhibi-tion impinging onto thalamic neurons from NRT synchronises the thal-amo-cortical oscillation, while the large LTCC present in thalamic neurons amplifies and drives the oscillation. The role of NRT-mediated inhibition in synchronising thalamo-cortical rhythms has been well established in sleep spindle-generation studies in vivo (reviewed in Steriade & Llinas, 1988), and in studies in thalamic slices (e.g. Huguenard & Prince, 1994; von Krosigk et al, 1993). This anomalous role of the inhibitory neurotransmitter GABA is probably responsible for most of the distinct pharmacological

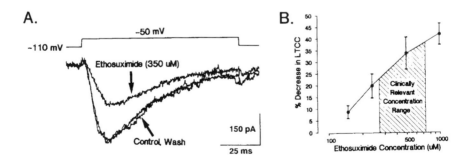

Fig. 3.2   Ethosuximide block of low-threshold calcium current (LTCC) in thalamic neurons. **A** Application of 350 μM ethosuximide resulted in a reversible reduction of the LTCC. Control, ethosuximide-blocked, and wash traces are super-imposed. **B** Concentration-dependence of ethosuximide block of LTCC in 5 neurons. Points are mean ±1 SEM. The 'clinically relevant concentration range' depicted in the hatched bar corresponds to free serum concentrations of 40–100 μg/ml (Coulter et al, 1989).

properties of typical absences relative to other forms of epilepsy.

Drugs which act through enhancement of GABA-mediated inhibition have inconsistent actions in the control of typical absences. Benzodiazepines such as diazepam and clonazepam control typical absences effectively, while anticonvulsant barbiturates are ineffective or may even exacerbate absences. Oh et al (1994) examined the activity of benzodiazepines and barbiturates in potentiating $GABA_A$-mediated responses in thalamic and cortical neurons.

To understand how drug effects can be interpreted, it is necessary to consider how inhibitory post-synaptic potentials (IPSPs) interact with the post-synaptic membrane properties of thalamic and cortical neurons. Cortical neurons have very little LTCC (Fig. 3.1), and so lack this large 'bursting' conductance de-inactivated by an IPSP-mediated hyperpolarisation. In thalamic neurons, with very large LTCC, IPSPs originating from NRT hyperpolarise the membrane potential, de-inactivate the calcium current and trigger a large low-threshold calcium burst on the decay phase of the IPSP, driving and synchronising subsequent thalamo-cortical rhythms (e.g. Fig. 3.4B, D; for review see Steriade & Llinas, 1988). Hence, regionally localised augmentation of GABA-ergic synaptic potentials would tend to promote oscillatory activity in thalamus and reduce activity in the cortex.

In studies with adult rat cortical and thalamic neurons, phenobarbital was equally effective in augmenting GABA responses in thalamic and cortical neurons (Oh et al, 1994). Clonazepam, in contrast, was much more efficacious in augmenting GABA responses in cortical rather than thalamic neurons (Fig. 3.3) (Oh et al, 1994), and would be a more effective anti-absence drug.

STUDIES ON SLICES

That SWDs require the presence of both the thalamus and cortex for expression has been demonstrated in the genetically epilepsy-prone rats of Strasbourg (Vergnes & Marescaux, 1982), and the feline generalised penicillin model (Prince & Farell, 1969), and has been studied in detail (e.g. Avoli et al 1983; reviewed in Gloor & Fariello, 1988). In both models, functional disconnection of cortex from thalamus, or inactivation of the cortex, stopped spike-wave discharges; other thalamo-cortical rhythms, like sleep spindles, only require intact thalamic/NRT connections for expression (e.g. Huguenard & Prince, 1994; von Krosigk et al, 1993; see review in Steriade & Llinas, 1988). Study of mechanisms underlying these rhythms requires a slice preparation (Agmon & Connors, 1991), which maintains reciprocal connections between thalamus and cortex and generates spontaneous thalamo-cortical oscillations when exposed to a medium without added Mg^{2+} (Coulter & Lee, 1993). These discharges resemble SWDs morphologically and pharmacologically.

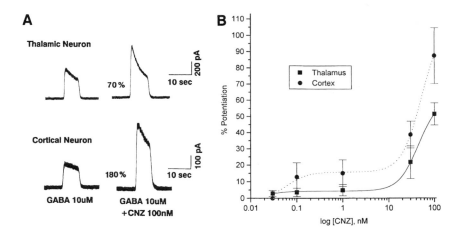

Fig. 3.3   Benzodiazepine augmentation of GABA$_A$ currents in adult rat cortical and thalamic neurons. **A** Representative traces illustrating the effects of the anticonvulsant benzodiazepine clonazepam on outward GABA-evoked chloride currents in adult rat thalamic and cortical neurons. Note the increased augmentation of GABA currents in cortical neurons (180% by 100 nM clonazepam) relative to thalamic neurons (70% under identical conditions). Both neurons are from the same animal, a 67-day-old rat. **B** Plot of the concentration-dependence of GABA current augmentation by clonazepam in adult cortical and thalamic neurons (all values mean ± 1 standard error). Note the significant increased effect of clonazepam in cortical neurons (modified from Oh et al, 1994).

CHARACTERISATION OF RHYTHMS

Perfusion of rodent thalamo-cortical slices with a medium without added Mg^{2+} results in generation of spontaneous generalised thalamo-cortical discharges consisting of 2–20 s periods of generalised activity, recurring every 10–120 s (Fig. 3.4A). Individual discharges usually begin with a large burst, which resembles a cortical paroxysmal depolarising shift (PDS). A period of smaller, rhythmic bursting occupies the remainder of the discharge, which builds from smaller initial bursts, undergoes a period of larger bursts and then wanes. The frequency of bursting varies from 3–12 Hz, usually in the range 7–10 Hz. Severing thalamo-cortical connections as they traverse the striatum results in loss of all activity in thalamus and severe truncation and disruption of the cortically recorded activity (Coulter & Lee, 1993).

Discharges recorded in somatosensory cortex in these conditions usually consist of a PDS, followed by an arrhythmic series of 2–5 small bursts lasting 1 s or less. Thus, intact thalamo-cortical connections are required for full expression of the low-Mg^{2+} spontaneous generalised activity in these slices, although neocortex alone is capable of sustaining some distinct types of activity. This thalamo-cortical oscillatory activity is distinct from the sleep spindle activity recorded in thalamic slices by Huguenard and Prince (1994) and von Krosigk et al (1993).

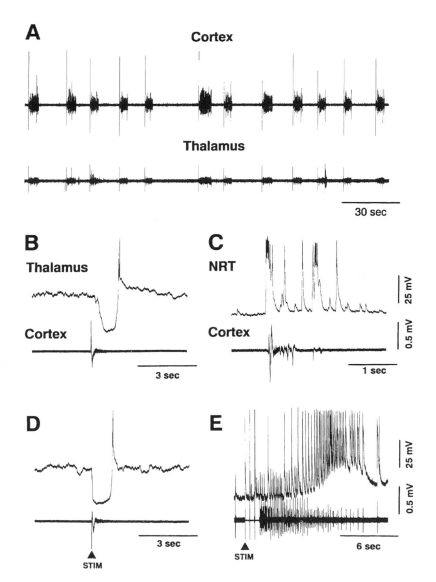

Fig. 3.4   Spontaneous generalised low-Mg^{2+} thalamo-cortical rhythms in vitro. **A** Extracellular field potential recordings of spontaneous thalamo-cortical rhythms induced by perfusion of a rat thalamo-cortical slice with medium containing no added Mg^{2+}. Note the tightly coupled activity in thalamus and cortex. **B** Patch recording from a thalamic ventrobasal complex neuron illustrating the response of this cell to a spontaneous burst recorded extracellularly in somatosensory cortex. Note the brief EPSP, followed by a large IPSP in this cell. **C** Patch recording from a nucleus reticularis thalami (NRT) neuron, illustrating the response of this cell to a short spontaneous rhythm, recorded extracellularly in somatosensory cortex. Note the large bursts of action potentials, with no sign of IPSPs. **D** Response of the thalamic neuron from **B** to extracellular stimulation of somatosensory cortex. Note the large IPSP elicited by this stimulus. **E** Response of an NRT neuron to a train of extracellular cortical stimuli, which triggered a seizure-like event. Note the large bursts and subsequent large sustained depolarisation elicited in this NRT neuron by the cortical stimulation.

CELLULAR CORRELATES OF THALAMO-CORTICAL SLICE RHYTHMS

Intracellular recording with conventional sharp or patch electrodes in slices exhibiting low-Mg^{2+} spontaneous thalamo-cortical rhythms discloses the cellular correlates of this extracellularly recorded activity. In thalamic somatosensory relay neurons, thalamo-cortical oscillations are usually accompanied by large initial IPSPs which trigger rebound low-threshold calcium spikes on the decay phase of the IPSP (Fig. 3.4B) (Coulter, 1992; Coulter & Zhang, 1994). Similar large IPSPs can be triggered in thalamic neurons by stimulating cortex (Fig. 3.4D) or by stimulating NRT, suggesting that these IPSPs may be mediated by cortical recurrent activation of NRT, which subsequently releases inhibitory neurotransmitter onto the thalamic neuron (Coulter & Zhang, 1994).

In contrast to the large IPSPs evident in thalamic relay neurons accompanying cortical activity, intracellular recordings in NRT neurons reveal large depolarisations and bursts of action potentials accompanying thalamo-cortical activity, with little or no evidence of IPSPs (Fig. 3.4C; Coulter and Zhang, 1994). Similarly, cortical stimulation elicits large EPSPs and burst firing in NRT neurons, with no evidence of inhibition (Fig. 3.4E) (Coulter & Zhang, 1994). These data suggest that these synapses do not play a major role in generating or expressing low-Mg^{2+} spontaneous thalamo-cortical activity (Jones, 1985; Steriade & Llinas, 1988). The role of inhibitory interconnections in generating absence seizures, or of sleep spindles in normal function, remains to be determined.

SENSITIVITY OF RHYTHMS TO ANTI-EPILEPTIC DRUGS

The anti-convulsant sensitivity of the low-Mg^{2+} spontaneous rhythms generated in rodent thalamo-cortical slices has begun to be characterised (Coulter, 1992; Coulter & Zhang, 1994). All drugs were applied in concentration ranges overlapping those achieved as free serum levels in effectively controlled patients. The anti-absence drugs ethosuximide, valproic acid and dimethadione were effective in reducing or blocking spontaneous thalamo-cortical rhythms in vitro. Phenytoin and carbamazepine were less effective, while phenobarbital was only effective in sedative concentrations. Their relative effectiveness was as follows: dimethadione > ethosuximide = valproate > phenytoin = carbamazepine > phenobarbital (Coulter, 1992; Coulter & Zhang, 1994).

Spontaneous oscillatory activity in rodent thalamo-cortical slices appears to constitute a potentially useful in vitro model of pathological thalamo-cortical oscillations like SWDs. Further studies examining important physiological and pharmacological factors critical in generating these discharges may prove valuable in understanding the pathophysiology of typical absences.

ACKNOWLEDGEMENTS

The contributions of Yun-Fu Zhang, Chang-Joong Lee, Kwang-Soo Oh and John W. Gibbs III at the Medical College of Virginia were instrumental in the experiments described in this chapter, as was the technical support of George P. Nanos, III. The contributions of Drs JR Huguenard and DA Prince of Stanford University Medical Center are also gratefully acknowledged. Supported by grants from the NIH-NINDS (R29 NS 31000), the Epilepsy Foundation of America, the Milken Family Foundation and the Sophie and Nathan Gumenick Neuroscience and Alzheimer's Research Fund.

REFERENCES

Agmon A, Connors BW 1991 Thalamocortical responses of mouse somatosensory (barrel) cortex in vitro. Neuroscience 41: 365–379

Avoli M, Gloor P, Kostopoulos G, Gotman J 1983 An analysis of penicillin-induced generalized spike and wave discharges using simultaneous recordings of single cortical and thalamic neurons. Journal of Neurophysiology 50: 819–837

Coulter DA 1992 Physiological studies of thalamo-cortical rhythms, recorded in vitro in a brain slice preparation. Soc. Neurosci. Abstr. 18: 1391

Coulter DA, Lee C-J 1993 Thalamocortical rhythm generation in vitro: Extra- and intracellular recordings in mouse thalamo-cortical slices perfused with low-Mg^{2+} medium. Brain Research 631: 137–142

Coulter DA, Zhang Y-F 1994 Thalamocortical rhythm generation studied in rat thalamo-cortical slices using whole cell patch techniques. Soc. Neurosci. Abstr. 20: (in press)

Coulter DA, Huguenard JR, Prince DA 1989a Specific petit mal anticonvulsants reduce calcium currents in thalamic neurons. Neuroscience Letters 98: 74–78

Coulter DA, Huguenard JR, Prince DA 1989b Calcium currents in rat thalamo-cortical relay neurones: kinetic properties of the transient, low-threshold current. Journal of Physiology 414: 587–604

Coulter DA, Huguenard JR, Prince DA 1989c Characterization of ethosuximide reduction of low-threshold calcium current in thalamic neurons. Annals of Neurology 25: 582–593

Coulter DA, Huguenard JR, Prince DA 1990 Differential effects of petit mal anticonvulsants and convulsants on thalamic neurones. I. Calcium current reduction. British Journal of Pharmacology 100: 800–806

Gloor P, Fariello RG 1988 Generalized epilepsy: Some of its cellular mechanisms differ from those of focal epilepsy. TINS 11: 63–68

Hirsch JC, Fourment A, Marc ME 1983 Sleep-related variations of membrane potential in lateral geniculate body relay neurons of the cat. Brain Research 259: 308–312

Houser CR, Vaugn JE, Barber RP, Roberts E 1980 GABA neurons are the major cell type of the nucleus reticularis thalami. Brain Research 200: 341–354

Huguenard JR, Prince DA 1994 Intrathalamic rhythmicity studied in vitro: nominal T current modulation causes robust antioscillatory effects. Journal of Neuroscience (in press)

Jones EG 1985 The thalamus. Plenum Press, New York

Kelly KM, Gross RA, Macdonald RL 1990 Valproic acid selectively reduces the low-threshold (T) calcium current in rat nodose neurons. Neuroscience Letters 116: 233–238

Oh K-S, Lee C-J, Gibbs JW, Coulter DA 1994 Postnatal development of GABA$_A$ receptor function in somatosensory thalamus and cortex: Whole-cell voltage-clamp recordings in acutely isolated rat neurons. Journal of Neuroscience (in press)

Prince DA, Farell D 1969 'Centrencephalic' spike-wave discharges following parenteral penicillin injection in the cat. Neurology 19: 309–310

Steriade M, Llinas RR 1988 The functional states of the thalamus and the associated neuronal interplay. Physiological Reviews 68: 649–742

Vergnes M, Marescaux C 1982 Cortical and thalamic lesions in rats with genetic absence
  epilepsy. Journal of Neural Transmission 35 (Suppl.): 71–83
Vergnes M, Marescaux C, Depaulis A, Micheletti G, Warter JM 1987 Spontaneous spike and
  wave discharges in thalamus and cortex in a rat model of genetic petit mal-like seizures.
  Experimental Neurology 96: 127–186
von Krosigk M, Bal T, McCormick DA 1993 Cellular mechanisms of a synchronized
  oscillation in the thalamus. Science 261: 361–364
Williams D 1953 A study of thalamic and cortical rhythms in petit mal. Brain 76: 50–69

DISCUSSION

Berkovic: Are the thalamic mechanisms for spindles identical to those for spike and wave discharges in absences as determined by measuring the properties of these channels? Is the fundamental abnormality in a rat or a human that generates spike waves in the cortex?

Coulter: Little is known about that. The problem is that it has not yet been possible to obtain spike-wave discharges in vitro. Getting spindle-like discharges in vitro has been possible and that is why I have discussed many spindle mechanisms. Most of the distinctions that have been seen in the animal models of absences, where there is a difference from normal function, seem to be cortical. Accordingly, I think it most likely that a cortical mechanism is activating the circuitry I have been discussing.

Van Luijtelaar: I am confused about this phasing bursting mode which we see in the thalamus and which is always present when a subject goes to sleep. When do spindles come in?

Coulter: In very deep stages of sleep we do not have spindles. One can move into a range of membrane potentials in thalamus which is too hyper-polarised to generate these kinds of rhythms. One has to be within a window of phasic activity and one cannot be too hyper-polarised so as not be be able to trigger the burst.

Spindles occur during spindle stages of sleep. Spike waves, on the other hand, tend to occur during periods of quiet wakefulness or sleep/wake transitions or drowsiness. One can move into a phasic mode of firing without being asleep.

4. Genetic mechanisms of spike-wave epilepsies in mouse mutants

Jeffrey L. Noebels

Defined single locus mutations in the mouse provide a coherent experimental framework for analysing the expression of excitability genes one at a time in the developing brain, and offer a powerful model system for the genetic analysis of spike-wave epilepsies (Noebels, 1979). A systematic search for these genetic models by electrophysiological screening has so far identified a subgroup of neurological mouse mutants with spontaneous epileptic phenotypes that has contributed to our understanding of basic mechanisms of spike-wave epileptogenesis in three essential ways. First, the mutants have permitted the correlation of specific murine gene loci with neurologically distinct absence epilepsy syndromes. Second, they have enabled detailed pathological studies of the developmental expression of mechanisms for spike-wave electrogenesis and of seizure-induced alterations in network excitability at the molecular and cellular levels. Third, they have provided reproducible biological test systems to explore the pharmacogenetics of this pattern of generalised epilepsy, and to experimentally correct the expression of the seizure phenotype prior to its clinical appearance.

In addition to their ongoing utility as phenotypic models, mouse mutants offer the substantial promise of contributing in a fourth way, namely, by providing specific points of departure in the search for human epilepsy genes. Attempts to identify these genes in man by chromosomal linkage analysis are presently hindered by the clinical heterogeneity of absence syndromes occurring in childhood, while the alternative strategy of testing pedigrees for individual candidate gene loci is burdened by the number and complexity of membrane mechanisms regulating thalamocortical synchronisation in the developing brain (Steriade et al, 1990). By taking advantage of the increasing resolution of restriction mapping of syntenic loci on the chromosomes of mouse and man, human absence epilepsies in small nuclear families can now be directly evaluated for linkage to markers corresponding to murine epilepsy genes. Will any of the mutations that arise spontaneously in mice actually coincide with those responsible for human absence syndromes? The answer to this question will come only once genetic testing is routine, since the homology that murine and human epilepsy genes might share is difficult to predict from clinical similarities alone.

While it is virtually certain that the entire set of molecular errors detected in epileptic mice will not be identical to those that currently prevail in the human clinical population, the basic cellular mechanisms of spike-wave epileptogenesis that are inherited in each are likely to converge on relatively specific circuits in the brain, and it will be surprising if several molecular steps in the intervening excitability disturbances that give rise to spike-wave synchronisation do not overlap between the two species. Most importantly, it will be invaluable to learn from the inherited mouse lesions which categories of molecules can give rise to these recurrent seizure syndromes. Are they membrane-bound channels or receptors that regulate rapid burst firing; cytoplasmic second messengers that control slower neuromodulatory processes; or releasable trophic molecules that mediate long-term changes in synaptic transmission and circuitry? Finally, in order to direct future studies toward novel molecular targets for therapy, it will be critical to learn from the mouse mutants whether epilepsy genes involve a gain or loss in function, at what temporal stage of brain development they act, and whether the inherited molecular error triggers a cascade of epileptogenic or anti-epileptogenic synaptic reorganisation. Such patterns of secondary neuronal plasticity could explain the appearance of a second clinical seizure type in the same patient, or (in 'benign' epilepsy syndromes) the subsequent disappearance of seizures.

GENETIC HETEROGENEITY IN MOUSE MODELS OF ABSENCE EPILEPSY

Along with the promise these models hold for our eventual understanding of the natural history of absence epilepsies, the comparative analysis of the nervous systems of mutant mice with spike-wave seizures has already begun to reveal the extent of genotypic and phenotypic diversity that is likely to be associated with this important category of childhood epilepsy. Electrophysiological survey of over 110 mapped murine mutants for cortical excitability defects has so far revealed 5 recessive gene loci (*lethargic*, chr 2; *tottering*, chr 8; *ducky*, chr 9; *mocha²ᴶ*, chr 10; *stargazer*, chr 15) expressing spontaneous, generalised 6 spikes/s discharges in the cortical EEG associated with arrest of movement (Fig. 4.1). The seizures typically begin in the third week of life, continue throughout adulthood, and are rapidly and effectively blocked by the antiabsence drug ethosuximide, but not by phenobarbital or phenytoin.

Initial studies of these mutants have revealed at least four fundamental properties underlying the heredity of the spike-wave cortical synchronisation trait in mice. First, a defect at a single gene locus is indeed sufficient to produce a spontaneous, generalised spike-wave seizure disorder. Second, the EEG trait itself is genetically heterogeneous, and can arise from recessive mutations at more than one chromosomal locus. Third, the intervening mutant cellular excitability mechanisms underlying the generation of spike-wave cortical synchronisation at these loci are not necessarily identical, and thus the cellular phenotype of genes for spike-wave epilepsy is also heterogeneous. Fourth, the mutant genes give rise to distinct neurological syndromes, each with a characteristic seizure frequency, sensitivity to antiepileptic drugs, and severity of the associated neurological phenotype. The specific elements of these epilepsy syndromes may vary according to the nature of the primary mutant molecular error, the time of onset in the developing brain, and the degree of secondary seizure-dependent plasticity in the affected neural circuits. Insight into these hereditary parameters is extremely useful in framing the search for related disease genes in human pedigrees.

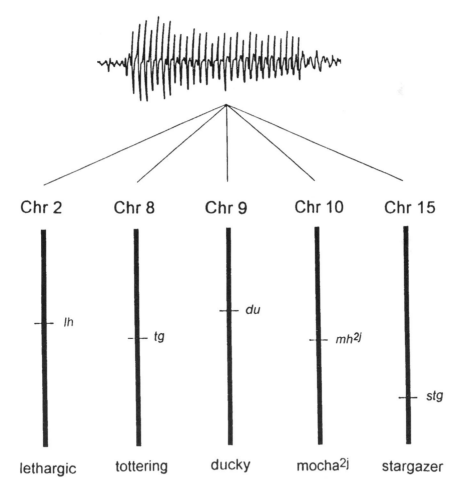

Fig 4.1 Genetic heterogeneity of the spike-wave EEG phenotype. Five recessive mutant loci mapped to independent mouse chromosomes demonstrate locus heterogeneity of the synchronous cortical excitability trait. EEG studies reveal additional gene-linked differences in seizure severity and cerebral localisation.

Continuing analysis of the spike-wave mutants has revealed a number of factors contributing to the variance of inherited absence epilepsy phenotypes. Locus heterogeneity and allelic heterogeneity are features of inherited absence syndromes that have now been clearly identified by the mapped mouse mutants. (Noebels, 1986). Gene dose, as well as the specific disease locus inherited, also contribute to the clinical severity of the spike-wave seizure disorder at certain murine loci (Qiao & Noebels, 1991). There is variability in the developmental onset of the seizure disorder when compared between genetic models; e.g. the *tottering* and *stargazer* mutant mice display seizures in the third postnatal week (Noebels and Tharp, 1994). However, seizures begin several weeks to months later in models derived from inbred rat strains (Coenen & Van Luijtelaar, 1987, Vergnes et al, 1990). The morphology of the spike-wave discharge can vary between genetic models, the most notable difference being the spike frequency (6–7/s in mouse mutants, 11/s in affected rat strains). Different regional cerebral synchronisation patterns have also been distinguished between these two sets of models; the *tg* and *stg* mouse mutants show hippocampal spike-wave discharges (Noebels, 1984, Qiao & Noebels, 1993a), a feature also described within human limbic structures (Angeleri et al, 1964, Niedermeyer et al 1969) that are absent in the inbred GAERS model (Vergnes et al, 1990). These data demonstrate that spike-wave synchronisation is a genetically heterogeneous EEG trait, and that differences in the clinical phenotype of generalised absence epilepsies in children may signal the existence of multiple disease genes.

DIVERSITY IN PRIMARY CELLULAR DEFECTS FOR SPIKE-WAVE EPILEPTOGENESIS

Neuropathological comparisons of the epileptic mouse mutants using anatomical and physiological studies provide clear evidence that different gene loci do not a share a single common mechanism favouring spike-wave epileptogenesis, although evidence is beginning to indicate that the various mutant gene actions may overlap at higher levels of neural organisation. For example, the *tottering* mutant shows a selective proliferation of noradrenergic axon terminals originating in the pontine Locus Coeruleus nuclei, and these fibres hyperinnervate the mutant forebrain (Levitt & Noebels, 1981). In vitro analysis of network excitability in *tg/tg* neurons reveals a reduction in neuronal afterhyperpolarisation under bursting conditions that is linked to the excess local release of noradrenaline (Helekar & Noebels, 1991,1994). In contrast, the *stargazer* mouse shows no noradrenergic hyperinnervation (Qiao & Noebels, 1991); nevertheless, in vitro intracellular recordings in *stg/stg* mice reveal that these neurons also show a reduction in burst-related afterhyperpolarisation (Keegan & Noebels, 1993) (Fig. 4.2). These findings demonstrate that two different gene mutations that give rise to cortical spike-wave epilepsy can act through separate intervening defects to produce similar decrements in cellular repolarisation. This pattern of network hyperexcitability may lower the threshold for aberrant thalamocortical oscillatory activity.

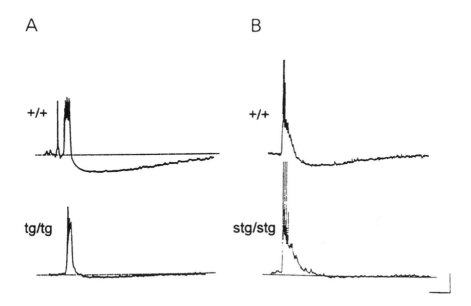

Fig 4.2 Two distinct genes for spike-wave seizures both reduce neuronal afterhyperpolarisation. Intracellular recordings in brain slices from *tottering* and *stargazer* mutants with generalised spike-wave epilepsy reveal in vitro repolarisation defect in bursting neural networks. **A** CA3 pyramidal neurons in +/+ and *tg/tg* hippocampal slices bursting in 10 mM $[K^+]_O$ bath solution demonstrate reduction of post-burst afterhyperpolarisation in the mutant compared to +/+ control. **B** Deep cortical neurons in +/+ and *stg/stg* thalamocortical slices bursting in 0 mM $[Mg^{2+}]_O$ bath solution show similar reduction in post-burst afterhyperpolarisation compared to the wild type (from Helekar & Noebels, 1991; Keegan & Noebels, 1993). Calibration: 10 mV, 100 ms.

Pharmacogenetic variation can also be used to distinguish between different genetic models of absence epilepsy, supporting the evidence for diverse mechanisms of spike-wave epileptogenesis. For example, spike-wave seizures in *lethargic* mice (Hosford et al, 1992) and GAERS rats (Marescaux et al, 1992) are blocked by the $GABA_B$ antagonist CGP 35348, while those in *stargazer* mutants are little affected by this compound (Qiao & Noebels, 1992), indicating varying degrees of dependence on functional $GABA_B$ receptor blockade for the abnormal expression of thalamocortical oscillations. While rodent models may or may not represent homologues of human epilepsy, these findings suggest an important approach toward further categorising clinical absence syndromes, but also predict that the useful antiepileptic spectrum of new drugs that are based on a specific molecular defect may be potentially limited to certain variants of generalised absence epilepsy syndromes in man.

MULTIPLE SITES FOR CORRECTING THE CELLULAR EXPRESSION OF EPILEPSY GENES

The inheritance of certain molecular defects in the nervous system may give rise to an easily identifiable, unitary, and stable cause of seizures, for example when a mutation alters the gene for a critical membrane ion channel or neurotransmitter receptor, resulting in abnormal synchronous bursting. Alternatively, the primary action of the mutant gene product may be several steps removed from the membrane instability producing the epileptic phenotype, for example when it encodes a growth factor that indirectly alters network excitability by modifying the balance of synaptic excitation and inhibition. To complicate matters, the inherited hyperexcitable signalling patterns can further modify synaptically-linked brain circuits by activity-induced gene transcription (Gall et al, 1991), and may play a role in the evolution of the clinical syndrome. These relationships, summarised in Fig. 4.3, evolve in both time and space during development of the epileptic brain. The spike-wave epilepsy mutants offer a highly reproducible model system to trace the biology of these inherited 'progressive' lesions, and to test the feasibility of modifying epileptic phenotypes at different temporal stages of the disease.

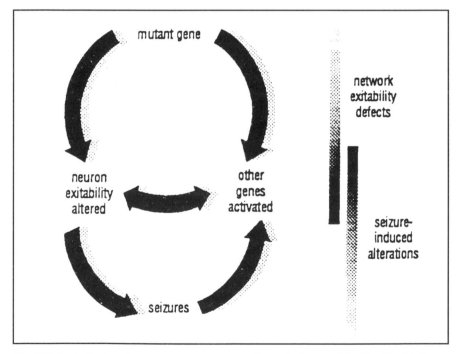

Fig 4.3 Intervening steps between mutant gene expression and seizure activity identify critical relationships underlying secondary plasticity in the epileptic brain, and new targets for antiepileptic therapy. Reciprocal relationship between abnormal synchronous discharges and evolving patterns of abnormal gene expression in the brain could underlie the changes in clinical seizure phenotype and severity during development.

One example of correctable gene-linked plasticity underlying the generation of spike-wave epilepsy is provided by the *tottering* mutant. Homozygous *tottering* mice show a proliferation of noradrenergic forebrain innervation in target regions involved in spike-wave epileptogenesis such as the thalamus, neocortex, and hippocampus. While the identity of the *tg* gene is not yet known, neonatal reversal of the inherited noradrenergic hyperinnervation using a selective neurotoxin permanently prevented the expression of spike-wave seizures in the adult mouse (Noebels, 1984). This treatment was subsequently found to be ineffective in blocking spike-wave seizure activity in the *stargazer* mouse brain where central noradrenergic systems are unaltered (Qiao & Noebels, 1991), demonstrating that the anti-epileptic effect in *tottering* mutants was due to a prevention of excess central noradrenergic signalling, rather than a non-specific effect on the developing brain. This selectivity demonstrates the potential for correcting gene-linked defects in excitability early in development by modifying endogenous neuromodulatory pathways.

The phenomenon of mossy fibre sprouting found in human focal hippocampal epileptic foci (Sutula et al, 1989) provides an example of the second type of plasticity in epileptic brain, namely seizure-induced synaptic reorganisation. Histochemical studies have revealed the presence of aberrant mossy fibre sprouting and neosynaptogenesis within the inner molecular layer of the *stargazer* dentate gyrus in a pattern identical to that found in human and experimental models of limbic epilepsy (Qiao & Noebels, 1993a). Developmental studies show clearly that the sprouting begins several weeks after the onset of seizures on postnatal days 16–18 in the mutant mouse, and recent data indicate that the level of mRNAs for a brain-derived growth factor, BDNF, is selectively elevated in *stargazer* granule cells at early stages of the seizure disorder (Qiao & Noebels, 1993b). Similar, but far less pronounced, patterns of axon sprouting were found in the *tottering* mutant, which shows a far less severe seizure disorder. These studies suggest that the spike-wave pattern of synchronisation found in generalised absence epilepsies is likely to be associated with progressive changes in cerebral excitability.

CONCLUSION

An experimental framework for identifying and analysing the cerebral expression of single epilepsy genes in the developing mouse brain is described. Within the coming decade, additional epilepsy genes in spontaneous mouse mutants will be phenotypically identified, and many will be cloned and sequenced, allowing the identification and mapping of their homologues to human chromosomes. A second set of epilepsy genes will emerge from a new generation of transgenic mouse mutations designed to test the contribution of specific candidate excitability molecules to spike-wave epileptogenesis. All of these loci should provide an entry point into the genetic analysis of human absence epilepsy pedigrees, as well as specific information regarding the molecular diversity of the underlying basic mechanisms. In parallel with these studies, molecular genetic analysis of human epilepsy pedigrees should begin to reveal (1) whether the various syndromes involve damage to a single gene or several contiguous ones; (2) whether the mutations determine a loss or gain in molecular function; and (3) whether absence epilepsy syndromes can be strongly influenced by multiple non-syntenic modifier genes. As this information becomes available, the naturally-occurring human genetic lesions can be precisely reproduced in transgenic mice by recombinant DNA techniques to create more faithful experimental models of the specific human diseases.

The reproducibility of neurological mouse mutants makes possible a controlled analysis of the evolution of cellular events leading to the expression of seizures in the developing brain. Once the affected cells are localised and the excitability changes pinpointed, subsequent seizure-induced aberrant gene expression can be assessed. The recent observations that spike-wave seizures trigger activity-dependent plasticity in the mouse brain raise important questions of whether similar changes may also take place in this category of childhood epilepsy. In the future, the ability to identify and regulate the expression of genes that can selectively minimise the likelihood of this pattern of aberrant synchronisation may point the way toward novel molecular approaches in antiepileptic therapy.

ACKNOWLEDGEMENT

I would like to thank S. Helekar, X. Qiao and W. Nahm for their contributions to this research. Supported by the NIH NS29709, Baylor Epilepsy Research Center NS11535, and the Blue Bird Circle Foundation for Pediatric Neurology.

REFERENCES

Angeleri F, Ferro-Milone F, Parigi S 1964 Electrical activity and reactivity of the rhinencephalic, pararhinencephalic and thalamic structures: prolonged implantation of electrodes in man. Electroencephalography and Clinical Neurophysiology 16: 100–129
Coenen AML, Van Luijtelaar ELJM 1987 The WAG/Rij rat model for absence epilepsy: age and sex factors. Epilepsy Research 1: 297–301
Gall CM, Lauterborn J, Bundman M, Murray K, Isackson P 1991 Seizures and the regulation of neurotrophic factor and neuropeptide gene expression in brain. In: Anderson E, Leppik I, Noebels J (Eds) Genetic Strategies in Epilepsy Research. Elsevier, Amsterdam
Helekar SA, Noebels JL 1991 Synchronous hippocampal bursting unmasks latent network excitability alterations in an epileptic gene mutation. Proceedings of the National Academy of Sciences (USA) 88: 4736–4740
Helekar SA, Noebels JL 1994 Analysis of voltage-gated and synaptic conductances contributing to a gene-linked prolongation of depolarizing shifts in the epileptic mutant mouse tottering. Journal of Neurophysiology 71: 1–10
Hosford DA, Clark S, Cao Z, Wilson W, Lin F-h, Morisett RA, Huin A 1992 The role of GABA$_B$ receptor activation in absence seizures of lethargic (lh/lh) mice. Science 257: 398–401
Keegan K, Noebels JL 1993 In vitro electrophysiology of spontaneous and induced

epileptiform discharges reveal increased cortical excitability in the mutant mouse, stargazer. Neuroscience Abstracts 19: 1031

Levitt P, Noebels JL 1981 Mutant mouse tottering: selective increase of locus coeruleus axons in a defined single locus mutation. Proceedings of the National Academy of Sciences (USA) 78: 4630–4634

Marescaux C, Vergnes M, Bernasconi R 1992 GABA$_B$ receptor antagonists: potential new antiabsence drugs. Journal of Neural Transmission (Suppl.) 35: 179–188

Niedermeyer E, Laws ER, Walker AE 1969 Depth EEG findings in epileptics with generalized spike-wave complexes. Archives of Neurology 21: 51–58

Noebels JL 1979 Analysis of inherited epilepsy using single locus mutations in mice. Federation Proceedings 38: 2405–2410

Noebels JL 1984 A single gene error in noradrenergic axon growth synchronizes central neurons. Nature 10: 409–411

Noebels JL 1986 Mutational analysis of the inherited epilepsies. In: Delgado-Escueta AV, Ward AA, Woodbury DM (Eds) Basic Mechanisms of the Epilepsies: Molecular and Cellular Approaches. Raven Press, New York

Noebels JL, Tharp B 1994 Absence Seizures in Developing Brain. In: Moshe S, Noebels JL, Schwartzkroin P, Swann J (Eds) Brain Development and Epilepsy. Oxford University Press, New York

Qiao X, Noebels JL 1991 Genetic heterogeneity of inherited spike-wave epilepsy: two mutant gene loci with independent cerebral excitability defects. Brain Research 555: 43–50

Qiao X, Noebels JL 1992 GABA$_B$ receptor-independent spike-wave epilepsy in the mutant mouse stargazer. Pharmacology Abstracts 18: 553

Qiao X, Noebels JL 1993a Developmental analysis of hippocampal mossy fiber outgrowth in a mutant mouse with inherited spike-wave seizures. Journal of Neuroscience 13: 4622–4635

Qiao X, Noebels JL 1993b Elevated BDNF mRNA expression in the hippocampus of an epileptic mutant mouse, stargazer. Neuroscience Abstracts 19:1030

Steriade M, Jones EG, Llinas RR 1990 Thalamic oscillations and signaling. Wiley, New York.

Sutula T, Cascino G, Cavazos J, Parada I, Ramirez L 1989 Mossy fiber synaptic reorganization in the epileptic human temporal lobe. Annals of Neurology 26: 321–330

Vergnes M, Marescaux C, Depaulis A, Micheletti G, Warter JM 1990 Spontaneous spike-wave discharges in Wistar Rats: A Model of Genetic Generalized Non-Convulsive Epilepsy. In: Avoli M, Gloor P, Kostopoulos G, Naquet R (Eds) Generalized Epilepsy: Neurobiological Approaches. Birkhauser, Boston, pp 238–253

DISCUSSION

Berkovic: I suggest that the model Dr Noebels has just described is not a model of human absence epilepsy but that the clinical features suggest it may be a better model of progressive myoclonus epilepsy. That condition, particularly Unverricht–Lundborg disease, is age-dependent. It lasts for ever and absence epilepsy does not. It is autosomal recessive which Unverricht–Lundborg disease is and absence epilepsy is not. In Unverricht–Lundborg disease the cerebellum is probably abnormal and there is dementia, which is not the case in absence epilepsy.

Noebels: Early on I tried to understand how to categorise these mutants and what to call them. The ones that have ataxia clearly are not in the typical category, but they do have something to teach us about the mechanisms of absence epilepsy.

Is the *stargazer* mouse a good model of Unverricht–Lundborg? It would not be too difficult to find out, since the Unverricht–Lundborg has been mapped to chromosome 21 and there has not been thought to be any genetic hetero-geneity for that diagnosis. I do not think that this region is homologous to areas of mouse genome that are responsible for the *stargazer* mutant. Perhaps there are other families that have similar phenotypes that have not been mapped yet and which will prove to be on different chromosomes, which may coincide with the mouse.

The important point about mouse genetics at this stage of our analysis of human diseases is that it encourages people to think, clinicians to work together with molecular geneticists, to define the peculiarities of these syndromes rather than lumping them together, because they may represent different diseases. The key thing about the mouse genes is they may help us find a human gene which is complicated and not common enough to find the right human pedigrees for analysis. When we identify that human gene, we can use transgenic technology to manufacture the same disease in the mouse and then study mice that actually do have Unverricht–Lundborg disease, for example.

5. Investigations in animal models – consensus statement

John Jefferys

The foundations for our understanding of absence seizures stem from clinical observations over many decades and from models such as the feline generalised penicillin epilepsy model pioneered by Gloor in Canada. These studies localised the problems to the thalamo-cortical system. More recently our understanding of the mechanisms of absence seizures has grown rapidly, in large part due to developments of new and better animal models. These can be divided in two broad categories: acute preparations which model seizure generation with convulsant drugs and chronic models of epileptogenesis, which are all genetically abnormal rodents. The latter were of particular interest in this session.

The GAERS rat (genetic absence epilepsy rat of Strasbourg), described by Marescaux, has many parallels with clinical absences. It is both predictive of pharmacological sensitivity and shows homology with absence seizures in physiology and other aspects of their expression. The mice described by Noebels have well-defined genetic defects and provide the prospect of developing more precise transgenic models of specific classes of human epileptic disorders. Chronic models have some disadvantages to balance their advantages in studying the mechanisms of absence epilepsies. Noebels described changes in neuronal circuitary secondary to the occurrence of spontaneous seizures in some mutant mice. Clearly this complicates the analysis. Several speakers commented that the presence of spike and wave discharges in nominally normal rats complicates the choice of controls in these studies. Nevertheless, animal models are uniquely good at giving insights into the cell mechanisms of disease processes.

There are some consistent differences between these animal models and typical absences in humans. Firstly, the frequency of the spike and wave discharges are always higher than 3 Hz in the animal models. Secondly, the genetic animal models fail to show the remission typical of human absences. Both differences may prove fruitful areas of research.

Our understanding of the cellular physiology and the neuronal networks of the thalamo-cortical system has grown substantially over the past few years. Coulter talked in some detail about the role of membrane currents in determining the intrinsic discharge pattern of thalamic neurons. The T channel, the low threshold, transient calcium channel, plays a critical role, providing the rebound excitation first promoted as a mechanism for thalamic spindles by Andersen & Sears over three decades ago. Divergent inhibitory connections from the reticular nucleus of the thalamus provide the synchronisation of the system.

It will be of great interest to see these new animal models analysed in terms of the detailed knowledge available on the cellular and network properties of both the thalamus and the neocortex. The large thalamo-cortical slice preparation described by Coulter may be one means of approaching this and work is in progress with this preparation on GAERS and other genetic models. The one question that occurred throughout these presentations is, where lies the primary lesion? Is it in the thalamus, the cortex, or the connections between the two? The jury is still out, but the betting is on the cortex as the primary site of the physiological lesion while the thalamus provides the oscillator that shapes the emergent population activity of spike and wave discharges.

Pharmacological treatments target specific cellular mechanisms in the thalamo-cortical system. Ethosuximide selectively affects the T channel, although there was some discussion of whether this was always the case. Other drugs affect the GABA system. The increasing diversity of the pharmacology and molecular structure of receptors provides the prospect of increased specificity of treatments for epilepsy. One particularly intriguing aspect is the distinction between the effects of benzodiazepine and barbiturates on absence seizures. This appears to be correlated with benzodiazepines being much more effective on $GABA_A$ receptors in the cortex than in the thalamus, while barbiturates have similar potencies in the two areas.

The rich variation of the molecular subunits of the $GABA_A$ receptor provide a mechanism for variations in receptor pharmacology and physiology. Bowery has pointed out that there could be up to 3500 distinct combinations of subunits in the pentameric assembly of the $GABA_A$ receptor, although no more than a dozen or two are likely to be functional. The diversity provides great scope for targeting drugs at particular diseases and particular parts of the brain.

The key question is how absence seizures emerge from the activity of these different populations of neurones within the thalamus, the multiple cell types within the neocortex and their interactions with each other. This kind of analysis is difficult enough in structures such as the hippocampus. It will be substantially more difficult for the thalamo-cortical system, but it will tell us much about both absences and normal function.

6. Action of anti-epileptic drugs in animal models: mechanistic framework of absence seizures with a focus on the lethargic (lh/lh) mouse model

David A. Hosford   Fu-hsiung Lin   Zhen Cao   Ying Wang
Diana L. Kraemer   John T. Wilson

There are numerous genetic and pharmacological models of absence seizures (Fisher, 1989; Green, 1989; Hosford et al, 1992; Löscher & Meldrum, 1984; Marescaux et al, 1992b; Mirsky et al, 1986; Noebels, 1986; Sidman et al, 1965; Snead, 1992). Each model has unique advantages and disadvantages for studying the diverse mechanisms that appear to underlie typical absence seizures in the hope that any new therapies will be applicable to the heterogeneous group of humans with absence seizures.

The goals of this chapter are: to review a general framework which suggests the mechanisms by which typical absence seizures may arise and the possible targets for anti-absence therapy; and to describe our use of the lethargic (lh/lh) mouse model to study some of these possibilities.

MECHANISTIC FRAMEWORK OF ABSENCE SEIZURES

The neuronal circuit that appears to generate the oscillatory thalamocortical burst-firing observed during typical absence seizures includes neocortical pyramidal neurons, thalamic relay neurons and neurons of the nucleus reticularis thalami (NRT) (Steriade & Llinás, 1988; Steriade et al, 1993) (Fig. 6.1). Central to this network is its ability to sustain a series of synchronised oscillatory burst-firings once triggered by a single stimulus (Steriade & Llinás, 1988).

A number of mechanisms appear to regulate its ability to undergo oscillatory burst-firing (Steriade & Llinás, 1988; Coulter et al, 1989; Crunelli & Leresche, 1991; von Krosigk et al, 1993; Steriade et al, 1993; Huguenard & Prince, 1994). Intrinsic mechanisms include those which subserve synaptic transmission within the circuit: reciprocal glutamate neurotransmission between thalamic relay cells and neocortical pyramidal cells and between neocortical pyramidal cells and NRT; and $GABA_A$ and $GABA_B$ neurotransmission between NRT and thalamic relay neurons. Other intrinsic mechanisms increase the ability of thalamic relay neurons to engage in burst-firing by de-inactivating T-channels in thalamic relay cells and NRT or by regulating the membrane potential of these neuronal populations (Fig. 6.1).

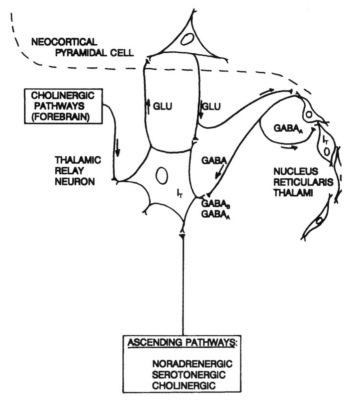

Fig. 6.1   Cartoon diagramming thalamo-cortical network that is proposed to generate absence seizures. Some of the key intrinsic neurotransmitters (GABA, glu [glutamic acid]), receptor subtypes (GABA$_A$, GABA$_B$), or cellular processes (I$_T$ = T-current) are labelled in appropriate parts of the network. Some of the extrinsic pathways which modulate membrane potential of thalamic relay neurons are also denoted.

Each of these intrinsic mechanisms represents a potential target for anti-absence drug therapy. Therefore, compounds interfering with these mechanisms would be predicted to have anti-absence effects. An interesting exception is that compounds which activate GABA$_A$ receptors in NRT (Fig. 6.1) may also have anti-absence effects by reducing NRT outflow to thalamic relay neurons (Liu et al, 1991; von Krosigk et al, 1993; Huguenard & Prince, 1994).

Extrinsic mechanisms that increase the pro-oscillatory tendencies of the circuit are also targets for anti-absence therapy. For example, extrinsic cholinergic and aminergic pathways activate specific neurotransmitter receptor sub-types to increase the membrane potential of thalamo-cortical cells, thereby decreasing the likelihood of burst-firing (McCormick, 1989; Steriade et al, 1993). Consistent with this idea, compounds which diminish the likelihood of thalamo-cortical burst-firing include dopaminergic and α_1-noradrenergic agonists (Marescaux et al, 1992b).

ACTIONS OF ANTI-EPILEPTIC DRUGS IN THE LETHARGIC (LH/LH) MOUSE MODEL

Characterisation of absence seizures in lh/lh mice

The lh/lh strain has a single-locus mutation on chromosome 2 (Sidman et al, 1965; Green, 1989) and expresses a phenotype of spontaneous seizures (Noebels, 1986), ataxia (Sidman et al, 1965) and a defect in cell-mediated immunity (Dung, 1977). An early study by Noebels et al (1986) suggested that lh/lh mice had spontaneous spike-wave discharges similar to those observed in the tottering (tg/tg) model.

We characterised seizures in lh/lh mice using behavioural, electroencephalographic (EEG) and pharmacological criteria. The seizures were characterised by brief (1–4 s) 5–6 Hz bursts of spike-wave discharges that arose from and returned to a normal EEG background. Seizures were accompanied by immobility and reduced responsiveness to external stimuli lasting the precise duration of the electrographic burst; no myoclonic twitches or clonic jerks were observed. These seizures were significantly suppressed in a dose-dependent way by anti-epileptic drugs effective against typical absence seizures in humans (ethosuximide, trimethadione, clonazepam and valproic acid), but not by phenytoin or carbamazepine (anti-epileptic drugs ineffective against absence seizures in humans). Together, these findings validate lh/lh mice as a model of typical absence seizures (Hosford et al, 1992). Interestingly, the behavioural features of seizures in lh/lh mice are reminiscent of childhood absence seizures in humans (Panayiotopoulos et al, 1989; Berkovic et al, 1993).

GABA$_B$ RECEPTORS AS TARGETS OF ANTI-ABSENCE THERAPY

Anti-absence effects of GABA$_B$ receptor antagonists

The mechanistic framework of typical absence seizures suggests the hypothesis that GABA$_B$ receptor activation helps to generate the underlying oscillatory burst-firing. To test this hypothesis, we examined the effect of GABA$_B$ receptor agonists and antagonists on seizure frequency in lh/lh mice. Administration of the GABA$_B$ agonist (–) baclofen produced a significant dose-dependent increase in seizure frequency in lh/lh mice (Fig. 6.2). The same doses of baclofen produced sedation but no seizures in matched, non-epileptic +/+ mice, providing evidence against a non-specific pro-absence effect. Administration of the systemically active GABA$_B$ receptor antagonists CGP 35348, 36742 or 46381 produced a dose-dependent abolition of seizures in lh/lh mice (Fig. 6.2). Administration of the structurally unrelated GABA$_B$ receptor antagonist 2-hydroxysaclofen (2-HS) (not systemically active; given i.c.v.) also produced a dose-dependent suppression of seizure frequency (Fig. 6.2) (Hosford et al, 1992).

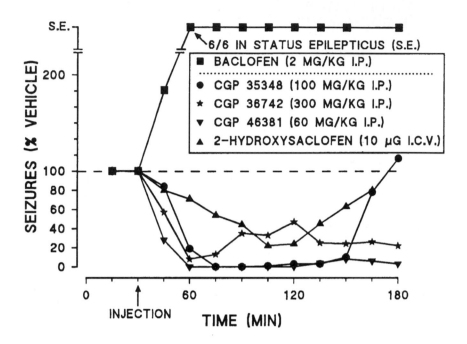

Fig. 6.2   Effects of GABAB receptor ligands [(-) baclofen, CGP 35348, CGP 36742, CGP 46381 and 2-HS] on seizure frequency in lh/lh mice, compared to effect produced by vehicle (dotted line). The seizure frequency during status epilepticus was arbitrarily assigned a score of 10 (a frequency 10 times that after vehicle); often the actual score was higher than 10.

Similar findings were obtained when GABA$_B$ antagonists were administered in two pharmacological models of absence seizures (Snead, 1992) and in the GAERS model (Marescaux et al, 1992a). Together, these findings offer the hope that GABA$_B$ receptor antagonists may represent a new class of anti-absence drugs for human patients.

Possible mechanisms underlying GABA$_B$ receptor regulation of absence seizures

The ability of baclofen to produce status epilepticus in lh/lh mice at doses that produced only sedation in matched, non-epileptic litter mates suggested the enhanced activation of GABA$_B$ receptors in lh/lh mice. In principle, enhanced activation could result from increased release of GABA from nerve terminals during synaptic transmission, an alteration of GABA$_B$ receptors favouring increased binding of GABA, enhanced coupling of GABA$_B$ receptors to GTP-binding proteins (G-proteins) or enhanced physiological responses to second messengers linked to $GABA_B$ receptor-mediated processes.

GABA release from nerve terminals   To test the possibility that enhanced release of GABA during neurotransmission underlies the enhanced effects of $GABA_B$ receptor activation in lh/lh mice, we measured depolarisation-evoked release of [^{3}H]-GABA from neocortical synaptosomes of 8-week-old male lh/lh and +/+ mice. Both K^+ (12 mM) and 4-aminopyridine (4-AP: 50 μM) evoked the release of [^{3}H]-GABA by 40–50% above basal levels of release. There was no difference in the amount of [^{3}H]-GABA release evoked by either method of depolarisation in neocortical synaptosomes from lh/lh and +/+ mice. This finding suggests that the amount of GABA released during neurotransmission in lh/lh mice does not play a factor in enhanced $GABA_B$ receptor activation in that strain (Lin & Hosford, 1994). However, we also examined the ability of $GABA_B$ receptors to inhibit the release of [^{3}H]-GABA evoked by K^+ (12 μM) in neocortical synaptosomes from both strains. Baclofen (50 μM) inhibited K^+-evoked [^{3}H]-GABA release to a significantly greater extent (p = 0.014) in lh/lh (51 ± 11%) than in +/+ (28 ±6%) synaptosomes. This effect of baclofen was fully reversed by the $GABA_B$ antagonist CGP 55845A. This finding supports the idea that $GABA_B$ receptors produce enhanced effects in lh/lh compared to +/+ mice. One possibility that could explain this effect is an alteration in $GABA_B$ receptors, resulting in enhanced binding of GABA in lh/lh mice (Lin & Hosford, 1994).

Receptor binding sites   To test the hypothesis that an alteration in either binding affinity or number (B_{max}) of $GABA_B$ receptors underlies the enhanced effects of $GABA_B$ receptor activation in lh/lh mice, we measured GABA-displaceable [^{3}H]baclofen binding in neocortical membranes from lh/lh and +/+ mice. Scatchard analyses revealed a small (26%) but significant increase in the number of $GABA_B$ binding sites from lh/lh mice compared to age-matched +/+ mice; there was no significant difference in the equilibrium dissociation constant (K_D) of $GABA_B$ receptors. Interestingly, the B_{max} of $GABA_B$ receptors was positively correlated with seizure frequency in lh/lh mice. This increased number of $GABA_B$ receptors was selective, because Scatchard analyses of NMDA and $GABA_A$ receptor binding revealed no differences in the binding characteristics of these receptors in lh/lh and +/+ mice (Hosford et al, 1992; Lin et al, 1993). The finding that $GABA_B$ binding sites are increased in number in neocortical membranes of lh/lh mice suggests a possible mechanism underlying the generation of absence seizures.

Coupling to G-proteins   To test the possibility that enhanced effects of $GABA_B$ receptor activation in lh/lh mice stems from increased coupling of the receptor to G-proteins, we examined the ability of GTP analogues to inhibit GABA$_B$ receptor binding in membranes from lh/lh and +/+ mice. There was no difference in the ability of a GTP analogue to reduce the binding affinity of the GABA$_B$ binding site for [^{3}H]-baclofen in membranes from lh/lh mice and matched controls (Lin et al 1993). Thus, there was no evidence of a further 'amplification' of GABA$_B$ receptor-mediated effects in lh/lh mice beyond that conferred by the increased numbers of binding sites (Lin et al, 1993).

Neuronal network in which GABA$_B$ receptors regulate absence seizures

To characterise further the regulatory role of GABA$_B$ receptors in absence seizures, it is important to identify the neuronal structures in which GABA$_B$ receptors exert their pro-absence effect. We used three sequential screening methods to identify the neuronal structures comprising this network in lh/lh mice. We accepted candidate neuronal structures if they met each of three criteria. These were: 1) structures with enriched density of GABA$_B$ binding sites in lh/lh compared to +/+ mice; 2) structures which satisfied criterion 1 and which generated absence seizures synchronously with neocortex; and 3) structures which satisfied criteria 1 and 2, and within which micro-injections of baclofen or CGP 35348 enhanced or suppressed absence seizures respectively (Hosford et al, 1993).

In the first screen we used autoradiographic techniques to compare the anatomical distribution of baclofen-displaceable [^{3}H]-GABA binding in slide-mounted sections of 8-week-old male lh/lh and +/+ mouse brain (Fig. 6.3), methods similar to Bowery et al (1987). Quantitation of the autoradiograms showed that the density of GABA$_B$ binding sites was significantly greater ($p < 0.05$) in neocortical layers, numerous thalamic subnuclei (particularly VAL, NRT and nucleus reuniens) and caudate-putamen of lh/lh mice (Hosford et al, 1993).

For the second screen we determined if the neuronal structures with enriched GABA$_B$ binding could also generate absence seizures by recording from bipolar EEG electrodes implanted into each candidate structure. EEG recordings of seizures in 8-week-old lh/lh mice showed synchronous spikewave discharges in neocortex and VAL thalamic nucleus (n = 6 of 6), NRT (n = 6 of 6) and nucleus reuniens (n = 6 of 6). As a negative control we also implanted electrodes into hippocampal formation and lateral amygdaloid nucleus; these structures have moderate GABA$_B$ receptor binding but would not be expected to generate absence seizures. As expected, we did not record absence seizures in hippocampal formation or lateral amygdaloid nucleus (n = 0 of 6), even when seizures were recorded in neocortex (Hosford et al, 1993).

For the third screen we began to identify if any of these structures had GABA$_B$ receptors that regulated absence seizures by micro-injecting baclofen or its vehicle bilaterally into the structures. Micro-injection of baclofen (3–300 ng/side in 0.25 μL) into VAL, NRT or nucleus reuniens of

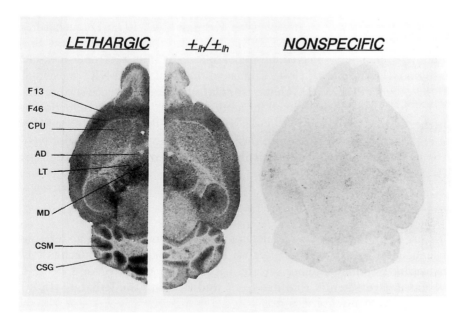

Fig. 6.3   Baclofen-displaceable [3H]-GABA autoradiograms in slide-mounted horizontal sections from 8-week-old male lh/lh and +/+ mice. Structures labelled include: F13 (superficial laminae, frontal neocortex), F46 (deep laminae, frontal neocortex), cpu (caudate-putamen), ad (anterodorsal thalamic nuc.), lt (lateral thalamic nuc.), md (mediodorsal thalamic nuc.), csm (stratum moleculare of cerebellum) and csg (stratum granulosum of cerebellum). Two left-hand autoradiograms show total binding in corresponding halves of lh/lh (left side) and +/+ brain (right side). Right-hand autoradiogram shows non-specific binding in lh/lh brain.

8-week-old male lh/lh mice produced a significant, dose-dependent increase in seizure frequency compared to vehicle. Conversely, micro-injections of CGP 35348 into any of these three thalamic nuclei significantly suppressed seizures. Studies are still underway in other sites (Hosford et al, 1993).

Interestingly, studies conducted in the GAERS model also suggested that lateral thalamic nuclei such as VAL are important to the generation of absence seizures in that model (Vergnes et al, 1990; Liu et al, 1991; Vergnes & Marescaux, 1992). It is important to continue to use these and other models to compare the neural networks which generate absence seizures and in which GABA$_B$ receptors regulate these seizures. The mechanisms underlying the behavioural and electrographic differences of these models must be examined in order to begin to understand possible mechanisms underlying the diversity of absence seizures in human patients.

GABA$_A$ RECEPTORS AS TARGETS OF ANTI-ABSENCE THERAPY

We hypothesised that activation of GABA$_A$ receptors in NRT would produce an anti-absence effect, based upon the effects of intra-NRT GABA$_A$ receptors in two in vitro models (von Krosigk et al, 1993; Huguenard & Prince, 1994) and in the GAERS model (Liu et al, 1991). To test this hypothesis, we micro-injected muscimol bilaterally into NRT of 8-week-old lh/lh mice (Hosford et al, 1994). Compared to vehicle, intra-NRT muscimol (10 ng/cannula in 0.25 µL volume/cannula) suppressed absence seizure frequency in a robust fashion in all lh/lh mice (n = 5). The mean reduction in absence seizure frequency (53%) was significant at the 0.05 level (Student's paired t-test). These data support the search for compounds that selectively activate GABA$_A$ receptor isoforms in NRT as potential anti-absence drugs (Hosford et al, 1994).

SUMMARY

The use of animal models facilitates the study of mechanisms underlying absence seizures. In this chapter we have summarised the mechanistic framework by which absence seizures appear to be generated, and we have presented experimental findings from studies using the lethargic (lh/lh) mouse model of absence seizures.

ACKNOWLEDGEMENTS

We thank Drs Nevin Lambert, Darryl V Lewis, James O McNamara, David Mott, H Scott Swartzwelder and Wilkie A Wilson, Jr for helpful discussions. We thank Betty Worrell and Sarah Sneed for administrative assistance. These studies were funded by grants to DAH from the Epilepsy Foundation of America, NIH (NINDS) and Veterans Administration; and by a grant to F-HL from NINDS.

REFERENCES

Berkovic SF 1993 Childhood absence epilepsy and juvenile absence epilepsy. In: Wyllie E (ed) The treatment of epilepsy: principles and practice. Lea & Febiger, Baltimore, pp 547–551
Bowery NG, Hudson AL, Price GW 1987 GABA$_A$ and GABA$_B$ receptor site distribution in the rat central nervous system. Neuroscience 20: 365–383
Coulter DA, Huguenard JR, Prince DA 1989 Characterization of ethosuximide reduction of low-threshold calcium current in thalamic neurons. Annals of Neurology 25: 582–593
Crunelli V, Leresche N 1991 A role for GABA$_B$ receptors in excitation and inhibition of thalamocortical cells. Trends in Neurological Sciences 14: 16–21
Dung HC 1977 Deficiency in the thymus-dependent immunity in 'lethargic' mutant mice. Transplantation 23: 39–43
Fisher RS 1989 Animal models of the epilepsies. Brain Research Reviews 14: 245–278.
Green MC 1989 Catalog of mutant genes and polymorphic loci. In: Lyon MF, Searle AG (eds) Genetic variants and strains of the laboratory mouse, 2nd edn. Oxford University Press, Oxford, pp 12–403

Hosford DA, Clark S, Cao Z, Wilson WA, Lin F-H, Morrisett RA, Huin A 1992 The role of GABA$_B$ receptor activation in absence seizures of lethargic (lh/lh) mice. Science 257: 398–401

Hosford DA, Lin F-H, Cao Z, Kraemer D, Huin A 1993 Neural network of absence seizures in lethargic (lh/lh) mice: use of GABAB autoradiograms, EEG recordings and microinjections. Society for Neuroscience 19: 1464

Hosford DA, Wang Y, Akawie E, Cas Z 1994 GABA$_A$ receptors in nucleus reticularis thalami (NRT) suppress absence seizures in lethargic (lh/lh) mice. Epilepsia 34 (Suppl.): in press

Huguenard J, Prince D 1994 Clonazepam suppresses GABA$_B$ inhibition in relay cells through actions in the reticular nucleus. Journal of Neurophysiology: in press

Lin F-H, Cao Z, Hosford DA 1993 Selective increase in GABA$_B$ receptor number in lethargic (lh/lh) mouse model of absence seizures. Brain Research 608: 101–106

Lin F-H, Hosford DA 1994 GABA$_B$ receptor-mediated inhibition of [^{3}H]-GABA release evoked by K$^+$ or 4-AP in neocortical synaptosomes of lethargic (lh/lh) and nonepileptic (+/+) mice. Society for Neuroscience 20: in press

Liu Z, Vergnes M, Depaulis A, Marescaux C 1991 Evidence for a critical role of GABAergic transmission within the thalamus in the genesis and control of absence seizures in the rat. Brain Research 545: 1–7

Löscher W, Meldrum BS 1984 Evaluation of anticonvulsant drugs in genetic animal models of epilepsy. Federation Proceedings 43: 276–284

McCormick DA 1989 Cholinergic and noradrenergic modulation of thalamocortical processing. Trends in Neurosciences 12: 215–221

Marescaux C, Vergnes M, Bernasconi R 1992a GABA$_B$ receptor antagonists: potential new anti-absence drugs. Journal of Neural Transmission [Suppl.] 35: 179–188

Marescaux C, Vergnes M, Depaulis A 1992b Genetic absence epilepsy in rats from Strasbourg – a review. Journal of Neural Transmission [Suppl.] 35: 37–69

Mirsky AF, Duncan CA, Myslobodsky MS 1986 Petit mal epilepsy: A review and integration of recent information. Journal of Clinical Neurophysiology 3: 179–208

Noebels JL 1986 Mutational analysis of inherited epilepsies. Advances in Neurology 44: 97–113

Panayiotopoulos CP, Obeid T, Waheed G 1989 Differentiation of typical absences in epileptic syndromes: a video EEG study of 224 seizures. Brain 112: 1039–1056

Sidman RL, Green MC, Appel SH 1965 Catalog of the neurological mutants of the mouse. Harvard University Press, Cambridge, Mass.

Snead OC 1992 Evidence for GABA$_B$-mediated mechanisms in experimental generalized absence seizures. European Journal of Pharmacology 213: 343–349

Steriade M, McCormick DA, Sejnowski T 1993 Thalamocortical oscillations in the sleeping and aroused brain. Science 262: 679–685

Steriade M, Llinás, R 1988 The functional states of the thalamus and the associated neuronal interplay. Physiology Reviews 68: 649–742

Vergnes M, Marescaux C 1992 Cortical and thalamic lesions in rats with genetic absence epilepsy. Journal of Neural Transmission [Suppl.] 35: 71–83

Vergnes M, Marescaux C, Depaulis A 1990 Mapping of spontaneous spike and wave discharges in Wistar rats with genetic generalized non-convulsive epilepsy. Brain Research 523: 87–91

von Krosigk M, Bal T, McCormick DA 1993 Cellular mechanisms of a synchronized oscillation in the thalamus. Science 261: 361–364

DISCUSSION

Gloor: Since GABA$_B$ blockers appear to inhibit spike-wave discharges in models that do not have increases in GABA$_B$ receptors, what evidence is there that the increase in lethargic mice is a causative change and not in consequence of the onset of seizures?

Hosford: The evidence that would favour GABA$_B$ receptors are related to seizures is the fact that everything is in the same direction. GABA$_B$ receptor agonists enhance absences. If the change in the number of GABA$_B$ receptors in these mice were an epiphenomenon, we would expect down-regulation rather than up-regulation.

Further, micro-injection into the different neuronal structures in which GABA$_B$ binding is increased actually enhances seizures, and GABA$_B$ antagonists injected into those structures inhibit absences. That is indirect proof, and I think it will await the cloning of a GABA$_B$ receptor, the exploration of its genetic regulation, and then the regulation of GABA$_B$ receptors in a naive mouse and the finding that up-regulation of those receptors in the appropriate structures results in absences. That kind of evidence would be necessary before we could conclude that abnormalities of GABA$_B$ receptors by themselves may underlie absence seizures.

Gloor: Could you not show that the increase precedes, or immediately coincides with, the onset of seizures in these mice?

Hosford: We have attempted to do that. Unfortunately the lethargic mice are a bit like the tottering and Stargazer strains. They express absence seizures very soon after birth. The earliest we have been able to hold them and implant electrodes is 14 days and they have the spike-wave discharges as early as that. We are unable to tell the difference between lethargics and non-epileptic litter mates earlier than 14 days because before that they do not express the phenotype of ataxic gait, which is how we segregate them out, so I cannot detect the phenotype early enough in order to investigate the ontogeny of the GABA$_B$ binding.

Bowery: I would expect a decrease in autoreceptors rather than an increase. Have GABA$_B$ receptors been quantified in the thalamus in tottering mice?

Hosford: We have only just started to analyse the thalamus. It takes many brains to get enough thalamic material to produce enough synaptosomes to study.

Bowery: If a GABA$_B$ agonist or antagonist is injected elsewhere, is the effect totally negative?

Hosford: We plan to implant the caudate . . . because there is enhanced binding there and the cerebellum because these structures have not been thought to be relevant in absence seizures. If injections of GABA$_B$ agonists and antagonists at those sites are effective, it would conflict with the theory that it is only the thalamic nuclei and neocortex where the increased binding is important. If we find negative results, it might partially support both our theories: in my case that GABA$_B$ binding is important, and in Professor Bowery's case that this genetic mutant may have up-regulation of GABA$_B$ receptors everywhere, but that these receptors produce different effects in different sites. For example, up-regulation in the cerebellum may produce the ataxic gait, but not seizures because the cerebellum is not a site that generates absence seizures.

7. GABA transmission in absence epilepsy

N. Bowery   D. A. Richards   T. Lemos   P. S. Whitton

GABA (γ-aminobutyric acid) is one of (if not the) most important inhibitory neurotransmitters in the mammalian central nervous system. Application of this simple amino acid to most neurons of the CNS, in vivo or in vitro, reduces their excitability in a manner identical with synaptic inhibition (Krnjevic & Schwartz, 1967). This fast action of GABA is mediated via a selective increase in membrane Cl⁻ conductance following activation of a membrane-bound receptor. The structure of the receptor responsible, termed $GABA_A$ (Hill & Bowery, 1981) has been elucidated by receptor cloning techniques (Burt & Kamatchi, 1991) and appears to comprise 5 sub-units of peptide residues each of which is configured with 4 membrane-spanning domains. A variety of sub-units have been elucidated to give a multitude of possible compositions of the $GABA_A$ receptor. A current listing of the sub-unit classification, α, β, γ, ∂ and ρ, together with their potential role is summarised in Table 7.1. In theory, any combination of 5 sub-units could

Table 7.1 $GABA_A$ Receptor Sub-Unit Classification

	Sub-unit	Amino acid residues	Suggested functional role
alpha	α_1	428	Defines benzodiazepine
	α_2	423	pharmacology
	α_3	465	Type I or Type II
	α_4	521	Responsible for GABA
	α_5	433	affinity
	α_6	434	
beta	β_1	449	
	β_2	450	Determines GABA response
	β_3	448	amplitude
	β_4	459	Responsible for desensitisation
	$\beta_{4'}$	463	
gamma	γ_1	430	Responsible for benzodiazepine
	$\gamma_2 S$	428	functional action
	$\gamma_2 L$	436	Sites for modulation –
	γ_3	450	protein kinase C & tyrosine kinase
delta	δ	433	
rho	ρ_1	458	Novel retinal receptors –
	ρ_2	465	bicuculline insensitive

form a GABA$_A$ receptor to give many thousands of receptor sub-types. In reality this seems unlikely and perhaps only 10–20 forms of the receptor will prove to be important, but this is pure speculation at present. Evidence exists to suggest that the sub-units may provide a locus for the modulatory actions of compounds such as the benzodiazepines which mediate their neuropharmacological effects via the GABA$_A$ receptor complex (Haefely, 1994). Facilitation of GABA$_A$ receptor function by benzodiazepine agonists suppresses neuronal firing activity. Agents which depress activation of the GABA$_A$ receptor by blocking the action of GABA, directly or indirectly, facilitate the production of epileptiform seizures. Thus competitive GABA$_A$ receptor antagonists provide no potential as therapeutic agents. This is not the case for GABA$_B$ receptor antagonists.

GABA$_A$ receptors are not the only group of sites through which GABA mediates its physiological and pathological effects. A second type of receptor quite distinct from GABA$_A$, termed GABA$_B$ (Hill & Bowery, 1981) has been described in the mammalian brain and, while its location compares with GABA$_A$ sites, the alignment is by no means absolute. Using receptor autoradiography in rat brain sections, distinct locations for each receptor sub-type binding site have been demonstrated (Bowery et al, 1987). The characteristics of this second receptor class differ widely from those attributed to the GABA$_A$ receptor (Table 7.2). In particular, GABA$_B$ receptors are not coupled to the Cl$^-$ channels but instead appear to gate Ca^{2+} and/or K$^+$ channels, and are coupled via GTP binding proteins to these channels and to adenylyl cyclase (Bowery, 1993). The neuronal response to GABA$_B$ receptor activation can be described as 'slow', in contrast to the 'fast' GABA$_A$-linked events. As a consequence, GABA$_B$-mediated synaptic inhibition is associated with late hyper-polarisation of prolonged duration and

Table 7.2 GABA$_A$ and GABA$_B$ receptor characteristics in mammalian brain

	GABA$_A$	GABA$_B$
Predominant locations	Frontal cortex Cerebellar granule Cell layer Olfactory bulb	Thalamic nuclei Frontal cortex Cerebellar molecular layer
Channel conductance	Cl$^-$	Ca$^{2+}\downarrow$ K$^+\uparrow$
Coupling to channel	Direct	via G-protein
Synaptic event	Fast IPSP	Slow IPSP
Modulation by benzodiazepines	Yes	No
Selective agonist	Isoguvacine	(–)Baclofen
Selective antagonist	Bicuculline	CGP 35348 CGP 36742
Effects of antagonists on neuronal activity	Convulsive seizures (general CNS)	Suppression of absence seizures (thalamus)

it is this characteristic which has recently been attributed to the mechanism underlying the generation of non-convulsive seizures within the thalamus.

Despite the prevalence and clinical significance of absence epilepsy, research into the underlying causes of absence seizures has been hindered by the scarcity of animal models available. However, the selective inbreeding of GAERS, with characteristic spike and wave discharges (SWDs) on the EEG (7–11 Hz), together with a valid control strain in which all evidence of SWDs has been bred out over a large number of generations, fulfils the basic requirements for an animal model of absence seizures (Marescaux et al, 1992a; see Ch. 6) in terms of neurophysiology, behavioural features, pharmacology and genetics. With the possible exception of absences induced in primates, this probably represents the best model available of this type of epilepsy.

As long ago as 1953 EEG recordings in man demonstrated a simultaneous and synchronous rhythmic activity in both cortex and thalamus during absence seizures, often appearing first in the latter structure (Williams, 1953). The involvement of thalamo-cortical pathways in the generation of SWDs has now been confirmed in animal models, including GAERS (Vergnes et al, 1987; Gloor & Fariello, 1988; Crunelli & Leresche, 1991).

While most neurotransmitters, including noradrenaline, dopamine and glutamate (acting at NMDA receptors), appear to be involved in the control of SWDs in GAERS (Marescaux et al, 1992a), there is convincing evidence that an excess of GABA-mediated inhibition may underlie its genesis (Liu et al, 1991). $GABA_A$ agonists such as muscimol and THIP exacerbate experimental absence seizures, although $GABA_A$ antagonists do not protect against these seizures (Micheletti et al, 1985). Other GABA-mimetics, such as γ-vinyl-GABA (vigabatrin), an inhibitor of GABA transaminase, and SKF 89976, a GABA re-uptake inhibitor, also exacerbate absence seizures in GAERS (Marescaux et al, 1992a). The $GABA_B$ agonist, (–) baclofen, increases SWDs in GAERS in a dose-dependent fashion (Vergnes et al, 1984) and, in contrast to $GABA_A$ antagonists, the selective $GABA_B$ antagonist, CGP 35348, and other $GABA_B$ antagonists (Bittiger et al, 1990), dose-dependently decrease both spontaneous SWDs, as well as those potentiated by (–)baclofen (Marescaux et al, 1992b).

Taken together, these results suggest that increased $GABA_B$ receptor function may underlie episodes of SWD in GAERS (Liu et al, 1992). In view of the marked similarities between the GAERS model and patients with absence seizures, this implies that $GABA_B$ antagonists may have therapeutic value as potential new anti-absence drugs. The need for a new class of absence drugs is clear, since neither ethosuximide nor valproate are effective in all cases of absence epilepsy (Rogawski & Porter, 1990), and both have a spectrum of side effects, some of which are potentially serious and may occasionally be life-threatening.

Although an increase in $GABA_B$ receptor binding site density has been reported by Hosford and colleagues in the lethargic mouse model of absence epilepsy (see Ch. 6), a difference in $GABA_A$ or $GABA_B$ receptor density or affinity in the thalamus, or other brain structures in GAERs has been excluded using autoradiographic techniques (Knight & Bowery, 1992). However, modified transduction of these receptors at the second messenger level, or abnormal extracellular concentrations of GABA in the vicinity of thalamic $GABA_B$ receptors remain as possible mechanisms by which abnormal GABA function might be expressed. Furthermore, $GABA_B$ receptors on presynaptic terminals also have a major pharmacological influence on synaptic processing, reducing release of other neurotransmitters, including glutamate (Morrisett et al, 1991) and monoamines (Bowery et al, 1980), and it is possible that mechanisms involving these transmitters may also be implicated in the genesis of SWDs in GAERS. Indeed, glutamatergic synapses are involved in the thalamo-cortical circuitry underlying SWDs and systemic and intracerebroventricular administration of N-methyl-D-aspartate (NMDA) induced a dose-dependent decrease in SWDs in GAERS (Marescaux et al, 1992a).

Although the GAERS strain has been extensively validated as a model of human absence epilepsy, there has been no in vivo characterisation of the neurotransmitter changes that might underlie the incidence of absences in these animals.

Using in vivo microdialysis in the ventrolateral thalamus of GAERs and control rats we have obtained data to support the possible involvement of GABA in the mediation of absences. Rats were anaesthetised with chloral hydrate (400mg/kg i.p.) and implanted with concentric dialysis probes as well as bipolar electrodes for EEG monitoring from the surface of the cerebral cortex. Probes were perfused with artificial CSF (0.5 μl/min) after a recovery period of 24 h following implantation of the probes.

Drugs were administered systemically or via the microdialysis probe in the perfusion solution. Analysis of dialysate fractions for GABA and other amino acids was performed by HPLC with fluorescence detection following pre-column derivatisation with o-phthalaldehyde. One problem in the interpretation of data obtained from microdialysis in relation to the electrographic state of the animal is the difference in the time resolution of the two measurements. In the mature GAERs the mean cumulative duration of the spike and wave discharges has been reported to be 24.3 ± 7.5 spikes/min (Marescaux et al, 1992a) and we concur with this in our laboratory. Thus a significant period of time ($\sim 40\%$) is spent in the absence state, which is sufficient to allow a gross correlation to be made between EEG and neurochemical changes during 30-min sampling periods.

We have observed that basal extracellular levels of GABA were increased by approximately 60% in the ventrolateral thalamus of GAERs when compared to control rats (Fig. 7.1). Levels of the structurally related amino acid taurine were also increased, although to a lesser extent (Fig. 7.1), whereas glutamine, aspartate and glutamate were unaltered.

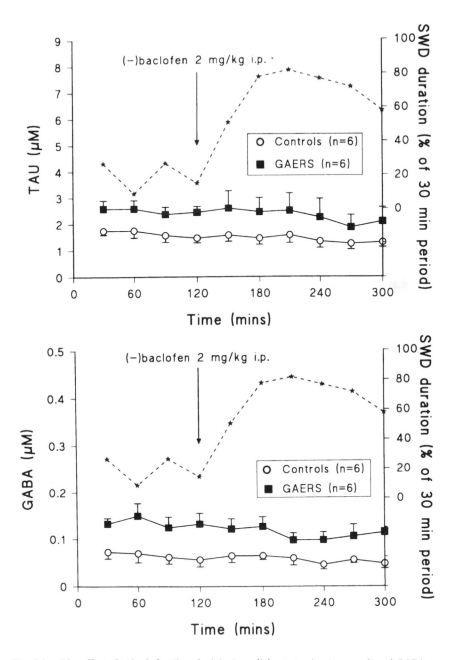

Fig. 7.1   The effect of (–)baclofen (2mg/kg⁻¹, i.p.) on dialysate taurine (top panel) and GABA (bottom panel), and on the duration of SWDs (broken line) in GAERS and control rats. Amino acid concentrations in microdialysates collected from ventrolateral thalamus of 12 rats were determined by HPLC as described in the text. Mean concentrations (± s.e. mean, vertical bars) of GABA were significantly greater (p<0.05) in GAERS(■) than in control rats (o) throughout the collection period. No muscle relaxant activity was noted following the injection of (–)baclofen.

Systemic administration of (–)baclofen (2 mg/kg i.p.) did not alter the GABA level (or the level of the other amino acids), suggesting that any possible activation of $GABA_B$ autoreceptors within the thalamus could not be observed as a decrease in GABA release. However, (–)baclofen administered in this manner did exert an effect in the thalamus as evidenced from the increase in spike and wave discharge frequency which occurred (Fig. 7.1). This supports the original observations by Marescaux et al (1992b). We are currently considering the possibility that a change or lack of autoreceptors in the thalamus might provide an explanation for the raised GABA levels and thus seizure activity in the thalamus of GAERS. However, many more studies will be required to validate or refute this hypothesis.

The $GABA_B$ antagonist, CGP 35348 (100 mg/kg i.p.) which suppressed the spike and wave discharge frequency also produced no change in the GABA level, which is not surprising since it can be assumed that the reduction in spike and wave discharges is due to $GABA_B$ receptor blockade independent of the GABA level. Perfusion via the microdialysis probe with K^+ (100 mM) produced an increase in the extracellular GABA level but no difference between GAERS and control could be detected, indicating that the size of the pool available for release does not underlie the difference in basal levels.

The data reported here are clearly of a preliminary nature and further studies are in progress. The types of questions we are attempting to answer are whether the increase in basal GABA levels is restricted to the thalamus, whether GABA autoreceptors play any part in the mechanism and whether $GABA_B$ receptor-linked second messenger systems are altered in the GAERS model. Answers to these questions may help us to understand the underlying role of the $GABA_B$ receptor system in the generation of absence epilepsy.

In summary, evidence has accumulated from animal models to indicate that absence epilepsy may arise from excessive GABA-mediated inhibition in the thalamus and pharmacological studies have indicated that the $GABA_B$ receptor may play an important role. $GABA_B$ receptor antagonists may represent a novel class of anti-absence drugs. Evidence from the GAERS model suggests that raised extracellular GABA levels rather than any change in receptor density may be responsible.

REFERENCES

Bittiger H, Froestl W, Hall R et al 1990 Biochemistry, electrophysiology and pharmacology of a new $GABA_B$ antagonist: CGP 35348. In: Bowery NG, Bittiger H, Olpe HR (eds) $GABA_B$ receptors in mammalian function. Wiley, Chichester, pp47–80
Bowery NG 1993 $GABA_B$ receptor pharmacology. In: Cho AK, Blaschke TF, Loh HH, Way JL (eds) Annual reviews in pharmacology and toxicology 33. Annual Reviews, Palo Alto, pp109–147
Bowery NG, Hill DR, Hudson AL et al 1980 (–)Baclofen decreases neurotransmitter release in the mammalian CNS by an action at a novel GABA receptor. Nature 283: 92–94

Bowery NG, Hudson AL, Price GW 1987 GABA$_A$ and GABA$_B$ receptor site distribution in the rat central nervous system. Neuroscience 20: 365–383

Burt DR, Kamatchi GL 1991 GABA$_A$ receptor subtypes: from pharmacology to molecular biology. FASEB Journal 5: 2916–2923

Crunelli V, Leresche N 1991 A role for GABA$_B$ receptors in excitation and inhibition of thalamocortical cells. Trends in Neuroscience 14: 16–21

Gloor P, Fariello RG 1988 Generalized epilepsy: some of its cellular mechanisms differ from those of focal epilepsy. Trends in Neuroscience 11: 63–68

Haefely W 1994 Allosteric modulation of the GABA$_B$ receptor channel: a mechanism for interaction with a multitude of central nervous system functions. In: Möhler H, da Prada M (eds) The challenge of neuropharmacology. Editions Roche, Basel, pp15–39

Hill DR, Bowery NG 1981 ^{3}H-Baclofen and ^{3}H-GABA bind to bicuculline-insensitive GABA$_B$ sites in rat brain. Nature 290: 149–152

Knight AR, Bowery NG 1992 GABA receptors in rats with spontaneous generalized nonconvulsive epilepsy. Journal of Neural Transmission (Suppl.) 35: 189–196

Krnjevic K, Schwartz S 1967 The action of γ-aminobutyric acid on cortical neurones. Experimental Brain Research 3: 320-326

Liu Z, Vergnes M, Depaulis A, Marescaux C 1991 Evidence for a critical role of GABAergic transmission within the thalamus in the genesis and control of absence seizures in the rat. Brain Research 545: 1–7

Liu Z, Vergnes M, Depaulis A, Marescaux C 1992 Involvement of intrathalamic GABA$_B$ neurotransmission in the control of absence seizures in the rat. Neuroscience 48: 87–93

Marescaux C, Vergnes M, Depaulis A 1992a Genetic absence epilepsy in rats from Strasbourg: a review. Journal of Neural Transmission (Suppl.) 35: 37–69

Marescaux C, Vergnes M, Bernasconi R 1992b GABA$_B$ receptor antagonists: potential new anti-absence drugs. Journal of Neural Transmission (Suppl.) 35: 179–188

Micheletti G, Marescaux C, Vergnes M, Rumbach L, Warter JM 1985 Effects of GABA-mimetics and GABA antagonists on spontaneous non-convulsive seizures in Wistar rats. In: Bartholini G, Bossi L, Lloyd KG, Morselli ML (eds) Epilepsy and GABA receptor agonists. Raven Press, New York, pp129–137

Morrisett RA, Mott DD, Lewis DV, Swartzwelder HS, Wilson WA 1991 GABA$_B$ receptor-mediated inhibition of the N-methyl-D-aspartate component of synaptic transmission in the rat hippocampus. Journal of Neuroscience 11: 203–209

Rogawski MA, Porter RJ 1990 Antiepileptic drugs: pharmacological mechanisms and clinical efficacy with consideration of promising developmental stage compounds. Pharmacology Reviews 42: 223–286

Vergnes M, Marescaux C, Micheletti G, Depaulis A, Rumbach L, Warter JM 1984 Enhancement of spike and wave discharges by GABAmimetic drugs in rats with spontaneous petit-mal like epilepsy. Neuroscience Letters 44: 91–94

Vergnes M, Marescaux C, Depaulis A, Micheletti G, Warter JM 1987 Spontaneous spike and wave discharges in thalamus and cortex in a rat model of genetic petit mal-like seizures. Experimental Neurology 96: 127–136

Williams D 1953 A study of thalamic and cortical rhythms in petit mal. Brain 76: 50-69

DISCUSSION

Chapman: In your microdialysis study would you not expect the baclofen to raise GABA levels? If some of the spiking is due to elevated thalamic extracellular GABA levels, surely that should have been affected by the administration of baclofen?

Bowery: Baclofen acts directly on the GABA$_B$ receptors when we inject it, to produce spike-wave discharges. In addition, baclofen binds to presynaptic autoreceptors to suppress GABA release, so that, although the baclofen causes the increase in spike-wave discharges, there would also be a reduction in GABA levels because of the action on autoreceptors.

Duncan: Is there yet any work on $GABA_B$ receptors in humans with typical absences?

Bowery: Nobody has done this. It would be nice to get some post-mortem tissue. The only studies in humans I know of is some work in the brains of Alzheimer's patients. We now have the facility for doing whole-brain autoradiography in the human brain. If we were ever to get post-mortem material from a patient with typical absences that would form a very important study.

Duncan: Does Professor Marescaux have any experience on $GABA_B$ studies in humans with epilepsy?

Marescaux: I do not know of any trials of $GABA_B$ antagonists in humans with epilepsy.

8. The role of the opioid system in absence epilepsy in rats

W. Lason   B. Przewlocka   A. M. L. Coenen   R. Przewlocki
E. L. J. M. van Luijtelaar

The majority of endogenous opioid peptides are products of an enzymatic cleavage of one of three distinct pro-peptide molecules: pro-encephalin (PENK), pro-opiomelanocortin (POMC) and pro-dynorphin (PDYN). The neurons synthesising and releasing peptides deriving from these pro-hormones form three independent endogenous opioid systems with different distributions in the central nervous system. The primary sites of action of opioid peptides are multiple opioid receptors, classified as mu, delta and kappa types. In recent years substantial progress has been made in their pharmacological and molecular characterisation, as well as in cloning genes coding for types and sub-types of opioid receptors.

The opioid-induced changes in membrane conductance inhibit neuronal activity, although they can also induce excitation. These effects imply a role of opioids in epilepsy, since a disturbance in the balance of neuronal excitatory and inhibitory processes is one of the basic mechanisms underlying seizures.

A possible involvement of endogenous opioid peptides, particularly in convulsive epilepsy, was the subject of numerous experiments (Ramabadran & Bansinath, 1990). A role for opioids in non-convulsive epilepsy has also been suggested (Snead, 1983; Snead & Bearden, 1980a; 1980b; Lason et al, 1992; 1994a;1994b).

EARLY STUDIES

Two early rat models were developed for absence epilepsy: the administration of leu-encephalin in the lateral ventricle (Snead, 1983) and the peripheral administration of gamma-hydroxybutyrate (GHB) (Godschalk et al, 1976; Snead, 1988). Leu-encephalin, an endogenous peptide with high affinity for the delta opioid receptor, evoked absence-like seizures in rats which was antagonised by anti-absence drugs such as sodium valproate, ethosuximide, trimethadione, but not by diazepam or phenytoin (Snead & Bearden, 1980b). The leu-encephalin-induced seizures could be antagonised by naloxone, which points to the involvement of the opioid receptors in this model.

GHB-induced seizures are continous and long-lasting (Snead, 1988). They can also be antagonised with anti-absence drugs (Godschalk et al,

1976; Snead, 1988), as well as with the non-selective opioid receptor antagonists naloxone or naltrexone (Snead & Bearden, 1980a). It was also found that these seizures are accompanied by changes in opioid peptide levels, such as a decrease in the level of beta-endorphin in the hypothalamus, thalamus and pituitary and an increase in the level of dynorphin in the hippocampus (Lason et al, 1983). These effects, found a short time after GHB administration, may reflect an increased release of beta-endorphin which may lead to activation of mu and delta receptors.

These studies suggested an involvement of opioid mechanisms in absence epilepsy, but the role of the particular endogenous opioid systems and receptors could not be elucidated due to a lack of specific opioid agonists and antagonists.

A GENETIC MODEL

The fully inbred WAG/Rij strain of rats exhibits spontaneously occurring spike-wave discharges (SWDs) (van Luijtelaar & Coenen, 1986). Adult WAG/Rij rats show several hundred bursts of 7–11 Hz SWD per day, concurrent with behavioural manifestations: twitching of the vibrissae, small perioral movements, accelerated breathing and sometimes a change in body posture. The EEG paroxysms are bilateral, symmetrical and generalised and also invoke parts of the thalamus and the thalamic reticular nucleus. There is a circadian modulation in the number of SWDs, and they mainly occur during intermediate levels of vigilance (Coenen et al, 1991).

Cognitive studies have shown two main features of epilepsy in the WAG/Rij strain: the modulation of the number of SWDs by mental or physical activity and the disruption of cognitive activity by SWDs (van Luijtelaar et al, 1991a;1991b). Pharmacological studies with clinically effective anti-epileptic drugs have shown a close agreement in man and rat. SWDs in rats were suppressed by clinically effective anti-absence drugs such as trimethadione, ethosuximide, diazepam, valproate, but not by the anti-epileptic drugs carbamazepine and phenytoin. Studies with new compounds suggest that loreclozole and remacemide might be effective in suppressing SWDs. The role of the GABA-ergic and glutaminergic system has been extensively investigated in this model (Coenen et al, 1992; Peeters et al, 1994). There is also good evidence for an involvement of other neurotransmitters such as as noradrenaline and dopamine. Many aspects of this model, including the EEG paroxysms, clinical manifestations and reaction to drugs, closely mimic the Strasbourg epileptic rat model (see Ch 2).

OPIOID SYSTEMS IN THE WAG/Rij MODEL

The activity of the endogenous opioid systems was estimated by measuring the level of peptides representative of each of the three opioid systems (met-encephalin-arg[6]-gly[7]-leu[8] for PENK, beta-endorphin for POMC and alpha-neoendorphin for PDYN), the level of mRNA coding for PENK and PDYN, as well as the density of opioid receptors in various brain areas. The four groups chosen – male 6-month-old WAG/Rij (WAG-6) rats which show SWDs, 3-month-old WAG/Rij rats (WAG-3), which do not yet exhibit SWDs, as well as non-epileptic 3- and 6-month-old ACI (ACI-3 and ACI-6) rats – allow a two-factor analysis of variance in which strain and age effects can be established, as well as an interaction between the two main effects. A significant interaction together with a significant difference between WAG-6 and the three control groups can be more safely attributed to SWDs being the underlying causative factor.

Pro-encephalin system

Pro-encephalin (PENK) neurons have a wide distribution throughout the central nervous system. They are predominantly interneurons, some of which form local circuits and others form longer-tract projections. PENK neurons are abundant in the hypothalamus, striatum and cortex as well as in limbic structures. PENK is processed to a number of opioid peptides, among others met- and leu-encephalin and their elongated forms hepta and octapeptide (met-encephalin-arg^6-gly^7-leu^8, MEAGL). The PENK-derived peptides are thought to interact mainly with delta receptors, but some also have substantial affinity to mu receptors.

Our biochemical studies showed that in WAG-6 rats the level of MEAGL was increased in some brain areas, especially in the striatum, the frontal cortex and the mesencephalon (see Table 8.1).

The elevated level of PENK mRNA and PENK-derived peptide content (Lason et al, 1992; 1994b) in the striatum of these rats strongly suggests enhanced biosynthesis in encephalinergic neurons in this structure. Buzsaki et al (1990) postulated that the striatum is involved in the control of SWDs, possibly through the dopaminergic system. Since the striatum is one of the richest sources of PENK-derived peptides, the increased striatal PENK biosynthesis may lead to a higher release of PENK-derived peptides and, in consequence, influence – in a paracrine way – other structures involved in SWD generation, such as the thalamus or cortex. Since SWDs are generated by oscillations in thalamo-cortical circuits (Inoue et al, 1993), the elevation of the PENK-derived peptide level in the cortex may be functionally connected with the occurrence of SWDs. MEAGL was also enhanced in the mesencephalon in the WAG-6 rats. Changes in the mesencephalon are not surprising considering the intimate relationship between the presence of SWDs and the level of vigilance (Coenen et al, 1991).

Pro-opiomelanocortin system

POMC-derived peptides are present in the nucleus arcuatus of the mediobasal hypothalamus and the nucleus tractus solitarii of the caudal

Table 8.1 The level of the pro-encephalin (PENK) and pro-dynorphin (PDYN) mRNAs and their related peptides met-encephalin-arg^6-gly^7-leu^8 (MEAGL) and alpha-neoendorphin (ANEO) respectively in brain structures of 3 control groups: 3-month-old ACI (ACI 3), 6-month-old ACI (ACI 6), 3-month-old WAG/Rij (WAG 3), and the epileptic 6-month-old WAG/Rij (WAG 6). The results are presented as means ± s.e.m. Optical densities (OD) from film autoradiograms of coronal sections were measured. The slices were hybridised with a ^{35}S-labelled cDNA directed against PENK or PDYN mRNA. The peptide levels are expressed in pmol/g of wet tissue; n.d. means not done.

	PENK mRNA OD	MEAGL pmol/g	PDYN mRNA OD	ANEO pmol/g
Striatum				
ACI 3	42.4±1.2	143±20	30.1±1.9	48±4
ACI 6	41.6±2.0	126±11	23.4±1.5	41±2
WAG 3	48.7±2.6	208±29	25.6±0.7	53±4
WAG 6	57.3±1.8*	318±22*	24.6±0.6	80±12*
Cortex				
ACI 3	11.8±0.9	65±6	16.9±1.1	n.d.
ACI 6	11.2±1.4	67±3	10.9±2.1	n.d.
WAG 3	12.5±1.5	60±6	17.1±1.3	n.d.
WAG 6	14.3±0.8	82±7	14.3±0.8	n.d.
Hippocampus				
ACI 3	17.2±1.3	39±4	19.7±2.8	40±4
ACI 6	15.9±1.0	47±3	21.9±1.3	39±6
WAG 3	18.2±0.7	37±3	17.3±2.3	32±3
WAG 6	15.5±0.7	39±2	38.8±2.0 *	67±3 *

* = $p<0.05$, the WAG=6 group differs from all the 3 control groups; strain and age effects are not indicated.
Sources: Chavkin C, Neumaier JF, Swearengen E 1988 Opioid receptor mechanisms in the rat hippocampus. In: McGinty JF, Friedman DP (eds) Opioids in the Hippocampus, NIDA Research Monograph, 94–117; Lason W, Przewlocka B, van Luijtelaar ELJM, Coenen AML, Przewlocki R 1992 Opposite effects of mu and kappa opioid receptor agonists on absence epilepsy in WAG/Rij rats. Society for Neuroscience, Anaheim, CA, p 658.

medulla. Fibre systems originating in the nucleus arcuatus terminate in hypothalamic, limbic and raphe nuclei and in some pontine nuclei. Endocrine cells of the anterior and intermediate lobes of the pituitary also contain, synthesise and release POMC peptides. The POMC-derived opioid peptide beta-endorphin shows a high affinity towards both mu and delta opioid receptors. An interaction of this peptide with the epsilon opioid receptor has also been postulated. There were no differences in the levels of beta-endorphin in WAG-6 rats, although strain- and age-related changes were detected in both lobes of the pituitary (Lason et al, 1992). The POMC system does not seem to play a role in the control of SWDs, in marked contrast to findings in the GHB model (Lason et al, 1983).

Pro-dynorphin system

PDYN neurons are widely distributed in the hippocampus, striatum, cortex, thalamus and hypothalamus. The main representative peptides of this system, alpha- and beta-neoendorphin, dynorphin A and dynorphin B, display high affinities for kappa opioid receptors, but they also bind to mu and delta receptors.

An age-related decrease in the PDYN biosynthesis was observed in the frontal cortex and, to a lesser extent, in the striatum of ACI-6 and WAG-6 rats. Since the peptides derived from PDYN interact mainly with kappa receptors whose activation produces anti-epileptic effects in this animal model of absence epilepsy (Lason et al, 1992), the decrease in PDYN biosynthesis in these structures may be a factor controlling the occurrence of SWDs.

The levels of alpha-neoendorphin and PDYN mRNA (Lason et al, 1992; 1994b) were elevated in the hippocampus in WAG-6 rats, which points to an increase in the PDYN biosynthesis in this structure. Although the hippocampus is not involved in this kind of epilepsy (Inoue et al, 1993), its indirect influence on this phenomena could not be excluded. Electrophysiological evidence indicates that PDYN-derived peptides exert predominantly inhibitory effects on hippocampal neuron activity (Chavkin et al, 1988). Inhibitory effects of PDYN-derived peptides on hippocampal neurons may participate in preventing the spread of SWDs into the limbic system.

PHARMACOLOGICAL STUDIES

Naloxone, a non-selective opioid receptor antagonist, increased the number of SWDs in WAG/Rij rats, in agreement with Frey & Voits (1991). The naloxone-induced increase suggests that some endogenous opioids are tonically active and may act like endogenous anti-epileptics. The irreversible mu receptor antagonist β-FNA did not evoke changes in SWD, indicating that the mu system is not tonically active. The same result was obtained for the delta receptor antagonist naltrindole, suggesting that the delta endogenous system does not tonically control SWDs either. On the other hand, the selective kappa antagonist nor-binaltorphimine (Nor-BNI) increased the number of SWDs, suggesting that kappa receptors tonically control SWDs.

In further studies the influence of specific opioid receptor agonists on SWDs has been evaluated. The selective mu agonist D-ala^2-n,-methyl-phe^4-gly^5-ol-encephalin (DAMGO) significantly increased SWDs in a dose-dependent manner. The specificity of the effects of DAMGO was determined by experiments with β-FNA, an irreversible mu antagonist. With a dose of β-FNA that was without intrinsic effects it was possible to antagonise the effects of DAMGO (Lason et al, 1994a). The delta agonist DPDPE showed no effects on SWDs.

Central administration of the kappa agonists U50,488H, U69,593 or PD117,302 dose-dependently decreased SWDs. These effects were attenuated or reversed in animals pre-treated with the specific kappa opioid receptor antagonist Nor-BNI (Lason et al, in preparation). Moreover, the enhancement of SWDs induced by the mu opioid receptor agonist DAMGO was attenuated in rats pre-treated with kappa agonists. These data indicate that activation of the kappa opioid receptor exerts an inhibitory effect on SWDs. Furthermore, the ability of kappa agonists to attenuate DAMGO-induced effects supports the hypothesis that mu and kappa receptors are involved in an opposite way in the modulation of SWDs.

GENERAL DISCUSSION AND CONCLUSIONS

Our biochemical data showed that rats with SWDs have enhanced PENK peptides and mRNA levels in discrete brain areas. Similarly, Patel et al (1991) reported enhanced brain levels of met-encephalin in a mouse model of absence epilepsy, which confirms the involvement of encephalins in the pathophysiology of absences. Since PENK is thought to provide endogenous ligands predominantly to delta receptors with a lower affinity to mu ones, it is rather surprising that the most selective delta agonist DPDPE had no effects on SWDs. This is in contrast to the suggested role of delta receptors in encephalin-induced absence-like epilepsy (Snead, 1983). We cannot exclude the possibility that opioid-induced absence-like seizures are due to activation of a different sub-type of delta receptor than that activated by DPDPE.

Alternatively, the SWDs from the encephalin-induced model might have a different basis from the SWDs of this genetic model. Another reason for the lack of effects of DPDPE might be that numerous thalamic nuclei exhibit a very dense mu binding in the rat, with minimal, if any, delta binding (Mansour et al, 1987). Although our preliminary autoradiographic study showed no significant changes in thalamic mu receptor density in WAG-6 rats in comparison to non-epileptic controls, differences at the post-receptor level cannot be excluded since activation of the mu receptor easily triggers SWDs.

An age-related decrease in the PDYN mRNA level in WAG-6 rats was found and this deficiency of the endogenous ligands to kappa receptors may facilitate SWDs. This hypothesis is corroborated by findings that all the kappa agonists used in our study decreased the spontaneous and DAMGO-induced SWD. Nor-BNI, a specific kappa opioid antagonist, caused a long-term increase in SWDs. Also, naloxone promoted the occurrence of SWDs (Lason et al, 1994a). The latter effect was likely to be mediated by antagonism towards kappa receptors, since specific antagonists of mu and delta receptors (β-FNA and naltrindole) had no effect on SWDs. These facts suggest that endogenous opioids, which act through the kappa receptors (eg, PDYN-derived peptides), tonically control SWDs in WAG/Rij rats.

Kappa opioid receptor agonists are efficient anti-epileptic agents in spontaneous, electrically and chemically induced generalised tonic-clonic seizures (Tortella et al, 1986; von Voigtlander et al, 1987). Some drugs for the treatment of tonic-clonic seizures, such as phenytoin, have no effect on absence seizures or even aggravate them; kappa agonists could be effective in both types of epilepsy. The neurochemical mechanism of protective effects of kappa agonists in this model remains to be elucidated. One possibility is that kappa agonists inhibit excitatory amino acids (von Voigtlander et al, 1987), which are known to play an important role in the regulation of SWDs (Peeters et al, 1994). Stimulation of kappa receptors also has an inhibitory effect on voltage-dependent N-type calcium channels, but the significance of this mechanism in regulation of absence seizures is unknown.

Kappa receptor agonists also attenuate the DAMGO-induced increase in SWDs. This finding is consistent with the reports that kappa opioid receptor agonists can antagonise some effects of mu agonists. Similarly, U50,488H antagonises the effect of ethorphine on the fluorothyl-induced seizures threshold (Porreca & Tortella, 1987). Although it is unclear at present whether the observed antagonism of mu and kappa agonists is competitive or functional in nature, our data suggest that various endogenous opioid systems may influence absences in opposite ways.

Our data indicate that mu receptors are primarily involved in facilitation of SWDs, whereas kappa receptors participate in their suppression. Differences in the activity of PENK and PDYN opioid systems and resulting changes in mu and kappa receptor occupancy may be important for the mechanisms controlling the absence-like epilepsy in WAG/Rij rats. The clinical value of knowledge of opioid mechanisms in animal models of absence epilepsy is questionable. The failure of naloxone to produce clear-cut benefits in human absence seizures (Ramabadran & Bansinath, 1990) could have been predicted from our studies in the WAG/Rij model. Naloxone blocks the mu as well as the kappa opioid receptor and these two receptor systems regulate SWDs in opposite ways. A more promising class of drugs for suppressing absences in man could originate from kappa agonists. A new generation of kappa agonists free from adverse psychomimetic effects might be developed in the near future. This should be preceded by biochemical studies on opioid receptors in epileptic patients as well as on the activity of endogenous opioid systems.

The first elegant study using positron emission tomography demonstrated the release of endogenous opioids during typical absences in patients (Bartenstein et al, 1993; see also Ch. 11) and these studies will be continued when specific positron-emitting ligands for the kappa receptor become available. Further detailed study on characterisation of sub-types of human opioid receptors, especially the kappa sub-types in the brains of patients with epilepsy, may shed light on the pathogenesis of absences as well as help with the design of new, efficient anti-absence drugs.

ACKNOWLEDGEMENTS

This research was supported by TNO Research Committee on Epilepsy of the Division for Health Research. The biochemical work was performed at the Institute of Pharmacology in Cracow and the EEG and drug studies were performed in Nijmegen.

REFERENCES

Bartenstein PA, Duncan JS, Prevett MC, Cunningham VJ, Fish DR, Jones AKP, Luthra SK et al 1993 Investigation of the opioid system in absence seizures with positron emission tomography. Journal of Neurology, Neurosurgery, and Psychiatry 56: 1295–1302

Buzsáki G, Laszlovszky I, Lajtha A, Vadász C 1990 Spike-and-wave neocortical patterns in rats: genetic and aminergic control. Neuroscience 38: 323–333

Chavkin C, Neumaier JF, Swearengen E 1988 Opioid receptor mechanisms in the rat hippocampus. NIDA Research Monograph 82: 94–117

Coenen AML, Drinkenburg WHIM, Peeters BWMM, Vossen JMH, van Luijtelaar ELJM 1991 Absence epilepsy and the level of vigilance in rats of the WAG/Rij strain. Neuroscience and Biobehavioral Reviews 15: 259–263

Coenen AML, Drinkenburg WHIM, Inoue M, Van Luijtelaar ELJM 1992 Genetic models of absence epilepsy with an emphasis on the WAG/Rij strain. Epilepsy Research 12: 75–86

Frey HH, Voits M 1991 Effects of psychotropic agents on a model of absence epilepsy in rats. Neuropharmacology 30: 651–656

Godschalk M, Dzoljic MR, Bonta IL 1976 Antagonism of gamma-hydroxybutyrate-induced hypersynchronization in the ECoG of the rat by anti-petit mal drugs. Neuroscience Letters 3: 145–150

Inoue M, Duysens J,Vossen JMH, Coenen AML 1993 Thalamic multiple-unit activity underlying spike-wave discharges in anesthetized rats. Brain Research 612: 35–40

Lason W, Przewlocka B, Przewlocki R 1983 The effect of gamma-hydroxybutyrate and anticonvulsants on opioid peptide content in the rat brain. Life Sciences (Suppl 1) 33: 599–602

Lason W, Przewlocka B, van Luijtelaar ELJM, Coenen AML, Przewlocki R 1992 Endogenous opioid peptides in brain and pituitary of rats with absence epilepsy. Neuropeptides 21: 147–152

Lason W, Przewlocka B, Coenen AML, Przewlocki R, van Luijtelaar ELJM 1994a Effects of mu and delta opioid receptor agonists and antagonists on absence epilepsy in WAG/Rij rats. Neuropharmacology 33: 161–166

Lason W, Przewlocka B, van Luijtelaar ELJM, Coenen AML, Przewlocki R 1994b Proenkephalin and prodynorphin mRNA level in brain of rats with absence epilepsy. Neuropeptides: in press

Mansour A, Khachaturian H, Lewis ME, Akil H, Watson SJ 1987 Autoradiographic differentiation of mu, delta, and kappa opioid receptors in the rat forebrain and midbrain. Journal of Neuroscience 7: 2445–2464

Patel VK, Abbott LC, Rattan AK, Teiwani GA 1991 Increased methionine-enkephalin levels in genetically epileptic (tg/tg) mice. Brain Research Bulletin 27: 849–852

Peeters BWMM, Ramakers GMJ, Ellenbroek BA, Vossen JMH, Coenen AML 1994 Interactions between NMDA and nonNMDA receptors in nonconvulsive epilepsy in the WAG/Rij inbred strain. Brain Research Bulletin 33: 715–718

Porreca F, Tortella FC, 1987 Differential antagonism of kappa agonists by U50,488H in the rat. Life Sciences 41: 2511–2516

Ramabadran K, Bansinath M 1990 Endogenous opioid peptides and epilepsy. International Journal of Clinical Pharmacology, Therapy and Toxicology 28: 47–62

Snead OC 1983 Seizures induced by carbachol, morphine and leucine enkephalin: a comparison. Annals of Neurology 13: 445–451

Snead OC, Bearden L 1980a Naloxone overcomes the dopaminergic, EEG, and behavioral effects of gamma-hydroxybutyrate. Neurology 30: 832–838

Snead OC Bearden LJ 1980b Anticonvulsants specific for petit-mal antagonize epileptogenic effects of leucine-enkephalin. Science 210: 1031–1033

Snead OC 1988 Gamma-hydroxybutyrate model of generalized absence seizures: further characterization and comparison with other absence models. Epilepsia, 29: 361–368

Tortella FC, Robles L, Holaday JW 1986 U50,488H, a highly selective kappa opioid: anticonvulsant profile in rats. The Journal of Pharmacology and Experimental Therapeutics 237: 49–53

van Luijtelaar ELJM, Coenen AML 1986 Two types of electrocortical paroxysms in an inbred strain of rats. Neuroscience Letters 70: 393– 397

van Luijtelaar ELJM, Van de Werf SJ, Vossen JMH, Coenen AML 1991a Arousal, performance and absence seizures in rats. Electroencephalography and Clinical Neurophysiology 79: 430–434

van Luijtelaar ELJM, De Bruijn SFTM, Declerck AC, Renier WO, Vossen JMH, Coenen AML 1991b Disturbances in time estimation during absence seizures in children. Epilepsy Research 9: 148–153

von Voigtlander PF, Hall ED, Kamacho-Ochoa M, Lewis R, Triezenberg HJ 1987 U-54494A: a unique anticonvulsant related to kappa opioid agonists. The Journal of Pharmacology and Experimental Therapeutics 243: 542–547

DISCUSSION

Duncan: Have there been studies of opioids applied to the cortex or to the thalamus to see whether these have different effects on the spike wave in this model?

Van Luijtelaar: The majority of the data I presented were ICV injections. We have injected mu-agonist into the thalamus, and a very low dose results in an increase in spike-and-wave discharges immediately following intra-cerebral injection. Autoradiographic studies have shown a high density of mu receptors in the thalamus.

Duncan: Is it suggested that kappa-agonists are anti-convulsant?

Van Luijtelaar: They act as anti-absence drugs in this model. There is clearly a difference between anti-absence drugs and anti-convulsant drugs. Kappa agonists have also been shown to prevent seizures in the maximum electro-convulsive shock model and might be broad-spectrum anti-epileptic drugs.

Chapman: I agree. The kappa-agonists are interesting. Most drugs that have anti-absence action will not block convulsive seizures, but the kappa-agonists block maximal electro-shock and reflex-induced clonic seizures and also absence seizures. They fall into the same category as valproate and benzodiazepines; they seem to have a spectrum for both types of seizure.

You said that there is an absence model in which mu-agonists cause an increase in spike wave discharges. Did you not also say that in another absence model mu-agonists suppress absence seizures?

Van Luijtelaar: Snead found that leu-encephalin induced spike wave discharges, which is the opposite to what we see with a mu antagonist in the spontanous model.

Bowery: Can you explain the control experiments? You mentioned WAG-3 and WAG-6. In WAG-6 you were getting development of absences, but not in

WAG-3. Is it not possible that something else is developing at the same stage?

Van Luijtelaar: Yes, of course the rats are getting 3 months older. But it is possible to control for age effects. That's why we have included age-matched non-epileptic controls, ACI_3 and ACI_6. This leaves us with two strains and two age groups, and only the WAG_6 have a substantial amount of spike-wave discharges. The analysis of variance (2×2 design) will yield age and strain effect, and an interaction. A significant interaction and statistical difference between the WAG_6 (epileptic) and the three non-epileptic controls can be more safely interpreted as being caused by the presence of hundreds of spike-wave discharges per day.

9. Anti-epileptic drugs in animal models – consensus statement

Astrid G. Chapman

Rodents (GAERS and WAG/Rij rats; lethargic, tottering, Stargazer mice) with a genetic predisposition to spontaneous, synchronous spike-wave discharges (SWDs) share many of the features of typical absence epilepsy in humans: brief 5–10 Hz SWDs (3 Hz in humans) in the cortico-thalamic circuit, behavioural arrest with occasional myoclonus or vibrissal twitching during SWDs, partial suppression of SWDs during mental arousal, as well as a very similar pharmacological profile to that of human absence epilepsy. The genetic rodent absence models represent relatively 'pure' absence epilepsy, whereas a significant proportion of human typical absence epilepsy co-exists with (or developmentally leads to) clonic/tonic or myoclonic epilepsy with paroxysmal discharges, which affects the choice of optimal anti-epileptic therapy under the two conditions.

SWDs in rodents with genetic absence seizures are suppressed by anti-epileptic drugs (AEDs) used clinically against absence epilepsy (ethosuximide, valproate, trimethadione and benzodiazepines), as well as by experimental anti-absence drugs, such as $GABA_B$ antagonists, excitatory amino acid antagonists or kappa-opiate agonists. Phenytoin, GABA (A or B) agonists, GABA uptake inhibitors, GABA transaminase (GABA-T) inhibitors, or γ-hydroxy-butyrate, on the other hand, aggravate SWD in both rodent and human absence epilepsy. With the exception of AEDs with a very broad spectrum of anti-epileptic action, such as benzodiazepines and sodium valproate, or kappa-opiate agonists that suppress both absence and convulsive seizures, there is very little overlap between AEDs that protect against convulsive and against absence epilepsies. Indeed, many of the drugs that are anti-epileptic against convulsive seizures (GABA-T inhibitors, GABA uptake inhibitors, and low doses of $GABA_A$ and $GABA_B$ agonists) acerbate absences in absence seizure models when given systemically or focally into cortico-thalamic regions. It is interesting, however, that some of the drugs that increase absences in absence seizure models (eg, the $GABA_A$ agonist, muscimol, or the GABA-T inhibitor, γ-vinyl-GABA) have anti-absence activity when administered focally into basal ganglia areas such as the substantia nigra.

Several transmitter systems ($GABA_A$ and $GABA_B$, glutamatergic, kappa- and μ-opiate systems or dopamine) are directly or indirectly involved in generating and modulating SWDs in the cortico-thalamic circuit, which includes neocortical pyramidal neurons, thalamic relay neurons and neurons of the nucleus reticularis thalami.

The effects of manipulations of the opiate system have been investigated mainly in 2 rodent absence models: the genetic absence WAG/Rij rat model, and a chemical absence model where spontaneous, synchronous cortico-thalamic SWDs are generated following systemic administration of γ-hydroxy-butyrate to rats. A complex pattern of interactions emerges from these studies. The non-selective opiate antagonist, naloxone, facilitates the generation of SWDs in WAG/Rij and suppresses them in the γ-hydroxy-butyrate model; paradoxically, μ-agonists also facilitate SWDs in WAG/Rij while suppressing them in the γ-hydroxy-butyrate model. Kappa-agonists, on the whole, suppress SWDs, while neither delta-agonists nor delta-antagonists appear to be involved in the generation of SWDs in rodent absence models. Altered endorphin levels have been reported in these absence models and an increased level of opiate receptors (alpha-neoendorphin binding) is reported in WAG/Rij at a seizure-susceptible age (6 months). However, this increase (versus non-absence controls) occurs in the hippocampus and striatum, but not, as might be expected, in the thalamus.

Many studies have focused on the importance of the GABA-ergic system in controlling absence epilepsy and for providing a possible clue to the underlying aetiology of spontaneous SWDs in genetically susceptible rodents or humans. Most of the strains of rodents exhibiting spontaneous SWDs appear to have normal overall levels of $GABA_A$/benzodiazepine receptors or $GABA_B$ receptors, with the exception of the lethargic (LH/LH) mouse model: it has a significantly increased level of cortical $GABA_B$ receptors, which appear to correlate with the seizure frequency in this model. $GABA_B$ antagonists potently suppress SWDs in this absence model as well as in other rodent absence models (eg, GAERS) that exhibit normal levels of $GABA_A$ receptors.

Although overall $GABA_A$ and $GABA_B$ receptor levels appear normal in most of the absence models, an altered regional receptor sub-unit composition in the seizure-susceptible strains remains an interesting possibility. Another biochemical GABA-ergic marker that has been studied in rodent absence models is that of altered cortico-thalamic release of GABA. Although potassium-evoked release of GABA from cortical synaptosomes from the lethargic mouse strain LH/LH is similar to that of control synaptosomes, the inhibitory effect of baclofen on GABA release is greater in LH/LH synaptosomes than in controls. Changes in the release of GABA have also been reported for the GAERS rat model. In vivo basal release of GABA in the thalamus of GAERS is elevated compared to controls, however this release is not affected by baclofen.

One of the most dramatic developments in recent years in experimental absence epilepsy is the discovery of the potent anti-absence activity of selective $GABA_B$ antagonists such as CGP 35348. Although not utilised against human typical absence seizures at the present time, the $GABA_B$ antagonists have been shown to suppress potently SWDs and to normalise behavioural absence symptoms in most of the rodent genetic and chemical absence models investigated. Conversely, CGP 35348 has a moderate but consistent pro-convulsant effect in some convulsive seizure models (potentiating isoniazid seizures; accelerating the development of kindling).

DISCUSSION

Noebels: It is estimated that up to half of patients with typical absences go on to develop tonic-clonic seizures. Is there a single mechanism in the GABA receptor story that can account for this or is there a separate mechanism?

Hosford: You provided a possible answer earlier when you described the variety of $GABA_A$ receptor subunits. It is possible there are multiple sub-types of some factor, whether $GABA_B$ receptor or something else, say Factor X, and it develops at different times, and maybe Factor XA develops earlier and the children have absences and as they outgrow them 50% of them develop Factor XB in some different neuronal population. That would be one possibility.

Noebels: That would imply that these are two different genes.

Hosford: They would have a different phenotypic expression due to ontogeny of two different sub-types of one gene product. That is like two different diseases.

Bowery: That is not unreasonable because there is a mouse mutation that may span three GABA receptor sub-unit genes that are all next to each other, and there are some alleles at that locus where either one, two or three of the genes are missing, but it behaves as if it is a single gene mutation.

It is possible that you could have one mutation that knocks out two different receptors, one of which might appear early and one later.

Bowery: It would be useful to have an animal model in which the change occurs. Has any change been seen in the Strasbourg animals where the epilepsy disappears?

Marescaux: No. However, if we use a very small dose of a $GABA_A$ antagonist we get absences, and if we increase the dose we get tonic-clonic seizures. Conversely, if we induce absences using a $GABA_A$ agonist, they never progress to tonic-clonic seizures. One way to differentiate the different kinds of absence epilepsy is the occurrence or otherwise of tonic-clonic seizures. I do not believe that half the patients with absence epilepsy develop tonic-clonic seizures. I believe that a specific sub-set of patients have a different disease which associates a small number of tonic-clonic seizures and absence seizures, and this is completely different to the people with only absence seizures, who have a different pathophysiological mechanism and a different disease.

Van Luijtelaar: We do not have to assume that it is an indication of a different disease when absences occur in isolation, or in conjunction with generalised tonic-clonic seizures. I do not think we have to make this assumption. In some conditions one may lead to the other. In our model some cats that produce spike-wave discharges go on to have a generalised tonic-clonic seizure. In this case, we find that inhibition, as measured as a histogram of probability of neuronal discharge, breaks down before that. The inhibition keeps the system oscillating in the spike-wave mode. When it breaks down, the inhibition can no longer counteract the hyper-excitability, and a generalised tonic-clonic seizure occurs. It is the same condition, in this case pharmacologically induced.

Repetitive activation of GABA-ergic synapses will lead to a diminution of the effectiveness of that synapse, so when there is a lot of GABA activation within a short time interval, it is easy to imagine that in certain circumstances the effective brake may fail, without having assumed that this is now a different gene or a different disease coming into function.

Hosford: If that were true, one would expect absence status to result in tonic-clonic seizures.

Dreifuss: Drs Sato, Penry and I did a 25-year prospective study on the outcome of absence seizures and did not find that up to 50% developed generalised tonic-clonic or any other kind of seizure than absences. Looking at all the predictive factors and doing a multivariate analysis, mental retardation and a strong family history of generalised tonic-clonic seizures were the only two factors that related to the subsequent onset of generalised tonic-clonic seizures. Many of the patients previously regarded as absence patients who developed generalised tonic clonic seizures in point of fact had juvenile myoclonic epilepsy with the early presentation of juvenile absence, supporting the concept that the aetiology of the epilepsy determines its prognosis.

Panayiotopoulos: Generalised tonic clonic seizures in adults with absences is the rule rather than the exception. There were no more than five such patients (absences without GTCS) in over 50 adult patients that we have seen in the last 5 years. What is interesting is the relation of these GTCS to absences. In the majority of patients GTCS occur independently of absences but in others GTCS are preceded by clusters of absences and in others they always occur after a prolonged absence status. This different pattern of absences–GTCS sequence may be important regarding treatment. I wonder, but there is no answer to this, whether anti-absence drugs alone are sufficient to prevent GTCS in those patients who present with this absence–GTCS sequence.

Stephenson: Another point in relation to this question about tonic-clonic seizures and absences in relation to ontogeny. We have seen tonic-clonic seizures with fever occurring before what apparently is typical childhood absence epilepsy in about 15% of cases. The sequence then is not always tonic-clonic seizures after absences; they may occur beforehand.

Chapman: We heard in the first session that these absence models share many properties as far as EEG pattern and behavioural and anatomical results go but there have been some indications that they are pharmacologically diverse. Does anyone have any feeling for which is the best predictive model of these genetic or chemically induced absence models in predicting which drugs will be effective in typical absence seizures, and do they have any experience with drugs such as felbamate and lamotrigine which have recently been shown to be quite active, at least in Lennox–Gastaut.

Marescaux: Gabapentin was ineffective in our model and was a bit aggravative; it was effective against pentylenetetrazol-induced seizures. As Professor Chadwick will discuss later, gabapentin was ineffective against absences in humans. This kind of model is very predictive if we can induce a tremendous increase of spike-wave discharge and then we know that the drug will be bad for humans, or if we get complete suppression. But we have problems with drugs which are ineffective in our model. Lamotrigine, for example, was ineffective in rodents yet is effective in humans. However, in rodents spike-wave discharges do not reduce with age, some drugs act in humans only on the specific pathway that participates in the control of absence epilepsy in adolescents. Such a drug, which may be a very good one, could not act in rodents because rodents do not display the kind of circuitry that allows the control of absence epilepsy in primates and in children.

Felbamate, too, is completely ineffective in our model but I am not sure that felbamate is effective against spike-wave discharge in humans; it is effective against some components of the Lennox–Gastaut syndrome but I do not believe it is very effective against spike-wave discharges.

Van Luijtelaar: We have tested Loreclazole, a drug that will not come to the market, which suppressed spike-wave discharges in a dose-dependent way. Remacemide results in a dose-dependent suppression of spike-wave discharges, but the few spike-wave discharges which were left were extremely long.

Bowery: How do phenytoin and carbamazepine induce absences? What is the mechanism? Is it anything to do with the GABA system?

Marescaux: I think it is certainly related to inhibitory transmission, but I have no idea as to the actual mechanism.

10. Feline generalised penicillin epilepsy: extrapolations to neurophysiological mechanisms in humans

Pierre Gloor

Feline generalised epilepsy (FGPE) is a model of generalised epilepsy induced as a transient condition in cats having received an intramuscular injection of 300 000–500 000 IU of penicillin (Gloor, 1988). Among models of generalised epilepsy, FGPE probably most resembles the electrographic and behavioural manifestations of human absence epilepsy. The neurophysiological mechanisms of FGPE may thus illuminate some aspects of human idiopathic generalised epilepsy. The manifestations and mechanism of FGPE are summarised by Gloor (1988), Gloor & Fariello (1988), Gloor et al (1990), Avoli et al (1990), where references to the original publications on FGPE can be found.

VALIDITY OF FGPE AS A MODEL OF HUMAN ABSENCE EPILEPSY

- EEG features: In both conditions the ictal EEG shows bilaterally synchronous spike and wave discharges (SWDs) which are blocked by arousal; their changes during slow-wave sleep are also similar. SWDs in FGPE are sensitive to intermittent photic stimulation as in some humans.
- Clinical features: Arrest of ongoing behaviour during SW bursts associated with eye-blinking is seen in the cat and humans. In both species a seizure with SWD occasionally progresses to a generalised convulsion. Behavioural deficits during SWDs in FGPE are similar to those in human absences: the cat fails to respond to stimuli to which it has been trained to respond; or, if it does respond during a SW burst, the reaction time is prolonged.
- Pharmacological features: SW bursts in FGPE are significantly reduced by anti-absence drugs like ethosuximide and valproate, but not reliably so by phenytoin.

NEUROPHYSIOLOGICAL MECHANISMS UNDERLYING FGPE

The SWDs of FGPE evolve from spindles. Under the influence of penicillin each thalamo-cortical spindle-inducing volley becomes more effective in discharging cortical neurons. Shortly thereafter an increasingly strong inhibitory phase develops after each increased burst of pyramidal cell discharge and evolves into the slow-wave component of the SW complex. Thus an oscillatory pattern develops with a burst of action potentials discharging during the spike representing an enhanced spindle wave, and virtual neuronal silence during the slow wave of the SW complex (Fig. 10.1). The frequency of the SW oscillation is one-half or one-third that of spindles.

Every second or second and third spindle wave is suppressed while the first one is enhanced. Soon or almost simultaneously a similar oscillatory pattern develops in the thalamus. The thalamic oscillation, however, never develops before the cortical one. Also, within each SW burst the oscillatory pattern of neuronal discharge underlying the SW rhythm always precedes by 2–3 cycles that of the thalamic neuron with which that cortical neuron is interconnected (Fig. 10.1). It never begins with the thalamic neuron. The cortical and thalamic oscillatory mechanisms are closely interlocked and

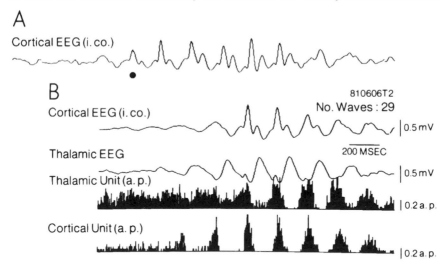

Fig. 10.1 During SWDs cortical and thalamic neurons undergo oscillations between increased excitation with the spike and increased inhibition with the wave. When the activity of 2 mutually connected neurons is recorded, one cortical, the other thalamic, the cortical neuron begins to oscillate 2–3 cycles earlier than the thalamic one. **A** Raw cortical EEG recorded intracortically (i.co), hence polarity reversed. **B** Computer-generated cortical and thalamic EEG averages and histogram of action potential (a.p.) discharges of a cortical and of a thalamic neuron which had been proved to be interconnected. The first EEG spike (dot) of successive SW bursts triggered the EEG averaging and the histogram computation for 1 s before and 1 s after the first EEG spike. Source: Avoli M, Gloor P, Kostopoulos G 1982 In: Akimoto H et al (eds) Advances in epileptology. XIII Epilepsy International Symposium. Raven Press, New York, pp493–496; with permission.

both are essential for the maintenance of the SW rhythm, since temporary suppression of neuronal function at the cortical or at the thalamic level by spreading depression confined to either cortex or thalamus abolishes SW discharge at both levels.

The thalamic oscillation is dependent on a de-inactivation of a low-Ca^{2+} current which occurs when the membrane potential of thalamic relay neurons is hyper-polarised (Steriade et al, 1993; von Krosigk, 1993). Since this is also a prerequisite for spindle generation, we suspect that the switch to the slower SW rhythm takes place as the membrane is hyper-polarised into the region which causes the cell to oscillate at the slower delta rhythm (Steriade et al, 1993) because more potent cortico-thalamic volleys activate the GABA-ergic thalamic nucleus reticularis neurons more strongly. The increased outputs of these neurons induce stronger inhibitory responses in the thalamic relay cells to which they are directed, thus hyper-polarising their membranes into the range at which the slow delta oscillation occurs. Thus in FGPE it is the cerebral cortex which initiates the chain of events that leads to SW oscillation in thalamo-cortico-thalamic networks. It seems that if the cortex is diffusely mildly hyper-excitable the thalamo-cortical spindle-generating mechanism can be switched to the SW mode.

EXTRAPOLATION OF PHYSIOLOGICAL MECHANISMS OF FGPE TO HUMAN GENERALISED EPILEPSY

Thalamo-cortical mechanisms

The thalamo-cortical mechanisms involved in SW genesis in FGPE also seem to operate in humans. Thus the incidence of SWDs in patients with absence attacks is highest during the phase of slow-wave sleep, normally dominated by spindles, and there is an inverse relationship between SW and spindles during that phase. The more SWs there are, the fewer spindles (Fig. 10.2) (Kellaway et al, 1990). This would be predicted if the two have a common generator that functions either in the spindle or in the SW mode, as is the case in FGPE. The underlying thalamo-cortical mechanism of SWs in human absence epilepsy thus seems to be the same as that in FGPE.

GABA-ergic mechanisms as a major factor sustaining SW genesis in human absence epilepsy

During absence attacks, as in FGPE, the GABA-ergic mechanisms ensure the maintenance of oscillations underlying SW discharge. This is in accord with the observation that, in humans as well as in animal models, GABA-ergic drugs increase SW discharge (Gloor & Fariello, 1988). The anti-absence drug ethosuximide seems to act by depressing the low-threshold thalamic Ca^{2+} current involved in promoting the thalamo-cortical oscillations underlying the SW rhythm (Coulter et al 1990).

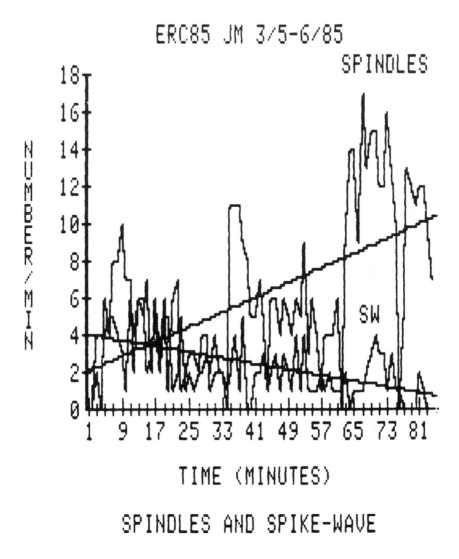

Fig 10.2   Trend analysis (straight lines) of the time distribution of spindles (upper line) and of SW bursts (lower line) in a single patient with absence seizures. The graph shows the reciprocal relationship between spindles and SWs (Kellaway, Frost & Crawley, 1990).

Cortical mechanisms in human SW discharge

In FGPE the prime mover setting into motion generalised SW discharge is a diffuse increase in the excitability of cortical neurons. If this is applicable to humans, one should find instances that support this view. Some clinical observations demonstrate the importance of cortical mechanisms in triggering SW discharge in humans.

● Photosensitivity: Intermittent photic stimulation is known to precipitate
SW discharge in FGPE as well as in some human patients with absence
seizures. Precipitation of SW discharge in both conditions is tied to a
dopaminergic mechanism that acts at the cortical level. Intermittent
photic stimulation reduces the release of dopamine in the cerebral cortex
(Reader et al, 1976). This increases cortical excitability and hence cortical
responsiveness to photic stimuli.

When the dopamine agonist apomorphine is administered to cats with
FGPE, intermittent photic stimulation no longer precipitates SW discharge (Quesney, 1981; Reader, 1990). In humans apomorphine also
abolishes epileptic photo-sensitivity without blocking spontaneous
SWDs (Quesney et al, 1980). Thus it is likely that in both FGPE and
photo-sensitive human epileptic patients reduction of cortical release of
dopamine in response to intermittent photic stimulation raises cortical
excitability enough to trigger SW discharge in response to intermittent
light stimuli. In FGPE, when the cortex is painted with 6-OH dopamine
(which eliminates dopaminergic transmission to cortical neurons), intermittent photic stimulation elicits SWDs even in cats that have not
received intramuscular penicillin (Quesney & Reader, 1990).

● Pattern sensitivity: In some patients SWDs and absence seizures are
triggered by looking at patterned visual stimuli such as stripes (Chatrian
et al, 1970; Wilkins et al, 1975; Wilkins, 1980). The critical stimuli are
parallel stripes. They are more effective than draughts board patterns,
even though the latter possess a larger number of brightness contours.
Unless binocular fusion of the striped pattern occurs, its potency to trigger SWDs is low (Wilkins et al, 1975; Wilkins, 1980). The only part of
the brain known to have neurons attuned to these visual features is the
striate cortex. Complex cells in this cortex would receive very powerful
stimulation by the pattern that is most effective in triggering SW bursts.
By manipulating the size and retinal distribution of stimuli, Wilkins
(1980) showed that a critical mass needs to be stimulated within striate
cortex to elicit a SW response. Stimulation of one visual hemifield by
these patterns elicits SWDs that predominate in the posterior quadrant
of the contralateral hemisphere (Wilkins et al 1981), which supports a
striate cortex triggering mechanism. Stimulation of a large enough population of striate cortex neurons thus raises the cortical excitability sufficiently to set in motion the cortico-thalamo-cortical oscillatory
mechanisms underlying SW discharge.

● Cognitive mechanisms and human SW discharge: The final example of a
likely cortical trigger mechanism of human SW discharge is that provided by stimuli resulting from engaging association cortex in cognitive
tasks (Goossens et al, 1990). There are patients in whom generalised
SWDs with absence attacks, often followed by generalised convulsions,
are specifically triggered by some cognitive endeavour. In some patients,

seizures only occur under such conditions. Activities that in susceptible individuals can trigger such seizures include playing cards, chess or draughts, performing arithmetic, making complex decisions, drawing complex figures, measuring, doing geometric problems, thinking about or performing complex movements and playing with a Rubik's cube. In all patients in whom such cognitive triggers were identified the epileptic EEG response consisted of generalised, bilaterally synchronous SW discharge. No focal epileptiform discharges were recorded in these patients. All these tasks engage large areas of association cortex, particularly that of the parietal lobe. It seems probable that in these susceptible individuals the excitability in a large enough population of association cortical neurons is raised enough to set into motion the cortico-thalamo-cortical oscillatory mechanism underlying SW discharge.

There is thus evidence that, at least in certain patients, it is the cortex that initiates the neuronal oscillations underlying generalised SW discharge. This is in line with experimental observation in FGPE where the cortex always seemed to initiate generalised SW bursts. This does not exclude the possibility that in some patients the oscillation may be initiated at the thalamic level. However, if the human brain produces generalised SW discharge by the same mechanism as the cat brain in FGPE, it is likely that the cortex is the site of the initiating trigger mechanism.

In all instances in which such cortical triggers are operating in humans, the cortex appears to be anatomically and functionally well preserved. Lesions of the cortex as they are commonly found in patients with partial epilepsy seem to be inimical to the operation of this mechanism, which has to engage an anatomically and functionally intact cerebral cortex.

SUMMARY

In FGPE spindle-inducing thalamo-cortical volleys elicit SWs instead of spindles in response to a diffuse increase in the excitability of cortical neurons. The increased output of these neurons impinging on the thalamus causes thalamo-cortical networks to oscillate at the SW frequency. GABA-ergic mechanisms in conjunction with the de-inactivation of a thalamic Ca^{2+}-conductance maintain this oscillatory pattern.

These findings explain the following features of human epilepsy associated with generalised SW discharge: the reciprocal relationship between spindles and SW discharge; the increase of SW discharge caused by GABA-ergic drugs and its reduction by ethosuximide which depresses the thalamic Ca^{2+}-conductance; and the triggering of generalised SW discharge by stimuli known to excite large populations of cortical neurons, as in photo-sensitive epilepsy, pattern-sensitive epilepsy and seizures precipitated by cognitive tasks.

REFERENCES

Avoli M, Gloor P, Kostopoulos G 1990 Focal and generalised epileptiform activity in the
    cortex: in search of differences in synaptic mechanisms, ionic movements, and long-lasting
    changes in neuronal excitability. In: Avoli M, Gloor P, Kostopoulos G, Naquet R (eds)
    Generalized epilepsy: neurobiological approaches. Birkhäuser, Boston, pp213–231
Chatrian GE, Lettich E, Miller LH, Green JR 1970 Pattern-sensitive epilepsy. Part I. An
    electrographic study of its mechanisms. Epilepsia 11: 125–149
Chatrian GE, Lettich E, Miller LH, Kupfer C 1970 Pattern-sensitive epilepsy. Part 2. Clinical
    changes, tests of responsiveness and motor output, alterations of evoked potentials and
    therapeutic measures. Epilepsia 11: 151–162
Coulter DA, Huguenard JR, Prince DA 1990 Cellular actions of petit mal anticonvulsants:
    implication of thalamic low-threshold calcium current in generation of spike-wave discharge.
    In: Avoli M, Gloor P, Kostopoulos G, Naquet R (eds) Generalized epilepsy: neurobiological
    approaches. Birkhäuser, Boston, pp425–435
Gloor P 1988 Neurophysiological mechanism of generalised spike-and-wave discharge and its
    implications for understanding absence seizures. In: Myslobodsky MS, Mirsky AF (eds)
    Elements of petit mal epilepsy. Peter Lang, New York, pp159–209
Gloor P, Avoli M, Kostopoulos G 1990 Thalamocortical relationships in generalised epilepsy
    with bilaterally synchronous spike-and-wave discharge. In: Avoli M, Gloor P, Kostopoulos
    G, Naquet R (eds) Generalized epilepsy: neurobiological approaches. Birkhäuser, Boston,
    pp190–212
Gloor P, Fariello RG 1988 Generalized epilepsy: Some of its cellular mechanisms differ from
    those of focal epilepsy. Trends in Neuroscience 11: 63–68
Goossens LAZ, Andermann F, Andermann E, Rémillard GM 1990 Reflex seizures induced by
    calculation, card or board games, and spatial tasks: a review of 25 patients and delineation of
    the epileptic syndrome. Neurology 40: 1171–1176
Kellaway P, Frost JD, Crawley JW 1990 The relationship between sleep spindles and spike and
    wave bursts in human epilepsy. In: Avoli M, Gloor P, Kostopoulos G, Naquet R (eds)
    Generalized epilepsy: neurobiological approaches. Birkhäuser, Boston, pp36–48
Quesney LF 1981 Dopamine and generalised photosensitive epilepsy. In: Morselli KG, Lloyd
    W, Löscher B, Meldrum B, Reynolds EH (eds) Neurotransmitters, seizures and epilepsy.
    Raven Press, New York, pp263–274
Quesney LF, Andermann F, Lal S, Prelevic S 1980 Transient abolition of generalised
    photosensitive epileptic discharge in humans by apomorphine, a dopamine-receptor agonist.
    Neurology 30: 1169–1174
Quesney LF, Reader TA 1990 Role of dopamine in generalised photosensitive epilepsy:
    electroencephalographic and biochemical aspects. In: Avoli M, Gloor P, Kostopoulos G,
    Naquet R (eds) Generalized epilepsy. neurobiological approaches. Birkhäuser, Boston,
    pp298–313
Reader TA, de Champlain J, Jasper HH 1976 Catecholamine released from cerebral cortex in
    the cat. Decrease during sensory stimulation. Brain Research 111: 95–108
Steriade M, McCormick DA, Sejnowski TJ 1993 Thalamocortical oscillations in the sleeping
    and aroused brain. Science 262: 679–685
von Krosigk M, Bal T, McCormick DA 1993 Cellular mechanisms of a synchronized
    oscillation in the thalamus. Science 261: 361–364
Wilkins AJ, Andermann F, Ives F 1975 Stripes, complex cells and seizures. An attempt to
    determine the locus and nature of the trigger mechanism in pattern-sensitive epilepsy. Brain
    98: 365–380
Wilkins AJ, Binnie CD, Darby CE 1980 Visually-induced seizures. Progress in Neurobiology
    15: 85–117
Wilkins AJ, Binnie CD, Darby CE 1981 Interhemispheric differences in photosensitive
    epilepsy. I. Pattern sensitivity thresholds. Electroencephalography and Clinical
    Neurophysiology 52: 461–468.

DISCUSSION

Marescaux: Photo-sensitivity in the feline model is correlated with an increase in cortical excitability. I have the same impression as a clinician. When we see a patient with typical absences who is also photo-sensitive, he is usually in the group at risk of developing generalised tonic-clonic seizures. I wonder if the degree of cortical excitability might predict the occurrence of spike-wave discharges or a combination of tonic-clonic seizures and absences.

Gloor: There are different sub-forms. Our discussions are not confined to a single monolithic condition and there are gradations. There is a common pathophysiological path that ties these things together. That does not mean that they are all exactly alike. On the other hand, to say that they are completely different is also wrong. It depends at what level we are talking. If we consider genetics, I would not be surprised if one day we found a very wide spread of different genetic conditions that produce a similar or even an identical phenotype, as well as other conditions that may lead to cortical hyper-excitability.

Fish: Many people with absences find that they have fewer absences when they concentrate on something. Are there any animals that have more (or less) seizures when they are performing tasks?

Gloor: Two things have to be taken into consideration. One is the non-specific arousal effect: being more attentive reduces spike and wave discharges. Blow in the face of a cat with FGPE and the spike and wave stops for a while because the cat has become aroused. That is the non-specific arousal effect.

Then there is the specific engagement of certain cortical areas. There must be something particular about these patients. Whether they have microsdysgenesis in these areas, as Professor Meencke will discuss, I do not know. But I think there are patients who have hyper-excitability in particular areas. My point is that it is very difficult to imagine this being mediated by the thalamus. It must involve the cortex.

Hosford: The nucleus reticularis of the thalamus connects large areas of the cortex. It could be that it is not the spreading around the cortex but the association of certain areas in the cortex, transferred at the level of the reticularis, which generates spike and wave discharges.

Gloor: I would not agree with that. The reticularis does not intervene at the cognitive level; it does not have the right connectivity. The reticularis has a very non-specific connectivity and is not able to act as the analyser of these things. Parietal and frontal cortex are able to do this and they feed into the reticularis, and the reticularis is probably a very important link. But it is not where discharges are triggered from.

Hosford: Could we agree that we do not necessarily need a particular stimulus in a particular place, but that we need some small movement somewhere in the whole system to trigger things off, and that that could happen anywhere?

Gloor: In some patients, maybe, but not necessarily in those that I was discussing.

11. Functional imaging studies in humans

M. C. Prevett   J. S. Duncan

Functional imaging in idiopathic generalised epilepsy has received relatively little attention compared with that in partial epilepsy. In those studies performed so far positron emission tomography (PET) has been the modality most commonly used. Lack of quantitation and inferior spatial resolution have limited the use of single photon emission computed tomography (SPECT) and the potential of functional magnetic resonance imaging has yet to be explored.

PET allows measurement of local tissue concentrations of injected radioactive tracers and provides a means of studying local cerebral physiology in vivo in humans (Phelps et al, 1982). The technique is analogous to tissue autoradiography in animals but uses external radiation detection and subsequent mathematical image reconstruction. Application of tracer kinetic models that describe the physiological process under study allow estimation of physiological parameters from the acquired data. PET depends on the use of tracers labelled with short half-life positron emitting isotopes, eg. [^{18}F], [^{15}O], and [^{11}C]. The first PET studies in patients with typical absence seizures used ^{18}F-labelled fluorodeoxyglucose (FDG) to measure cerebral glucose metabolism. Subsequently cerebral blood flow (CBF) has been studied using [^{15}O] H_2O and the roles of the benzodiazepine binding site of the GABA$_A$ receptor (BZ-GABA$_A$ receptor) and opiate receptors have been investigated using [^{11}C] flumazenil and [^{11}C] diprenorphine respectively.

CEREBRAL METABOLISM AND BLOOD FLOW

There have been three studies of cerebral glucose metabolism (CMRglu) in humans with idiopathic generalised epilepsy using FDG and PET. In the first, four children with typical absence seizures were studied before and after treatment (Engel et al, 1985). Treatment with ethosuximide or valproate resulted in suppression of spike-wave activity in three. In those three patients CMRglu was 2–3.5-fold higher before treatment, when generalised spike-wave activity occupied 32–61% of the EEG record. There was no clear correlation between the amount of spike-wave activity and CMRglu, and no focal increases or decreases were detected. A drug effect was unlikely to have accounted for the results because CMRglu did not decrease after treatment in the fourth patient, in whom spike-wave activity persisted.

In the second study, CMRglu was measured in six adults with typical absence seizures (Theodore et al, 1984). Inter-ictal CMRglu was normal in all six. Two patients were studied again during absence seizures. In one, generalised spike-wave occurred during 38% of the scan and was associated with a diffuse 60% increase in CMRglu. The other patient was in absence status and a global reduction in CMRglu was seen. In the third study, CMRglu was 30–36% higher in two adults during typical absence seizures compared with normal control data. In the same study, CMRglu was 10–44% lower during absence seizures in patients with atypical spike-wave and symptomatic generalised epilepsy compared with normal controls (Ochs et al, 1987).

In summary, variable diffuse increases in CMRglu have been recorded during typical absence seizures, the larger increases being seen in children. In the limited numbers of patients studied, symptomatic absence seizures and absence status were associated with a diffuse reduction in CMRglu. As has been observed in animal models (Nehlig et al, 1993), there was a lack of correlation between CMRglu and electro-encephalographic activity. Also, specific structures preferentially involved in the generation of absence seizures were not identified. 70–80% of FDG uptake by the brain occurs over the first 15 min following intravenous injection, during which time a combination of pre-ictal, ictal, and post-ictal events may be taking place. The poor temporal resolution of the FDG method may have contributed to the failure to identify any specific anatomical structures.

The temporal resolution of studies of cerebral activation can be improved by measuring CBF instead of CMRglu. In the 1960s non-tomographic methods were developed to measure regional CBF. These used either intra-carotid injection or inhalation of $[^{133}Xe]$ and external detectors. Using $[^{133}Xe]$ inhalation, cortical CBF was found to be on average 30% higher during typical absence seizures in four patients compared with normal controls (Sakai et al 1978). In another study, CBF was measured inter-ictally in 24 patients with idiopathic generalised epilepsy with $[^{131}Xe]$ and SPECT. No focal or global differences were found when compared with normal controls (Leroy et al 1987). SPECT data, however, is not quantitative and the spatial resolution of these techniques is poor compared to current PET.

Regional cerebral blood flow (rCBF) was measured in eight patients with idiopathic generalised epilepsy using a high resolution PET scanner (ECAT 953b, CTI/Siemens) and a bolus injection of $[^{15}O]$ H$_2$O (Prevett et al, 1994a). This technique achieved a spatial resolution of $8 \times 8 \times 4.3$ mm and a temporal resolution of ≤ 30 s. The patients hyperventilated to induce absence seizures during an intravenous injection of $[^{15}O]$ H$_2$O followed by a 90 s scan. The distribution of rCBF during absence seizures was compared with the distribution of rCBF when absence seizures did not occur. During absence seizures there was a mean global increase in blood flow of 15%.

After normalisation of global flow there was an additional selective 8% increase in blood flow in the thalamus (Fig. 11.1). There were no focal increases in blood flow in cortex and no focal decreases.

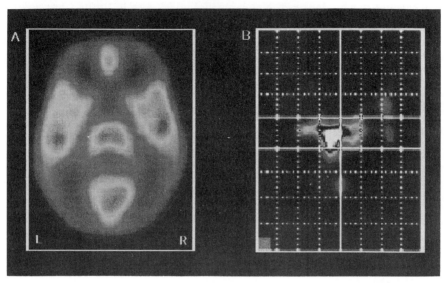

Fig. 11.1   Transverse PET images through the thalamus: **A** mean cerebral blood flow image to provide an anatomical reference; **B** map showing the areas in which cerebral blood flow selectively increased during absence seizures. White areas represent significant focal increases in cerebral blood flow.

The increase in rCBF seen in the thalamus reflects increased local neuronal activity (Raichle, 1987) and supports the hypothesis that the thalamus is involved in the generation of absence seizures in humans (Williams, 1953). The statistically significant focal increases in blood flow during absence seizures were on the left side. There was also a 3.9% (NS) increase in blood flow in the right thalamus. The apparent asymmetry may be a reflection of spontaneous variability in the small number of subjects studied and the limitations of spatial resolution. It was not considered likely that this asymmetry was relevant to the pathophysiology of generalised spike-wave activity.

Neurophysiological data in animal models suggests that spike-wave activity oscillates within thalamo-cortical circuits but the site of the primary abnormality remains uncertain (Avoli et al, 1983; Vergnes & Marescaux, 1992; Chs 3, 10). The preferential increase in thalamic rCBF may reflect a convergence of widespread synchronous cortical activity on the thalamus via thalamo-cortical connections. Alternatively the focal increase in thalamic rCBF may reflect a primary thalamic process. No significant increases in rCBF were detected in thalamus in the 30 s prior to the onset of generalised spike-wave activity on the scalp EEG and it was not possible to determine whether the thalamus was the site of initiation of absence seizures.

Temporal resolution was much better than with FDG and PET, but still not adequate to demonstrate the site of initiation of absences. An increase in rCBF in thalamus lasting for 5 s or less before spike-wave appeared on the EEG would not be detected. Neurophysiological data is limited but available evidence suggests that thalamic spike-wave may precede cortical activity by $\sim$ 1–2 s (Velasco et al, 1989). The blood flow response to a local alteration in neuronal activity occurs within 2 s. Thus any associated increase in thalamic blood flow is likely to occur only very briefly (at most <2 s) before the appearance of cortical spike wave activity.

BZ-GABA$_A$ RECEPTORS

Flumazenil, a specific benzodiazepine antagonist, binds reversibly to the majority of BZ-GABA$_A$ receptors (Olsen et al, 1990). Savic et al (1990) used [^{11}C] flumazenil and PET to quantify BZ-GABA$_A$ receptors in patients with generalised epilepsy who were receiving anti-epileptic medication but not valproate and found a 15% (NS) reduction in [^{11}C] flumazenil binding in cerebral cortex. The patients in this study, however, formed a heterogeneous group, many of whom had frequent generalised tonic-clonic seizures and the control values were obtained from 'non-focus' areas in patients with partial epilepsy.

In another study, PET was used to determine whether there was an abnormality of [^{11}C] flumazenil binding to BZ-GABA$_A$ receptors in patients with childhood and juvenile absence epilepsy (CAE/JAE), and to examine the effects of valproate on ^{11}C-flumazenil binding (Prevett et al, 1994c). The regional cerebral volume of distribution (V$_d$) of [^{11}C] flumazenil binding was used as a measure of specific receptor binding. V$_d$ was measured in 3 groups: 8 patients with CAE/JAE not treated with valproate, 8 patients with CAE/JAE treated with valproate and 8 age-matched normal subjects. There was no significant difference in [^{11}C] flumazenil V$_d$ between normal subjects and patients not on valproate but V$_d$ was on average 9% lower in patients on valproate than in normal subjects (p=0.03) and 9.5% lower than in the patients not on valproate (p=0.05). The normal subjects and the patients on valproate had a second [^{11}C] flumazenil scan performed in order to quantify receptor density and affinity. Receptor density (B$_{max}$) was on average 20% lower in the patients taking valproate (p=0.04) but there was no significant difference in receptor affinity (K$_d$).

In summary there was no evidence for a primary abnormality of the BZ-GABA$_A$ receptor in CAE/JAE but the data suggested that treatment with valproate was associated with a reduction in the number of BZ-GABA$_A$ receptors available for binding. There is no evidence from animal studies that valproate has a direct effect on the BZ-GABA$_A$ receptor and the mechanism of the reduction in the number of BZ-GABA$_A$ receptors is uncertain. One possibility is that valproate is acting pre-synaptically on GABA metabolism or release with secondary effects on the BZ-GABA$_A$ receptor.

Alternatively, postulated direct effects of valproate on neuronal membrane ion channels or on excitatory amino acid transmission may have secondary consequences on BZ-GABA$_A$ receptors. Although the mechanism is uncertain, the reduction in the number of BZ-GABA$_A$ receptors associated with valproate may be relevant to its action in CAE/JAE, perhaps by rendering the patient less sensitive to the spike-wave enhancing effects of GABA. Alternatively, reduced receptor availability may be a consequence of valproate treatment which is not directly related to its mode of action.

Five patients with CAE/JAE who were not taking valproate were studied with paired PET scans, performed at rest and with provocation of flurries of typical absences by voluntary hyperventilation (Prevett et al, 1993). Normalised regional cerebral time–activity curves from the resting and ictal scans were compared with each other and with computed simulations showing the effects of changes in cerebral blood flow and [^{11}C] flumazenil binding. No evidence was found for a change in [^{11}C] flumazenil binding at the time of absence seizures in any neocortical area or in the thalamus.

These studies do not support a primary abnormality of the BZ-GABA$_A$ receptor in idiopathic generalised epilepsy but do not exclude an abnormality of the GABA binding site. Currently there are no PET ligands suitable for the study of the GABA binding site of the GABA$_A$ receptor and an abnormality at this site or of coupling between the benzodiazepine and GABA binding sites remains a possibility. The results do, however, suggest that treatment with valproate is associated with a reduction in the number of BZ-GABA$_A$ receptors.

OPIATE RECEPTORS

In animal models, systemic administration of opiates tends to cause an increase in generalised spike-wave activity and absence seizures (Frey & Voits, 1991). This is in contrast to the anti-convulsant effects of opiates and endogenous opioids on generalised tonic-clonic seizures and suggests that an increase in endogenous opioid transmission may be involved in the generation of absence seizures.

Diprenorphine is a weak partial opiate receptor agonist with similar affinities for the three main receptor sub-types (μ, κ, and δ) and [^{11}C] diprenorphine has proved to be a useful PET ligand. There has been one inter-ictal PET study of regional cerebral [^{11}C] diprenorphine binding in patients with childhood and juvenile absence epilepsy (Prevett et al, 1994b). Eight patients and eight normal sujects had a single scan after a high specific activity injection of [^{11}C] diprenorphine. The cerebral volume of distribution (V_d) of [^{11}C] diprenorphine relative to plasma was used, on a pixel by pixel basis, as a measure of specific receptor binding. There were no significant differences in [^{11}C] diprenorphine V_d between patients and control subjects in any region studied, including cortex and thalamus, suggesting that there is no overall abnormality of opioid receptors in patients with childhood and juvenile absence epilepsy. Diprenorphine, however, labels μ, κ and δ receptor subtypes with similar affinity. In a group of patients with seizures of mesial temporal lobe origin [^{11}C] carfentanil binding to μ receptors was increased in lateral temporal cortex despite normal [^{11}C] diprenorphine binding. This finding was interpreted as reflecting a coincident decrease in the number of κ receptors available for binding (Mayberg et al, 1991). It is possible therefore that there is an imbalance of receptor subtypes in idiopathic generalised epilepsy and investigation with sub-type specific ligands is required to elucidate this.

A further study was carried out to determine whether there were any acute changes in cerebral opiate receptor occupancy at the time of absence seizures (Bartenstein et al, 1993). Five patients with idiopathic generalised epilepsy in whom hyperventilation reliably provoked serial absence seizures were studied with paired [^{11}C] diprenorphine PET scans. One scan was performed at rest and in the other absence seizures were precipitated by hyperventilation 30–40 min after injection of [^{11}C] diprenorphine. Absence seizures, with generalised spike-wave discharges on the EEG, occurred for 10–51% of the period of hyperventilation. Comparison of the inter-ictal and ictal normalised time-activity curves over 60–90 min showed increased tracer washout following the provocation of serial absences from association cortex (Fig. 11.2). There was no significant difference in tracer washout from thalamus or any other regions between the inter-ictal and ictal scans. There was no significant difference in tracer washout from association cortex in normal subjects who hyperventilated and patients studied inter-ictally, suggesting that the increase in tracer washout was associated with the occurrence of absence seizures and was not the result of the condition of epilepsy or of hyperventilation. The divergence of the ictal and inter-ictal time-activity curves appeared to follow the occurrence of serial absence seizures at 30–40 min and there was no evidence to suggest that this preceded the period of hyperventilation. The temporal resolution of the dynamic changes in diprenorphine binding was limited, however, and this precluded detailed analysis of the dynamic changes in diprenorphine binding from 30 to 40 min.

Computed simulation studies indicated that changes in CBF in relation to hyperventilation and typical absence seizures could not account for the changes observed. It was estimated that a 15–41% decrease in the specific tracer uptake rate constant in cortex would account for the observed increase in elimination. It was suggested that the most likely explanation of this finding was that endogenous opioids were released, which displaced bound [^{11}C] diprenorphine. While it is possible that endogenous opioid release may have been an epiphenomenon to the provocation of serial absence seizures, it was postulated that release of endogenous opioids has a role in the pathophysiology of absence seizures. There was no correlation between the number of absence seizures provoked and the extent of reduced diprenorphine retention in the association areas of the neocortex, suggest-

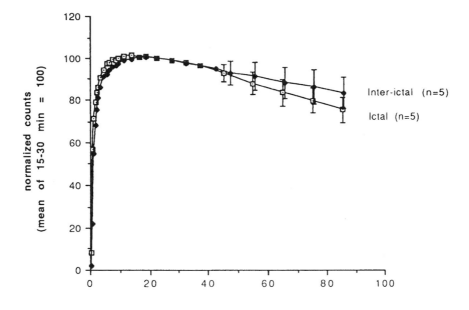

Fig. 11.2 Comparison of normalised inter-ictal and ictal [^{11}C] diprenorphine time-activity curves for association cortex showing more rapid tracer washout after induction of absence seizures at 30-40 min.

ing that opioid release may be one component of a multifactorial process. The limited temporal resolution of the study did not allow determination of whether opioid release preceded or followed the absence seizures, which occurred in flurries over the 10 min period of hyperventilation. Also, there was no evidence to suggest release of endogenous opioids in thalamus, suggesting that endogenous opioids may have an effect on thalamo-cortical circuits through association areas of cortex.

CONCLUSION

In vivo functional imaging studies allow the investigation of the anatomical and biochemical basis of typical absence seizures in humans. Functional imaging in typical absence seizures has to date been dominated by PET. These PET studies have produced data which indicate that the thalamus has a key role in the pathogenesis of absence seizures and that endogenous opioid transmission in association areas of cerebral cortex is also involved in the process. No evidence for a primary role for the BZ-GABA$_A$ receptor has been found. Limitations of temporal resolution may limit further use of PET in investigating the anatomy of absence seizures. Functional magnetic resonance imaging may offer an alternative.

The future role of PET lies in the investigation of mechanisms of neurotransmission. The development of ligands to study $GABA_B$ receptors and excitatory amino acid transmission will allow investigation of the role of these systems in vivo in the generation of typical absence seizures.

REFERENCES

Avoli M, Gloor P, Kostopoulos G, Gotman J 1983 An analysis of penicillin-induced generalised spike and wave discharges using simultaneous recordings of cortical and thalamic single neurons. Journal of Neurophysiology 50: 819–837

Bartenstein PA, Duncan JS, Prevett MC et al 1993 Investigation of the opioid system in absence seizures with positron emission tomography. Journal of Neurology, Neurosurgery, and Psychiatry 56: 1295–1302

Engel JJr, Lubens P, Kuhl DE, Phelps ME 1985 Local cerebral metabolic rate for glucose during petit mal absences. Annals of Neurology 17: 121–128

Frey HH, Voits M 1991 Effect of psychotropic agents on a model of absence epilepsy in rats. Neuropharmacology 30: 651–656

Leroy RF, Devous MD, Ajmani AK, Rao KK, Bonte FJ 1987 Regional cerebral blood flow determined by xenon 133 inhalation and SPECT scan among epileptics with primary generalised seizures. Neurology 37 (Suppl 1): 102

Mayberg HS, Sadzot B, Meltzer CC et al 1991 Quantification of mu and non-mu opiate receptors in temporal lobe epilepsy using positron emission tomography. Annals of Neurology 30: 3–11

Nehlig A, Vergnes M, Marescaux C, Boyet S 1993 Cerebral energy metabolism in rats with genetic absence epilepsy is not correlated with the pharmacological increase or suppression of spike-wave discharges. Brain Research 618: 1–8

Ochs RF, Gloor P, Tyler JL et al 1987 Effect of generalised spike-and-wave discharge on glucose metabolism measured by positron emission tomography. Annals of Neurology 21: 458–464

Olsen RW, McCabe RT, Wamsley JK 1990 $GABA_A$ receptor subtypes: autoradiographic comparison of GABA, benzodiazepine, and convulsant binding sites in rat central nervous system. Journal of Chemical Neuroanatomy 3: 59–76

Phelps ME, Mazziotta JC, Huang SC 1982 Study of cerebral function with positron computed tomography. Journal of Cerebral Blood Flow and Metabolism 2: 113–162

Prevett MC, Lammertsma AA, Brooks DJ, Fish DR, Duncan JS 1993 Investigation of benzodiazepine-$GABA_A$ receptor function during absence seizures using PET. Epilepsia 34 (Suppl 6): p126

Prevett MC, Duncan JS, Fish DR, Jones T, Brooks DJ 1994a Demonstration of thalamic activation during absence seizures using $H_2^{15}O$ positron emission tomography. Journal of Neurology, Neurosurgery, and Psychiatry 57: 245–246

Prevett MC, Cunningham VJ, Brooks DJ, Fish DR, Duncan JS 1994b Opiate receptors in idiopathic generalised epilepsy measured with ^{11}C-diprenorphine and PET. Epilepsy Research: in press

Prevett MC, Lammertsma AA, Brooks DJ et al 1994c Benzodiazepine-$GABA_A$ receptors in idiopathic generalised epilepsy measured with ^{11}C-flumazenil and PET. Epilepsia: in press

Raichle ME 1987 Circulatory and metabolic correlates of brain function in normal humans. In: Plum F (ed) Handbook of physiology: the nervous system. American Physiological Society Oxford University Press, New York, p643

Sakai F, Meyer JS, Naritomi H, Hsu MC 1978 Regional cerebral blood flow and EEG in patients with epilepsy. Archives of Neurology 35: 648–657

Savic I, Widén L, Thorell JO, Blomqvist G, Ericson K, Roland P 1990 Cortical benzodiazepine receptor binding in patients with generalised and partial epilepsy. Epilepsia 31: 724–730

Theodore WH, Brooks R, Sato S et al 1984 The role of positron emission tomography in the evaluation of seizure disorders. Annals of Neurology 15 (Suppl): 176–179

Velasco M, Velasco F, Velasco AL, Luján M, Vázquez del Mercado J 1989 Epileptiform EEG activities of the centromedian thalamic nuclei in patients with intractable partial motor, complex partial and generalised seizures. Epilepsia 30: 295–306

Vergnes M, Marescaux C 1992 Cortical and thalamic lesions in rats with genetic absence
   epilepsy. Journal of Neural Transmission 35 (Suppl): 71–83
Williams D 1953 A study of thalamic and cortical rhythms in petit mal. Brain 76: 50–69

DISCUSSION

Berkovic: I am puzzled about how to put together the human FDG data, the
human blood flow data and the Strasbourg data about exactly what is hap-
pening to blood flow and metabolism during absence attacks. The FDG
PET data reported by Engel suggest there is a two- to threefold increase in
glucose metabolism and I appreciate that the temporal resolution of glucose
studies is very long. Dr Prevett found a much smaller increase in CBF and
Professor Marescaux suggests that much of the increase may be a post-ictal
effect. I wonder if there is any way to put all of this together.

Prevett: I find it difficult. The larger increases reported by Engel were in
young children and all the other FDG studies in adults showed increases of
the order of 30%. The few blood flow studies that have been performed in
humans, other than those described today, showed a similar 30% increase in
CBF. Our study showed a global increase of about 15%, as well as a selective
focal increase in the thalamus. The temporal resolution probably accounts
for the FDG technique not being able to pick out specific structures. One
explanation as to why there should be no clear correlation between amount
of spike-wave and the blood flow or glucose metabolism is that we might be
observing mechanisms that are switching on or suppressing the spike-wave
activity but not active during its continuation.

Panayiotopoulos: What is the time resolution of your technique?

Prevett: Thirty seconds is probably the worst. There have been studies at
the Hammersmith using this technique which have detected cerebral activations associated with hand movements for periods as short as 5 s. Even so
that is a long time in electrophysiological terms.

Panayiotopoulos: Could the fact that usually people stop breathing during
absences, particularly if they hyperventilate, affect the data?

Prevett: We monitored end-tidal CO_2 throughout the studies. There was no
clear increase in the PCO_2 at the time of the absence seizures and it
remained constant during the period, so we felt that that was not a factor.

12. Clinical neurophysiology in humans

S. J. M. Smith

The 3 Hz spike wave discharge of a typical absence seizure was among the first electrographic seizure patterns to be recognised (Gibbs et al, 1936) using the electroencephalogram (EEG). Gibbs et al distinguished the 3 Hz spike wave pattern from the slow spike and wave abnormality seen in petit mal variant (later known as the Lennox–Gastaut syndrome).

EEG CHARACTERISTICS

The characteristic EEG accompaniment of a typical absence seizure is rhythmic bilaterally synchronous generalised spike wave (SW) activity, maximal over the frontal regions. The discharge has an abrupt start and end, arising from (and returning to) normal background activity. Although the frequency of the SW discharge is often described as 3 Hz, it may range between 3–4.5 Hz, slowing to 2–2.5 Hz towards the end of the discharge, particularly in longer-duration bursts. Weir (1965) proposed that the SW consisted of four components: an initial surface positive transient, of abrupt onset and duration 100–150 msec; two surface negative spikes, the first of low voltage and short duration (15 msec) with a centrotemporal maximum, and the second, the 'classical spike', of longer duration with a frontal maximum; and a final surface negative wave which emerges from the second spike. The first negative spike was seen in only 44% of patients, but occurred in >90% of bursts lasting 5 s or longer. A prolonged surface negative direct current potential change (paroxysmal DC shift) accompanies the SW burst, with a similar frontal field to the negative wave (Chatrian et al, 1968). The DC shift begins at the onset of the SW burst and reaches maximum voltage after 1–5 s.

The apparent symmetry and synchrony of the bursts may be an anomaly of the temporal resolution of the written EEG tracing. Electro-encephalographers have long recognised that the SW discharge can arise randomly in either hemisphere, preceding the discharge in the other hemisphere by a few msec. Measurement of small time differences (STD) between hemispheres (Gotman, 1983) shows STD of 5 msec or less in idiopathic generalised epilepsy, in contrast to seizures with lateralised epileptogenicity, where STD are usually 5–30 msec. However, there may be overlap between idiopathic and secondary generalised epilepsies (Fig. 12.1) (Allen et al, 1991). Rapid

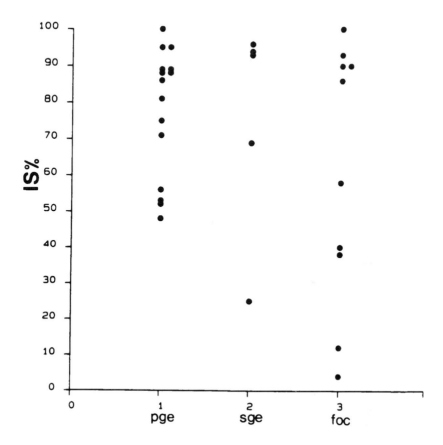

Fig. 12.1 Inter-hemispheric synchrony (IS%; proportion of inter-hemispheric time difference measurements of ≤5 msec) in patients with idiopathic generalised epilepsy (IGE), secondary generalised epilepsy (SGE) and focal seizure disorders. Each point refers to an individual patient.

synchronisation is presumed to occur through the major inter-hemispheric commissural pathways, the corpus callosum and anterior commissure.

The amplitude, morphology and duration of the SW discharge can vary considerably among individual patients and between bursts in the same patient. The voltage of the spikes may reach 600 µV, with the highest amplitude at the start of the discharge. Ictal discharges last a few s, but very brief bursts (1 s or less) also occur. These short-duration SW bursts tend to be frontal rather than generalised.

In analysis of the cerebral electrical fields of the SW discharge during absence seizures, Rodin & Onchetta (1987) found that, although the maximum negativity and positivity of individual complexes was mainly frontal and consistent, the way the maxima were reached was highly variable, with different origins and spread of fields. Spread could be discontinuous, with appearance and disappearance of preliminary peaks over posterior and frontal head regions, suggesting that several intra-cortical generators could contribute to the formation of the SW complex.

The topographic distribution of the SW discharge may have prognostic significance. Dondey (1983) analysed the transverse patterns of paroxysmal bursts and found two types: a lateral distribution (13 of 46 patients), with two symmetrical maxima 7.5 cm from the midline and a medial distribution (30 of 46 cases), with one midline maximum. Three patients showed a mixed pattern. The lateral pattern was typically associated with simple absence seizures and early remission, whereas patients with the medial distribution had mixed seizure types (absences, generalised tonic clonic seizures and myoclonus) without remission.

ASSOCIATED EEG FINDINGS

Additional features may be seen in the EEGs of patients with typical absences. Background rhythms are characteristically normal. Although Gibbs & Gibbs (1952) noted marked slowing in 1% of cases, slow background activity is much more likely to indicate atypical absence seizures. In addition to the variable lateralised onset of SW bursts, focal spikes may be seen, rarely, and their occurrence should lead to reassessment of the diagnosis. In 137 cases of absence epilepsy, Gibbs & Gibbs (1952) found frontal spikes in 1.4%, occipital spikes in 2.2% and multiple spikes in 0.7%, with some increase in focal spiking during sleep. Runs of rhythmical 2.5–3 Hz slow waves, often with a posterior distribution (occipital intermittent rhythmic delta, OIRDA) are seen in 15% of cases (Fig. 12.2). Holmes et al (1987) found OIRDA only in typical absences, not in patients with atypical absences. Children with OIRDA tend to have, in addition to classical SW,

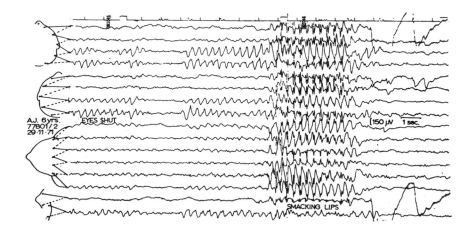

Fig. 12.2 Bilateral occipital intermittent rhythmical delta (OIRDA) preceding a clinical absence seizure with 3 per s generalised spike wave.

pure absence epilepsy and are unlikely to develop generalised tonic-clonic seizures (Loiseau et al, 1983).

BIOLOGICAL FACTORS

The activation of SW discharge with hyperventilation is one of the best-known features of typical absences, so much so that if hyperventilation does not induce SW or a clinical seizure, some would consider the diagnosis to be virtually excluded. Photic stimulation induces SW bursts in 20% of cases (Wolf & Gooses, 1986). The state of alertness and sleep have marked effects on the SW bursts. Greater alertness and eye opening abolish discharges. In non-REM sleep, there is an increased number of bursts of shorter duration, with a greater irregularity of the discharge, sometimes with multiple spikes. In REM sleep, the morphology of the discharges is similar to that in the waking state, with a slightly greater incidence of bursts. There may be marked diurnal variation in the occurrence of SW bursts (Fig. 12.3), which can have implications for the timing of anti-epileptic drug administration.

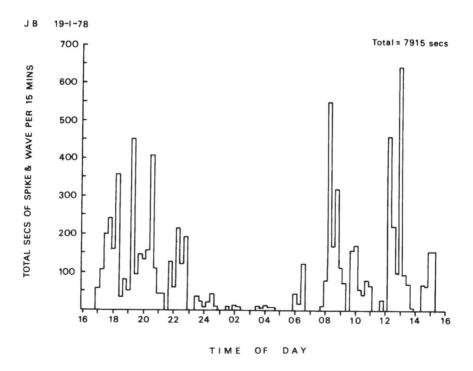

Fig. 12.3 Diurnal variation in spike wave discharge in 14-year-old girl with typical absences treated with sodium valproate and ethosuximide.

PATHOPHYSIOLOGICAL AND CLINICAL CORRELATIONS

The underlying pathophysiological mechanisms of bilaterally synchronous generalised spike wave discharge have long been debated. Although Gibbs et al (1936) originally mooted a diffuse cortical disturbance, the centrencephalic theory of Penfield & Jasper (1947) achieved greater prominence. It was believed that deep brainstem and diencephalic structures entrained cortical regions in generation of the SW discharge. However, studies in animal models of epilepsy, particularly feline generalised penicillin epilepsy, and in man, indicate that the cortex is the primary site of abnormality (see Ch. 10).

There is clinical and experimental evidence that the spike component of the SW complex is excitatory and the slow wave inhibitory. Electro-clinical correlations from video-EEG recordings have shown that the myoclonic components of absence seizures occur synchronously with the second spike of the discharge. Phasic loss of tone in neck or arm muscles may be observed with each slow wave. Time locking of magnetic cortical stimulation to the wave component shows a significant reduction in the size of the motor evoked potential (MEP), suggesting reduced cortical excitability (Gianelli et al 1994), although no enhancement of amplitude of the MEP was seen when the stimuli were delivered during the spike phase of the discharge.

The duration of the SW discharge may affect seizure semiology. Automatisms tend to occur with bursts of longer duration, appearing in approximately 50% of seizures of >6 s duration and 90% of absences lasting 12 s or longer (Penry et al, 1975). There is no variation in the morphology of the SW with variable clinical phenomena. If there is slowing of the frequency during the burst, the clinical seizure is likely to be of longer duration (Holmes et al, 1987), perhaps reflecting less effective inhibition.

The clinical significance of very brief SW bursts is uncertain. Gibbs & Gibbs (1952) noted 'larval' discharges of duration 1 s or less in 61% of cases, which were considered to be sub-clinical episodes. However, although it may be difficult to discern clinical change during brief SW bursts, cognitive testing of reaction time and performance has shown that transient cognitive impairment occurs when a stimulus is presented during the burst, including SW paroxysms of short duration (Fig. 12.4) (Aarts et al, 1984; Ch. 14). Thus it is arguable that any of the EEG abnormality in idiopathic generalised epilepsies is truly sub-clinical.

DIFFERENTIAL DIAGNOSIS

The EEG in atypical absences shows slow (2–2.5 Hz) irregular spike wave; there may be focal or multifocal inter-ictal spikes and the background activities are usually abnormal, with widespread slow activity. Although this combination of electrographic features is unlikely to be confused with those of typical absences, there may be a continuum between typical and atypical absences. Holmes et al (1987) found no single EEG or clinical feature which allowed accurate distinction between these two syndromes.

Bifrontal spike wave discharges or paroxysmal bursts occur in frontal lobe epilepsies, particularly those arising from mesial frontal foci. Electrical stimulation of the mesial frontal structures may also evoke bilaterally synchronous SW discharge. The variable clinical seizure patterns of frontal lobe epilepsy, which include brief complex partial seizures or absences, may make distinction from typical absences difficult. However, the EEG in mesial frontal epilepsy shows only slight similarities with that of typical absences. There may be SW or slow activity, usually less than 3 Hz, irregular and clearly frontal rather than generalised with frontal predominance.

Three Hz SW, electrographically indistinguishable from that seen in idiopathic generalised epilepsy, has been reported in a patient with cortical dysplasia whose MRI showed subependymal heterotopia (Ali et al, 1994).

SPECIFIC SYNDROMES

Childhood absence epilepsy

The electrographic characteristics of typical seizures in childhood absence epilepsy (CAE) have been described above. Panayiotopoulos et al (1989) found the mean duration of ictal paroxysms in CAE to be 12.4 s, with the average frequency at the start of the burst being 3.4 Hz and 2.5 Hz in the terminal phase. When absence seizures persist into adulthood, the ictal electrographic pattern remains similar to that seen in childhood, with no deterioration in background; the classical SW discharge was maintained in 84% of cases (Gastaut et al, 1986).

Juvenile absence epilepsy

Juvenile absence epilepsy has a later age of onset than CAE and there are both similarities and differences of the EEG features in comparison with CAE. Spikes may be multiple and the relationship between the spike and wave of the complex is less fixed than in CAE (Panayiotopoulos et al, 1989). Mean duration of SW paroxysms is longer (16 s), but the frequency of the SW slows during the paroxysm in the same way. Hyperventilation induces SW and clinical seizures, but photo-sensitivity is less common in JAE: 7.5% compared with 18–20% in CAE (Wolf, 1985).

Juvenile myoclonic epilepsy with absences

Multiple spikes and slow waves are the characteristic feature of juvenile myoclonic epilepsy (JME) with absences. Up to 8 spikes per complex may be seen, with considerable variation in amplitude and number within SW bursts. The polyspikes may precede or be superimposed on the slow wave

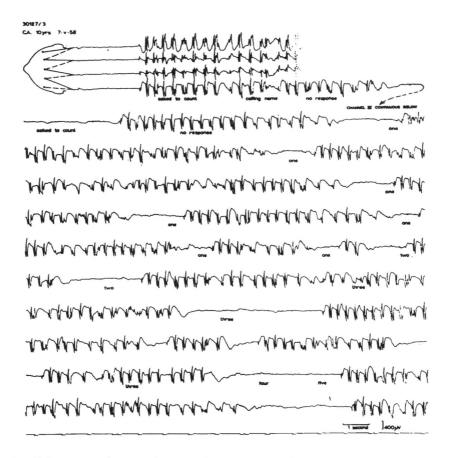

Fig. 12.4 Interrupted sequential counting during an episode of repeated absence seizures; some bursts show fragmentation or slowing in frequency of the spike wave discharge, during which counting aloud continues.

(Panayiotopoulos et al, 1989). Mean duration of bursts is shorter than in CAE or JAE (6.6 s), but slowing of frequency of the discharge in the terminal phase of the burst occurs in JME as in the other absence syndromes. Fragmentation of the SW complexes may occur in older patients.

Myoclonic absence epilepsy

The SW complexes are similar to those of JME, although variation in the amplitude of the polyspikes within bursts does not occur and fragmentation is not seen in older children.

Eyelid myoclonia with typical absences

This recently described syndrome (Appleton et al, 1993) comprises absence seizures and eyelid myoclonia associated with high-amplitude SW or polyspike discharges. The discharges may be induced by eye closure and disappear in darkness. Photo-sensitivity occurs, with generalised SW activity evoked by a wide range of flash frequency.

Perioral myoclonus with absences

The ictal EEG of this absence syndrome with rhythmical myoclonic jerking of perioral muscles shows generalised short irregular spikes, or, more often, polyspike and wave discharges at 3 Hz (Panayiotopoulos et al, 1994). Photo-sensitivity does not occur.

ABSENCE STATUS

Although non-convulsive status is more common in atypical absence epilepsy, absence status may occur in children with typical absences (3% of cases, Gibbs & Gibbs, 1952). Absence status may also present de novo in middle-aged or elderly patients without a previous history of epilepsy, often

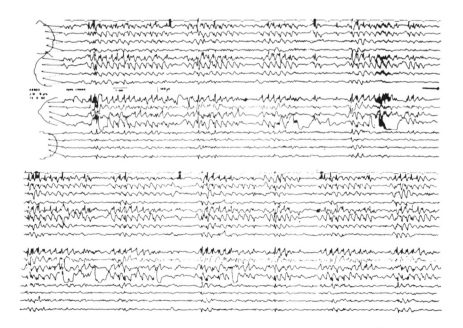

Fig. 12.5 Absence status in a 9-year-old boy.

resulting from acute drug withdrawal or metabolic disturbances (see Ch. 31). In typical absence status, the EEG shows repeated or continuous SW bursts, with similar characteristics to those of the ictal discharge during a typical absence, although the SW may be less regular (Fig. 12.5). The electrographic features of de novo absence status of late onset are highly variable, with SW, polyspike and wave, repetitive spikes or generalised irregular slow activity (Thomas et al, 1992).

CONCLUSIONS

The 3 Hz SW discharge of typical absences is the most characteristic of all EEG phenomena. Differences exist between the electrographic features of absence syndromes in idiopathic generalised epilepsy, but there is overlap as well, both between the individual syndromes and the ictal patterns of typical and atypical absences. The differences are of value for precise diagnosis, prognosis and treatment. The variations in the electrographic patterns of absence syndromes may be a reflection of the balance between excitatory and inhibitory mechanisms, resulting perhaps from differential expression of polygenes.

REFERENCES

Aarts JHP, Binnie CD, Smit AM, Wilkins AJ 1984 Selective cognitive impairment during focal and generalised epileptiform activity. Brain 107: 293–308
Ali R, Fish DR, Sisodiya S, Alsanjari N, Stevens JM, Shorvon SD 1994 Subependymal heterotopia: a distinct neuronal migration disorder associated with epilepsy. J Neurol Neurosurg Psychiatry: in press
Allen PJ, Smith SJM, Scott CA 1991 Measurement of interhemispheric time differences in generalised spike and wave. Electroenceph Clin Neurophysiol 82: 81–84
Appleton RE, Panayiotopolous CP, Acomb BA, Beirne M 1993 Eyelid myoclonia with typical absences: an epilepsy syndrome. J Neurol Neurosurg Psychiatry 56: 1312–1316
Chatrian GE, Somasunduram M, Tassinnari CA 1968 DC changes recorded transcranially during 'typical' 3 per second spike and wave discharges in man. Epilepsia 9: 185–209
Dondey M 1983 Transverse topographical analysis of petit mal discharges: diagnostical and pathogenic implications. Electroenceph Clin Neurophysiol 55: 361–371
Gastaut H, Zifkind BG, Mariani E, Puig JS 1986 The long term course of primary generalised epilepsy with persisting absences. Neurology 36: 1021–1028
Gianelli M, Cantello R, Civardi C, Naldi P, Bettuci D, Pia Sciavella M, Mutani R 1994 Idiopathic generalised epilepsy: magnetic stimulation of motor cortex time-locked and unlocked to 3 Hz spike and wave discharges. Epilepsia 35: 53–60
Gibbs FA, Davis H, Lennox WG 1936 The EEG in epilepsy and in conditions of impaired consciousness. Arch Neurol and Psychiatry 34: 1133–1148
Gibbs FA, Gibbs EL 1952 Petit mal. In: Gibbs FA, Gibbs EL (eds) Atlas of electroencephalography Vol 2. Addison-Wesley Press, Cambridge, Mass, pp55–65
Gotman J 1983 Measurement of small time differences between EEG channels: method and application to epileptic seizure propagation. Electroenceph Clin Neurophysiol 56: 501–514
Holmes GL, Mckeever M, Adamson M 1987 Absence seizures in children: clinical and electrographic features. Ann Neurol 21: 268–273
Loiseau P, Pestre M, Dartigues JF, Commenges D, Barberger-Gateau C, Cohadon S 1983 Long term prognosis in two forms of childhood epilepsy: Typical absence seizures and epilepsy with rolandic (centrotemporal) EEG foci. Ann Neurol 13: 642–648
Panayiotopoulos CP, Obeid T, Waheed G 1989 Differentiation of typical absence seizures in epileptic syndromes. Brain 112: 1039–1056

Panayiotopoulos CP, Ferrie CD, Giannakodimos SE, Robinson RO 1994 Perioral myoclonia with absences: a new syndrome. In: Wolf P (ed) Epileptic seizures and syndromes. John Libbey, London (in press)

Penfield W, Jasper H 1947 Highest level seizures. Assoc Res Nerv Ment Dis 26: 252–271

Penry JK, Porter RJ, Dreifuss FE 1975 Automatisms associated with the absence of "petit mal" epilepsy. Arch Neurol 21: 142–149

Rodin E, Ochetta O 1987 Cerebral electrical fields during petit mal absences. Electronceph Clin Neurophysiol 66: 457–466

Thomas P, Beaumanoir A, Genton P, Dolisi C, Chatel M 1992 'De novo' absence status of late onset: report of 11 cases. Neurology 42: 104–110

Weir B 1965 The morphology of the spike wave complex. Electroenceph Clin Neurophysiol 19: 284–290

Wolf P 1985 Juvenile absence epilepsy. In: Roger J, Dravet C, Bureau M, Dreifuss FE, Wolf P (eds) Epileptic syndromes in infancy, childhood and adolescence. John Libbey, London, pp242–246

Wolf P, Gooses R 1986 Relation of photosensitivity to epileptic syndromes. J Neurol Neurosurg Psychiatry 49: 1386–1391.

DISCUSSION

Panayiotopoulos: The differentiation between typical and atypical absences has often been based on the frequency of the first second of the generalised spike and slow wave discharge. If it was <2.5 Hz the patient was classified as atypical and >2.5 Hz would be classified at typical. This is an arbitrary criterion. The first second is also the most unreliable factor in these discharges. In the same patient the frequency of the discharge may be 2.5 Hz, 2.0 Hz or 5.0 Hz.

Smith: The difficulty is knowing what criteria can be used to separate them. The clinical criteria are not reliable either, and one needs to use a combination.

Marescaux: What percentage of patients with typical absence epilepsy are photo-sensitive? We find that it is very rare and have almost never seen patients with childhood absence epilepsy and a good prognosis who have photo-sensitivity.

Smith: In our experience 10 or 20% may be photo-sensitive.

Tassinari: By typical absence we mean the pattern of the absence, not of the spike and wave discharge. We are not able to define as typical a single spike and wave but the pattern of typical absences is identifiable.

Genton: What is the percentage, in Dr Smith's population of typical absences, of patients with focal findings, excluding delta waves? When we reviewed recent cases in our own population, about 3% had rolandic spikes, which is not more than the general population.

Smith: We have seen focal spikes in up to 10% of children with typical absences. I think if they have benign rolandic spikes that may be an associated finding, not related to the absence epilepsy per se.

13. Transcranial magnetic stimulation in idiopathic generalised epilepsies

Samuel F. Berkovic   David C. Reutens
Richard A. L. Macdonell

CORTICAL HYPER-EXCITABILITY IN GENERALISED EPILEPSIES

There is persuasive animal experimental data that a permanent state of diffuse cortical hyper-excitability is present in certain animal models of idiopathic generalised epilepsy. Unlike the well-recognised spike-and-wave discharges, which are evanescent, such cortical hyper-excitability is persistent. It probably relates to the fundamental neurophysiological deficit in generalised epilepsies that allows the episodic ictal clinical and electroencephalographic (EEG) changes to appear (see Ch. 10).

There is no direct evidence for persistent cortical hyper-excitability in human idiopathic generalised epilepsies. Methods to test for such an abnormality are few. Routine scalp EEG is normal in patients with idiopathic generalised epilepsy, except for sub-clinical and clinical ictal discharges and the occurrence of intermittent rhythmic delta activity with an occipital or frontal predominance in certain patients (see Ch. 12). However, EEG does not reveal evidence of a stable ongoing disturbance of physiological function. Evoked potentials are altered during spike-and-wave discharges (see Ch. 14), but inter-ictal evoked potential studies have not shown evidence of persistent hyper-excitability. Inter-ictal studies using visual evoked potentials have shown some enlargement of visually evoked potentials (VEPs) in patients with photo-sensitivity (Broughton et al, 1989) but the interpretation of this uncertain. No consistent findings have been reported in patients using somatosensory evoked potentials or brainstem auditory evoked potentials. In patients with progressive myoclonus epilepsies, however, which perhaps represent a more extreme state of cortical hyper-excitability, giant somatosensory evoked potentials are often seen (Shibasaki et al, 1985).

TRANSCRANIAL MAGNETIC STIMULATION

Transcranial magnetic stimulation (TMS), first described by Barker et al (1985), permits painless stimulation of the cerebral cortex. A brief time-varying magnetic field is generated over the scalp, which induces an electrical field in the cerebral cortex. Cortical neurons, particularly cortico-cortical interneurons are depolarised, exciting descending motor pathways. As a result of spatial and temporal summation of the descending impulses at the spinal motor neurons an evoked motor response is produced in limb muscles which can be easily recorded in small muscles of the hand. Increased cortical excitability could be reflected by an enlarged motor response, decreased latency or decreased central conduction time, reflecting more rapid recruitment of cortical neurons. It could be manifested also by a decreased threshold to stimulation. Like all neurophysiological measures there is considerable variability in these parameters and determination of abnormalities therefore needs a large control group and standardisation of condit-ions in subjects and controls.

TMS: EARLY STUDIES IN EPILEPSY

Safety

TMS was initially used to study disorders affecting central motor conduction. Studies in the epilepsies were first reported by Michelucci et al (1989). There was initial concern that TMS could activate epileptic seizures. There have been some isolated reports of seizures occurring in proximity to TMS, usually in patients with structural brain lesions (Homberg & Netz, 1989; Hufnagel et al, 1990a) but larger studies and increasing experience have shown that TMS is safe and does not activate seizures in the vast majority of patients with epilepsy (Tassinari et al, 1990; Dhuna et al, 1991; Gates et al, 1992; Michelucci & Tassinari, 1992).

TMS in partial epilepsies

Hufnagel et al (1990a) reported that TMS activated inter-ictal discharges in 12/13 patients with sub-dural electrodes. Subsequent work using scalp and intra-cranial electrodes has failed to replicate this finding, and interest in the role of TMS for localisation of seizure foci has waned (Dhuna et al, 1991; Schuler et al, 1991; Jennum et al, 1994). Anti-epileptic drugs have been shown consistently to increase the threshold for stimulation and, in some studies, there has also been prolongation of the peripheral latency of the motor evoked response (Hufnagel et al, 1990b; Michelucci & Tassinari, 1992).

TMS in generalised epilepsies

In early studies no abnormalities were noted in patients with treated generalised epilepsies during the inter-ictal state (Michelucci et al, 1989). Two groups have attempted to study ictal changes during spike-and-wave discharges. Michelucci & Tassinari (1992) and Tassinari et al (1993) reported no significant change in latency or amplitude of the motor evoked potential (MEP) when stimulation occurred during spike-and-wave discharges compared with the inter-ictal state. More recently, Gianelli et al (1994) reported a consistent reduction of the MEP when it was induced during the wave portion of generalised spike and wave discharges, but variable changes when it was time-locked to the spike.

We attempted to take a more critical look at TMS in the inter-ictal state of idiopathic generalised epilepsies by avoiding the confounding effects of anti-epileptic drugs, minimising the variability in measurements by extensive studies in controls and by excluding the potential effect of alterations of segmental excitability by measuring F wave and H reflex parameters. We searched for evidence of persistent cortical hyper-excitability in human generalised epilepsies. Detection of this would not only be of theoretical interest but also could potentially provide a stable inter-ictal neurophysiological marker for idiopathic generalised epilepsy.

SUBJECTS AND METHODS

We selected adolescent and adult patients with idiopathic generalised epilepsy, all of whom had documented spike and wave discharges on inter-ictal EEG. There were 20 untreated patients (mean age 20 years, range 11–41). These patients had various combinations of tonic-clonic (17), myoclonic (10) and absence (12) seizures. In addition, there were 36 patients with treated idiopathic generalised epilepsy (mean age 27 years, range 40–45) who suffered with tonic clonic (34), myoclonic (17) and absence (24) seizures. The majority (30) of these cases were on sodium valproate. There were 89 neurologically normal controls (mean age 28 years, range 12–55).

TMS was performed using a Magstim 200 with a circular coil and a maximum flux density of 2.0 tesla. Motor evoked potentials (MEP) were recorded from the abductor digiti minimi of the dominant hand. Complete relaxation was ensured by monitoring real time surface EMG. The maximum output of the stimulator was designated at 100% and threshold was determined by progressive 5% increments in intensity. Threshold was defined as the lowest intensity where at least three out of five MEPs were recorded with an amplitude of 100 μvolts (peak to peak) or more. Peripheral latencies were measured by cervical stimulation (Reutens, 1992; Reutens et al, 1993a).

RESULTS

Onset latency, central conduction time and amplitude

There was no significant difference in onset latency and amplitude of the evoked motor potential in untreated patients compared to controls (Table 13.1). However, in treated patients there was slight but significant prolongation of the latency. Central conduction time was longer in treated patients, but this result was not significant at the $p < 0.05$ level (Reutens, 1992). It is likely that these effects relate to the anti-epileptic drugs and these observations are consistent with reports in focal epilepsies (Hufnagel et al, 1990b; Michelucci & Tassinari, 1992). These measures, therefore, did not reveal any evidence of increased excitability in the idiopathic generalised epilepsies.

Table 13.1 Motor evoked potential parameters in idiopathic generalised epilepsies (IGE)

	Onset latency (ms; mean ± 95% CI)	Central Conduction (ms; mean ± 95% CI)	Amplitude (mV; median)
Untreated IGE	21.7 ± 0.7	8.9 ± 0.7	0.22
Controls	22.1 ± 0.3	8.9 ± 0.3	0.23
Treated IGE	22.9 ± 0.7*	9.5 ± 0.4	0.17

* Onset latency was greater in treated IGE patients compared to the other two groups ($p<0.05$, ANOVA with multiple pairwise comparisons).

Threshold intensities

Threshold intensities in untreated patients were significantly less than in controls; chronically treated patients had thresholds that were significantly higher than controls (Fig. 13.1). The effect of anti-epileptic drugs was further explored by retesting untreated subjects after they had been commenced on sodium valproate. There was a significant increase in their threshold, whereas retesting normal subjects revealed no change (Fig. 13.2). It was of interest that the mean threshold in the newly treated patients was similar to the control values and did not reach the high levels seen in the more chronically treated subjects.

In treated patients there was a weak correlation between the threshold and the plasma level of sodium valproate suggesting that it does have a direct effect on altering threshold intensity (Fig. 13.3). We studied the relationship between threshold and the degree of control in treated subjects, but no definite relationship emerged. This may have been due to the small numbers of poorly controlled subjects and the confounding effects of different doses and levels of anti-epileptic agents.

Sub-groups of idiopathic generalised epilepsy

Analysis of threshold in untreated adolescent and adult patients according to clinical sub-group revealed some apparent differences but these were not statistically significant, possibly due to small numbers (Table 13.2). Patients with myoclonic seizures (juvenile myoclonic epilepsy) had lower thresholds than those with absence seizures (juvenile absence epilepsy), whereas those with both seizure types had intermediate threshold values. We did not

Threshold Intensity (%)

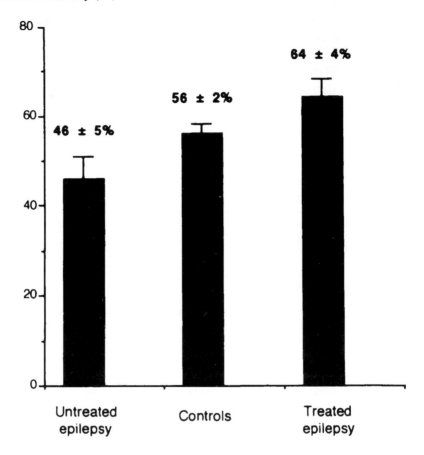

Fig. 13.1 Mean threshold intensities in control subjects and patients with idiopathic generalised epilepsy. The error bars indicate 95% confidence intervals for the mean. For all pairwise comparisons, $p < 0.01$ (ANOVA with multiple pairwise comparisons using Student–Newman–Keuls test). From Reutens et al (1993a) with permission.

Table 13.2 Threshold intensities in clinical sub-groups of untreated patients with idiopathic generalised epilepsies

Clinical Subgroup	Threshold (% of maximum; mean ± 95% CI)
Myoclonus (n=6)	41 ± 7%
Myoclonus & absence (n=4)	44 ± 9%
Absence (n=8)	50 ± 14%
Controls (n=89)	56 ± 2%

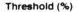

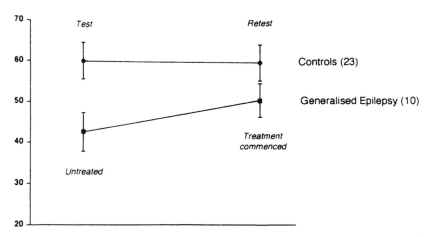

Fig. 13.2 Threshold intensity increased significantly in untreated patients with idiopathic generalised epilepsy after commencement of treatment (p< 0.01; paired t test). This was not a practice effect as threshold did not alter after retesting control subjects (p>0.05; paired t test). From Reutens et al (1993a) with permission.

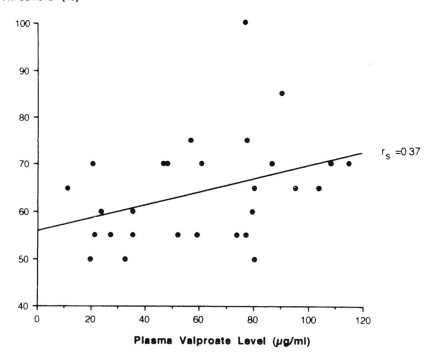

Fig. 13.3 Correlation between threshold intensity and plasma valproate level in chronically treated patients. From Reutens et al (1993a) with permission.

study subjects with untreated childhood absence epilepsy due to technical difficulties in performing TMS in young children and because thresholds are higher in normal children.

Segmental excitability

As reduced threshold could reflect increased excitability at cortical or segmental (spinal) levels, measures of segmental excitability were performed using the F wave and H reflexes. In control subjects there was no correlation between threshold measurements and measurements of segmental excitability (H_{max}/M_{max}; F_{mean}/M_{max} and F_{max}/M_{max}). Similarly, there was no significant difference in these measurements in the treated and untreated patients compared to control values (Reutens, 1992). These studies strongly suggest that the alterations in threshold observed were not due to spinal mechanisms but rather to alterations in supra-segmental and, presumably, cortical excitability.

DISCUSSION

The differences we observed in TMS threshold in untreated patients and controls were relatively subtle but nonetheless reproducible. We initially reported the reduction in threshold in a series of 10 untreated patients (Reutens & Berkovic, 1992) and this was subsequently confirmed in the total series of 20 patients (Reutens et al, 1993a). The lack of change in segmental excitability is consistent with the interpretation that the reduced threshold indicates increased cortical excitability, as is observed in animal models of idiopathic generalised epilepsy.

While we were able to show group differences in our patients the sensitivity and specificity of these findings do not appear sufficient to allow TMS to become a routine diagnostic test. Using a threshold of 45% or less we found a sensitivity of 0.75 and specificity of 0.79 (Reutens et al, 1993a). Treatment with anti-epileptic drugs reversed the lowered threshold in newly diagnosed patients and was even higher in chronically treated subjects. It remains to be determined if rising threshold can be used to predict therapeutic response.

There was a non-significant trend for lower thresholds in patients with myoclonus compared to those with absence (Table 13.2). It has been observed experimentally in the monkey that when epileptogenic lesions are made in the cortex, lesions in the pre-central areas evoke myoclonus, whereas premotor lesions cause absence-like seizures (Marcus et al, 1968). If this applies in man, it may be that TMS is more sensitive to the increased excitability in myoclonic patients because we are examining the motor areas.

Previous studies of TMS in generalised epilepsies have concerned treated patients and the differences described here had not been appreciated. Recently Gianelli et al (1994) described a small series of cases with absence seizures with findings differing from ours. In eight untreated patients with absence epilepsy they found a slightly higher mean threshold compared to their controls. Unfortunately they only had ten control subjects and there was considerable variability in their measurements in comparing right and left hemisphere thresholds. The conflicting results between their study and ours may relate to methodological differences, small numbers and inclusion of cases with very frequent epileptiform discharges in the Gianelli study, and our observation that threshold differences between control subjects and absence patients may be less than those between controls and patients with myoclonus. Further studies with larger groups of absence patients will be needed to resolve this issue.

FUTURE STUDIES

More sophisticated measurements of cortical excitability, such as analysis of silent periods and generation of excitability curves, may improve separation of measurements between controls and patients and between patients with different sub-syndromes of idiopathic generalised epilepsy. Studies with larger patient groups might be used to see whether change in TMS threshold has a relationship to therapeutic response.

Studies of the symptomatic generalised epilepsies have only just begun. We reported evidence for an exaggerated effect of afferent input on motor cortical excitability in patients with progressive myoclonus epilepsy (Reutens et al, 1993b), but there has been no work on patients with slow spike-and-wave discharges. Further studies of the technically difficult issue of examining ictal discharges may also shed light on the differences between the ictal and inter-ictal states in patients with a variety of forms of generalised epilepsy.

REFERENCES

Barker AT, Jalinous R, Freeston IL 1985 Non-invasive magnetic stimulation of human motor cortex. Lancet 1: 1106–107
Broughton R, Meier-Ewert KH, Ebe M 1969 Evoked visual, somatosensory and retinal potentials in photosensitive epilepsy. Electroencephalography and Clinical Neurophysiology 27: 373–386
Dhuna A, Gates JR, Pascual-Leone A 1991 Transcranial magnetic stimulation in patients with epilepsy. Neurology 41: 1067–1071
Gates JR, Dhuna A, Pascual-Leone A 1992 Lack of pathological changes in human temporal lobes after transcranial magnetic stimulation. Epilepsia 33: 504–508
Gianelli M, Cantello R, Civardi C, Naldi P, Bettuci D, Schiavella MP, Mutani R 1994 Idiopathic generalised epilepsy: magnetic stimulation of motor cortex time-locked and unlocked to 3-Hz spike-and-wave discharges. Epilepsia 35: 53–60
Homberg V, Netz J 1989 Generalised seizures induced by transcranial magnetic stimulation of motor cortex. Lancet 2: 1223
Hufnagel A, Elger CE, Durwen HF, Böker DK, Entzian W 1990a Activation of the epileptic focus by transcranial magnetic stimulation of the human brain. Annals of Neurology 27: 49–60
Hufnagel A, Elger CE, Marx W, Ising A 1990b Magnetic motor evoked potentials in epilepsy: effect of the disease and of anticonvulsant medication. Annals of Neurology 28: 680–686

Jennum P, Winkel H, Fuglsang-Frederiksen A, Dam M 1994 EEG changes following repetitive transcranial magnetic stimulation in patients with temporal lobe epilepsy. Epilepsy Research 18: 167–173

Marcus EM, Watson CW, Simon SA 1968 An experimental model of some varieties of petit mal epilepsy. Epilepsia 9: 233–248

Michelucci R, Rubboli G, Plasmati R, Salvi F, Forti A, Tassinari CA 1989 Trancranial magnetic stimulation of the cerebral cortex in epilepsy. Neurology 39 (Suppl. 1): 414

Michelucci R, Tassinari CA 1992 Clinical applications of magnetic transcranial stimulation in epileptic patients. In: Lissens MA (ed) Clinical applications of magnetic transcranial stimulation. Uitgeverij Peeters, Leuven, p 219–226

Reutens DC 1992 Aspects of the nosology and pathophysiology of the idiopathic generalised epilepsies of adolescence. Unpublished MD thesis, University of Melbourne

Reutens DC, Berkovic SF 1992 Increased cortical excitability in generalised epilepsy demonstrated with transcranial magnetic stimulation. Lancet 339: 362–363

Reutens DC, Berkovic SF, Macdonell RAL, Bladin PF 1993a Magnetic stimulation of the brain in generalised epilepsy: reversal of cortical hyperexcitability by anticonvulsants. Annals of Neurology 34: 351–355

Reutens DC, Puce A, Berkovic SF 1993b Cortical hyperexcitability in progressive myoclonus epilepsy: a study with transcranial magnetic stimulation. Neurology 43: 186–192

Schuler D, Claus D, Neubauer V, Stefan H 1991 Transcranial magnetic stimulation: not a useful tool to reduce monitoring time in preoperative evaluation of epilepsies. Epilepsia 32 (Suppl. 1): 117–118

Shibasaki H, Yamashita Y, Neshige R, Tobimatsu S, Fukui R 1985 Pathogenesis of giant somatosensory evoked potentials in progressive myoclonic epilepsy. Brain 108: 225–240

Tassinari CA, Michelucci R, Forti A et al 1990 Transcranial magnetic stimulation in epileptic patients: usefulness and safety. Neurology 40: 1132–1133

Tassinari CA, Valzania F, Santangelo M et al 1993 Transcranial magnetic stimulation in epilepsy: effects during seizures. Epilepsia 34 (Suppl. 2): 175

DISCUSSION

Tassinari: An interesting point is that in untreated generalised epilepsy the brain is more excitable. Cortical stimulation may be a useful tool by which to assess the efficacy of anti-epileptic drugs against myoclonus.

Janz: Has any attempt been made to determine the threshold under different conditions? One can imagine that the threshold in juvenile myoclonic epilepsy, for instance, is different during the morning and the evening or after sleep deficit. Also, does the threshold change after repeated stimulations?

Berkovic: We had considered looking at the threshold immediately after waking, but we have not done it. As far as the reliability of the measurements, certainly in control patients tested by the same investigator the measurements are very similar when separated by days or even weeks or months. We have certainly repeated the measurements in patients on the same day and they seem to remain stable, but one would imagine that there would be diurnal variations and we have not measured that.

Panayiotopoulos: How does age affect the threshold?

Berkovic: The threshold is quite high in the under-10s. If one wanted to look at children under 10 years of age with childhood absence epilepsy, one would need very tight age-matched controls. In the older patients I do not think it changes greatly through adolescence or adult life.

Meencke: Do you have developmental data about the threshold? Could this decreased threshold reflect some developmental state?

Berkovic: The higher threshold in children may in part be due to physical factors such as skull and brain orientation, and there may be a neurophysiological factor, but the details are unclear.

Fish: If tests are to be of use clinically, they need to be robust and quick to administer. I presume these data were acquired in an extremely careful fastidious way and took a long time. Is that correct?

Berkovic: At the moment this is not a clinical test but it only takes about 20 minutes. We are exploring other measures of excitability to see whether we can get a better separation from normals, but so far no luck.

Mirsky: Of the three measures presented, amplitude and latency of evoked responses did not seem to fit with the notion of increased cortical excitability. Should those be dismissed, or not considered?

Berkovic: The data suggest there that they do not differ between patients and controls. Were the latency shorter or the amplitude greater, then one might suggest that was showing hyper-excitability. The absence of a finding is not proof that there is not increased excitability. I suspect that the threshold is just a more sensitive measure.

14. Neuropsychological and psychophysiological aspects of absence epilepsy

Allan F. Mirsky   Connie C. Duncan   Miriam L. Levav

Since beginning the study of patients with typical absences in 1953, we have been intrigued with the phenomenon of the absence and with the insights that it might reveal into the nature of consciousness. Our research has involved neuropsychological and electrophysiological studies in patients, as well as extensive modelling of the signs and symptoms of the disorder in animals. We have conducted research, as well, on the familial aggregation of the cognitive signs of the disorder.

Schwab was the first to ask patients to perform simple reaction time tasks during EEG recording (Schwab, 1939). Brief disturbances in attentiveness (as indexed by longer response times) accompanied paroxysmal bursts of symmetrical and synchronous 3 Hz spike-wave EEG activity.

Many investigators have confirmed the observation that brief interruptions of consciousness accompany spike-wave bursts, although the correlation between EEG and behavioural signs of the absence is not perfect (Browne & Mirsky, 1983). Thus, stimuli presented in earlier portions of a spike-wave burst are less likely to be detected than are those presented later in the burst. Moreover, patients with absence epilepsy were more likely than controls to make errors on tests of sustained attention even when spike-wave bursts were excluded. That finding, which has been replicated several times, raised the question of whether the cognitive processing of patients with typical absence seizures is normal between spike-wave episodes (Mirsky & Duncan, 1990). Relevant to this question are EEG data that have been recorded in inter-ictal periods in such patients; such periods may be characterised by a periodic build-up of low-frequency EEG activity, which may be a harmonic of the fundamental 3 Hz frequency. This build-up may be prodromal for ictal discharges (Siegel et al, 1982; Mirsky & Grady, 1988).

These findings support the view that the transitory bursts of spike-wave activity represent the tip of an iceberg. Below the surface there may be a more or less continuously active pathophysiological process which is reflected in impaired performance on tests of attention and in alterations in event-related brain potentials (ERPs) (Duncan, 1988; Mirsky, 1988).

Thus, in addition to the impairment of attention that may accompany EEG spike-wave bursts, there are effects on attention associated with inter-ictal periods in patients with typical absences. This paper focuses on the work on attention during the inter-ictal period.

SENSORY AND COGNITIVE EFFECTS OF SPIKE-WAVE BURSTS

Studies of the effects of spike-wave bursts on information processing, some of which made use of animal models of the disorder, indicate that sensory input is altered during bursts (Mirsky, 1988; Mirsky & Duncan, 1990). Such alterations have been seen in visual evoked potentials, including effects measurable just prior to the onset of bursts (Orren, 1978), and in brainstem auditory evoked potentials (Mirsky, 1988; Mirsky & Duncan, 1990).

Moreover, we have modelled the sensory as well as the behavioural effects seen during bursts by disrupting brainstem functioning in monkeys (Mirsky & Duncan, 1990). This has involved the placement of irritative aluminium cream lesions in sub-cortical structures, as well as electrical stimulation of these structures in monkeys while they perform attention tasks. A significant finding in the work with monkeys has been the discovery of what is presumed to be a network of 'attention cells' in the brainstem (Bakay Pragay et al, 1978; Ray et al, 1984). If the brainstem comprises a key component of the attention system (Mirsky et al, 1991), then disturbance of this portion of the system could provide the basis for the effects that have been observed during spike-wave bursts.

THE INTER-ICTAL ATTENTION DISTURBANCE IN ABSENCE EPILEPSY

Evidence from three lines of investigation helps specify the inter-ictal characteristics of patients with typical absences. The first line describes the type of attention deficit seen in these patients, in contrast with that seen in a more 'focal' seizure disorder (ie, complex partial seizures). The second line concerns investigation of ERPs. The third has to do with the influence of gender and familial factors on the expression of the attentional deficit.

Specifying the deficit in attention in absence epilepsy

To study cognitive impairment in absence epilepsy, we administered a battery of tests (Mirsky et al, 1991) and used a comparison group of patients with focal disorders as well as non-seizure controls. This allowed us to identify the tests that are sensitive to the underlying pathophysiology of the disorder and to establish whether the impairment is specific to absence epilepsy (Mirsky et al, 1960; Lansdell & Mirsky, 1964; Fedio & Mirsky, 1969; Mirsky & Duncan, 1990; Mirsky, 1992).

In a recent study comparing two groups of patients with seizure disorders with a group of normal control subjects we used a model of attention linked to a series of tests that had been identified by statistical methods as tapping distinct aspects or functions of attention (Mirsky et al, 1991). What the model proposes can be summarised by the following statements:

1. Attention is a complex process or set of processes that can be sub-divided into a number of distinct functions, including shift, focus-execute, sustain and encode.
2. These functions are supported by different brain regions which are organised into a system.
3. Each function is tapped by one or more specific neuropsychological tests.
4. Damage or disturbance in one of these brain regions leads to deficits in a specific attention function.

The scores from neuropsychological tests assessing each of these four attention functions (shift, focus-execute, sustain and encode) were combined statistically into four component scores, each of which represents a more robust measure than that derived from a single measure or test (Mirsky et al, 1991). In this study, we compared the component scores derived from normal controls with those derived from patients with complex partial epilepsy, absences and closed head injuries. The groups appear to be distinct in terms of their profiles of differences from the normal controls; no two groups showed the same pattern of component score differences from controls (Fig. 14.1).

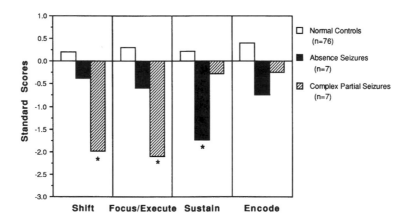

Fig. 14.1 Component scores extracted by principal components analysis of attention tests on normal control subjects (white columns), patients with absence seizures (black columns) and complex partial seizures (cross-hatched columns). The asterisks appearing below the columns indicate that the group so designated differed significantly from the other two groups on that component. The absence group performed significantly worse than the other two groups on the sustain component, whereas the complex partial group was impaired, in comparison with the other groups, on the shift and focus/execute components. (Reproduced with permission from Mirsky et al, 1991).

Examining the individual group component scores indicated the following significant differences: on the shift and focus-execute functions, the group with complex partial seizures had scores that were significantly lower than those of the other two groups; on the sustain function, the group with absence seizures differed from the other groups.

The profile of the group with complex partial seizures (Fig. 14.1) suggests functional impairment of those cerebral structures subserving the shift and focus-execute functions (ie, pre-frontal, anterior cingulate, inferior parietal cortices, corpus striatum) (Mirsky et al, 1991). In contrast, the system sub-serving the sustain attention function is less involved in the pathophysiology of this disorder. In striking contrast, the group with absences shows the greatest impairment of the sustain function. Elsewhere, we have argued that sustained attention represents the functional involvement of a thalamo-mesopontine system (Mirsky et al, 1991).

The distinctive profiles seen in complex partial and absence epilepsy are consistent with the concept of dysfunction of the thalamus or reticular formation underlying absence seizures. In contrast, complex partial epilepsy is usually thought to arise from focal cortical disturbances. Finally, the attentional differences seen here in the sustain function are consistent with previous research on sustained attention in patients with seizure disorders (Fedio & Mirsky, 1969; Lansdell & Mirsky, 1964; Mirsky et al, 1960; Mirsky & Duncan, 1990), which has indicated significantly greater impairment of this function in absence than in focal epilepsy.

Event-related brain potential (ERP) studies of absence epilepsy

Duncan (1988) used cognitive ERPs to study information-processing in the inter-ictal period in patients with absence epilepsy. The task used to elicit ERPs was the Continuous Peformance Test (CPT), which requires sustained attention and a push-button response to targets in a series of visual or auditory stimuli. In the visual task, the target was the letter X if it followed the letter A (AX task). In the auditory task, it was the highest of three tones if it followed the lowest tone (equivalent to the visual AX task). Figure 14.2 presents the ERPs elicited by the targets in the two tasks.

The P300 component is the prominent positive wave occurring at approximately 400 msec in the visual version of the CPT, and at approximately 300 msec in the auditory version of the task. P300 is a manifestation of cognitive activity, invoked by task-relevant stimuli, and is considered to reflect the updating of current working memory. Its amplitude reflects the amount of attention allocated to stimuli. Little group difference is apparent between the P300 components elicited by visual targets, whereas the P300 to auditory targets was significantly reduced in amplitude in the absence group.

The slow-wave component, very prominent in these averages, overlaps and follows the P300; it is elicited by stimuli for which continued processing occurs, subsequent to their identification. The presumption is that the aud-

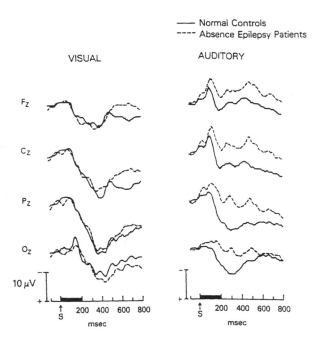

Fig. 14.2 Event-related potentials (ERPs) elicited by visual (left) and auditory (right) target stimuli in the 'AX' version of the Continuous Performance Test. The data collected from the two groups (matched for sex, age and educational level) were averaged over subjects: the grand-mean ERPs for the normal controls (solid lines, n=7) and patients with absence epilepsy (dashed lines, n=8) are superimposed at four midline scalp locations. Whereas the visual ERPs did not distinguish the two groups, the prominent P300 and slow-wave components that characterise the auditory ERPs of the controls were virtually absent in the auditory ERPs of the absence patients. (Adapted from Duncan, 1988).

itory slow wave in this task reflects the need for the subject to keep traces of the tones, and their identification as 'high', 'medium' or 'low', continuously active in memory.

The results indicate that patients with absence seizures tend to have reduced amplitude cognitive ERP components (P300, slow wave) in comparison with normal control subjects, an effect that is especially marked on tests of auditory sustained attention. The visual task did not discriminate between the groups. The findings thus suggest that auditory and visual information-processing systems may be impaired differentially in absence epilepsy, although we cannot rule out the interpretation that the auditory task was simply more difficult, requiring more of a mnemonic effort and/or greater allocation of attention. The possible implication is that the impairment in attention in these patients is enhanced by increased attentional demands.

Duncan and co-workers have recently extended this work to include a group of patients with complex partial seizures (Duncan et al, in preparation). The results indicate that absence patients tend to have reduced amplitude P300 and slow-wave components in comparison with both control and complex partial subjects, an effect that was especially marked on tests of auditory sustained attention.

The ERP data agree with the neuropsychological data presented in Fig. 14.1. The results in both instances emphasise the impairment in sustained attention in the inter-ictal period in the absence patients as well as the distinctive character of their impairment. The reduced auditory P300 is consistent with the altered brainstem auditory evoked potentials seen in spike-wave bursts (Mirsky, 1988) and emphasises the impaired auditory processing seen in absence epilepsy.

Gender and familial factors in the attention deficit in absence epilepsy

Whereas the existence of a genetic component in absence epilepsy is documented (Anderson & Hauser, 1988; Chs 36, 37), the specific mode of inheritance remains unknown. Studies of the relatives of probands have used as genetic markers the occurrence of spike-wave bursts in the EEG. We are studying impaired attention as a potential vulnerability marker in the relatives of persons with absence epilepsy (Levav et al, in preparation).

Levav (1991) found that probands with absence epilepsy were unimpaired on most tests of attention, although significant impairment (in comparison with their unaffected siblings) was seen on tests of sustained attention (tapped by the CPT); moreover, female probands tended to be more affected than males (Fig. 14.3). Greater impairment in the female than the male proband was first reported by Lansdell & Mirsky (1964).

Levav's finding of no attention impairment in the siblings of probands is consistent with the results of genetic studies summarised by Anderson & Hauser (1988): the prevalence of absence epilepsy in non-proband members of dizygotic twin pairs is significantly lower than the comparable figure for monozygotic non-probands.

Another gender-related difference was seen in the performance of the parents of the probands: mothers tended to perform more poorly on the CPT (which assesses the sustain function of attention) than fathers. This difference, which was apparent in measures of response speed and accuracy, was not seen in the sample of normal controls. These results are also summarised in Fig. 14.3, which presents mean reaction time scores (top bar graph) and percentage of correct responses (bottom bar graph) averaged over the four CPT tasks employed (Visual X, AX and Degraded X, Auditory X). Data for the four groups of subjects (probands, siblings, parents and adult controls) are presented separately by sex.

Although these data are preliminary, they are consistent with previous reports that point to a maternally transmitted influence on seizure susceptibility (Ottman et al, 1988). The present information suggests that measures of attention provide additional markers of vulnerability to the disorder that may enhance and enrich the sensitivity of genetic investigations.

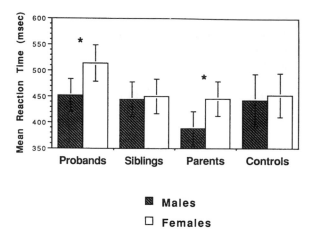

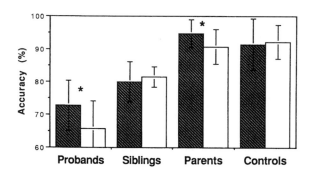

Fig. 14.3 Mean CPT scores (averaged across four CPT tasks) of four groups of male (cross-hatched columns) and female (white columns) subjects. Groups include probands with absence epilepsy (n=14, 8 females), unaffected siblings (n=15, 6 females), parents of the probands (n=16, 9 females) and adult control subjects (n=23, 15 females). The average age of the probands was 10.6 years, of the siblings 12.1 years. The mean age of the parents was 39 years, of the controls 32 years. The two adult groups had similar levels of education. Top graph, reaction times; bottom graph, accuracy scores. The asterisks above the columns indicate that the male and female subjects within that group differed significantly. Note that the female probands performed significantly worse than the male probands and the mothers of the probands performed significantly worse than the fathers. (Data from Levav, 1991.)

SUMMARY

Neuropsychological and ERP studies of absence epilepsy have found deficits in sustained auditory and visual attention that are distinct from those seen in other seizure disorders. These findings appear to implicate a disturbance in brainstem-mediated attention functions in the pathophysiology of the disorder. The ERP studies indicate impaired sensory input during spike-wave bursts. Moreover, there is evidence for a pathophysiological mechanism in absence epilepsy that results in reduced attentional capacity, seen primarily in the auditory modality, during inter-ictal periods as well. Female probands appear to have greater deficits in sustained attention than male probands, and mothers of probands may have a mild form of the attention deficit that is not evident in the fathers.

REFERENCES

Anderson VE, Hauser WA 1988 Genetics of absence seizures and related epileptic syndromes. In: Myslobodsky MS, Mirsky AF (eds) Elements of petit mal epilepsy. Peter Lang, New York, pp37–70

Bakay Pragay E, Mirsky AF, Ray CL, Turner DF, Mirsky CV 1978 Neuronal activity in the brain stem reticular formation during performance of a 'go-no go' visual attention task in the monkey. Experimental Neurology 60: 83–95

Browne T, Mirsky AF 1983 Absence seizures. In: Browne T, Feldman RG (eds) Epilepsy: diagnosis and management. Little, Brown, Boston, pp61–74

Duncan CC 1988 Application of event-related brain potentials to the analysis of interictal attention in absence epilepsy. In: Myslobodsky MS, Mirsky AF (eds) Elements of petit mal epilepsy. Peter Lang, New York, pp341–364

Duncan CC, Mirsky AF, Theodore WH The effects of absence epilepsy and complex partial epilepsy on information processing: an ERP study. (in preparation)

Fedio P, Mirsky AF 1969 Selective intellectual deficits in children with temporal lobe or centrencephalic epilepsy. Neuropsychologia 7: 287–300

Lansdell H, Mirsky AF 1964 Attention in focal and centrencephalic epilepsy. Experimental Neurology 9: 463–469

Levav ML 1991 Attention performance in children affected with absence epilepsy and their first-degree relatives. Unpublished PhD dissertation, University of Maryland

Levav ML, Mirsky, AF, Amir N Familial factors in the behavioral impairment in absence epilepsy (in preparation)

Mirsky AF 1988 Behavioral and psychophysiological effects of petit mal epilepsy in the light of a neuropsychologically based theory of attention. In: Myslobodsky MS, Mirsky AF (eds) Elements of petit mal epilepsy. Peter Lang, New York, pp311–340

Mirsky AF 1992 Neuropsychological assessment of epilepsy. New Issues in Neurosciences 4: 25–39

Mirsky AF, Anthony BJ, Duncan CC, Ahearn MB, Kellam SG 1991 Analysis of the elements of attention: a neuropsychological approach. Neuropsychology Review 2: 109–145

Mirsky AF, Duncan CC 1990 Behavioral and electrophysiological studies of absence epilepsy. In: Avoli N, Gloor P, Kostopoulos G, Naquet R (eds) Generalized epilepsy: cellular, molecular and pharmacological approaches. Plenum, New York, pp254–269

Mirsky AF, Grady C 1988 Toward the development of alternative treatments in absence epilepsy. In: Myslobodsky MS, Mirsky AF (eds) Elements of petit mal epilepsy. Peter Lang, New York, pp285–310

Mirsky AF, Primac DW, Ajmone Marsan C, Rosvold HE, Stevens JA 1960 A comparison of the psychological test performance of patients with focal and nonfocal epilepsy. Experimental Neurology 2: 75–89

Orren MM 1978 Evoked potential studies in petit mal epilepsy: visual information processing in relation to wave-spike discharges. In: Cobb WA, Duijn HV (eds) Contemporary clinical neurophysiology. Elsevier, Amsterdam (EEG Suppl. 34): 251–257

Ottman R, Annegers JF, Hauser WA, Kurland LT 1988 Higher risk of seizures in offspring of mothers than of fathers with epilepsy. Am J Human Genetics 43: 257–264

Ray C, Mirsky AF, Bakay Pragay E 1982 Functional analysis of attention-related unit activity in the reticular formation of the monkey. Experimental Neurology 77: 544–562

Schwab 1939 Method of measuring consciousness in attacks of petit mal epilepsy. Arch Neurol Psychiatr 41: 215–217

Siegel A, Grady CL, Mirsky AF 1982 Prediction of spike-wave bursts in absence epilepsy by EEG power spectrum signals. Epilepsia 23: 47–60.

DISCUSSION

Van Luijtelaar: There were a lot of tests for determining sustained attention. I was wondering whether there were any other tests apart from those presented to look at continuous A-X tasks and whether any effects on sustained attention were found.

Is there any explanation for the differences between visual and auditory tasks during the inter-ictal periods?

Mirsky: In the familial aggregation study I reported we used four versions of the continuous performance test. One was the letter X as the target, the other was one I described: X if it follows A. Then there was a degraded image version of the task, in which the letter is more difficult to discern, and finally an auditory version of the task. The data I presented represented the summation of those four different kinds of tasks.

The auditory is a more difficult cognitive task than the visual. The patient has to keep in mind that he or she just heard a high tone: was it a low tone that came immediately before and what is a low tone after all? The patient must keep a kind of a model of what the tones are, what the stimuli are, in order to know whether a response is indicated on the next trial. Normal subjects can carry out this task without much difficulty.

Van Luijtelaar: It is just a subjective impression that this auditory task was more difficult. There is no data to back that up.

Mirsky: I cannot rule out the possibility that it is something specific to the auditory modality as opposed to a difficulty level. Difficulty level, however, is extremely important in these tests. When comparing some groups of subjects using simple reaction time tasks and ERPs elicited by simple reaction time tasks one will see no differences. In contrast, a more complex attention-demanding task separates out the groups very clearly. The level of effort required is extremely important and so far we cannot rule that out, although I think there is something more to it. I think there is something about auditory processing although I could not prove it on the basis of these data alone.

Duncan: There were differences in the pattern of attention deficit in people with typical absences and those with complex partial seizures. What medications were they taking and is it possible that different medications could have different effects on the tests used?

Mirsky: It is possible, but unlikely. Ideally we would have these patients without medication but that is just not possible. It is something we need to be concerned about but the medication effects would not easily account for the differences we saw between the groups.

Berkovic: I should like some clarification on the family data. The mothers did worse on the reaction time than the fathers, but, looking at the controls, it seemed to me that the mothers did as well as the controls, but the fathers were doing better.

Mirsky: For some reason the fathers of that group of probands did extremely well on the test. The mothers clearly did worse than the fathers who were like the control adults. We are in the process of trying to replicate those data.

Gloor: There is a possible explanation for the dip of the performance curve before the spike and wave starts. The scalp EEG is a poor measure to tell us exactly when the disturbance that underlies spike and wave activity starts. We became aware of that when we looked at the cat model. The EEG in the cat, recorded from the skull, shows the same kind of abrupt onset of spike and wave discharge as we see in humans. When we record from the cortex directly the onset is not as crisp; it builds up a little, and there is obviously something before it really comes on. If we then go to the microphysiological level we see that some individual cortical cells begin to oscillate before anything is visible in the EEG, and I think that what happens is that a few cells begin to do this, and then more and more, and then suddenly there is a big population and that is what we see in the scalp EEG. There is something going on beforehand at a low level that is not recordable from the skull.

Mirsky: That is probably quite correct.

If we divide the patients into two groups A and B, Group A was the group in which there was a very abrupt, clear onset that is symmetrical, synchronous in all channels. In that group there was a very clear correlation between the onset of erroneous performance and the beginning of the spike wave discharge; it was practically perfect. However, if we looked at the group in which the spike-wave form was more irregular, in which it might have been somewhat asymmetrical between the sides, then that is the group that was contributing the appearance of early errors before the spike-wave burst and it may be that it is extremely difficult to tell when the spike-wave burst begins in such a group. Sometimes, particularly with patients who have an abnormal background activity, there is a slow transition from the abnormal background into what we would accept as spike-wave activity. It could be that it is just a matter of defining when the spike wave onset occurs.

Fish: Can I clarify the time Dr Gloor was talking about with this build-up in the cats.

Gloor: It is of the order of a second or so.

Tassinari: If we look at absences, from time to time we are able to pick up some synchronising of the EEG before the onset of the spikes. I wonder if these small changes that happen just before are not due to some lowering of vigilance, which in turn could trigger the absence. It is difficult to know what is going on but it could be that there is some small change that takes a fraction of a second. I do not know if this is due to absence or if it is a condition that triggers off the absence, but it does exist.

15. Pathological findings in childhood absence epilepsy

H. J. Meencke

Following our first report of pathological findings in eight cases of idiopathic generalised epilepsy, including six cases with childhood absence epilepsy (CAE) (Meencke & Janz, 1984), we have analysed six additional cases with CAE. At present we have a total of 12 brains from patients with CAE out of 650 brains from patients with epilepsy. In the literature there are so far only single case reports with an additional two cases (Cohen; 1968; Bridge, 1949).

The neuropathological findings in CAE represent a distinct sub-group of autopsy findings in 650 cases with unselected epilepsies (Tables 15.1, 15.2). Contrary to the term idiopathic, the brains of patients with CAE do have pathological changes: predominantly slight developmental disturbances

Table 15.1 Autopsy findings in 650 unselected patients with epilepsy

Malformation	63.0%
Hippocampal sclerosis (HS)	30.5%
Parenchymal necrosis (extra HS)	21.0%
Meningo-encephalitis	5%
No pathology	18.0%

Table 15.2 Neuropathological findings in 12 patients with childhood absence epilepsy

Patient No.	Age	Brain weight (g)	Microdysgenesis	Malformation	Ischaemic lesions	Systematic atrophy	Trauma
1	17	1470	+				
2	23	1400	+				
3	23	1470	+				
4	25	1295	+				
5	39	1410	+			+	
6	41	1830	+				
7	41	1490	+				+
8	47	1330	+	+		+	
9	57	1390	+		+		
10	71	1250	+	+		+	
11	72	1130	+	+	+		+
12	72	1450	+	+	+		

summarised under the term microdysgenesis. In addition, three cases had mild aetiologically irrelevant malformations (microangioma). Three cases had ischaemic lesions, two of these with complete necrosis with microangiopathy and one with neuronal necrosis after cardiac arrest and resuscitation. Cerebellar cortical atrophy was seen in two cases and was of para-neoplastic origin. One patient, who developed a Parkinsonian syndrome in late life, had atrophy of the caudate nucleus.

HIPPOCAMPAL SCLEROSIS

No case with CAE had hippocampal sclerosis. In general, hippocampal sclerosis is seen in around 30 per cent of cases with epilepsy, most commonly in temporal lobe epilepsy followed by the West syndrome and Lennox–Gastaut syndrome (Meencke & Veith, 1985) (Table 15.3). The morphometric analysis of neuronal density in the stratum pyramidale of the hippocampus

Table 15.3 Hippocampal sclerosis (HS) in different epilepsy syndromes

Syndrome	N	HS	% with HS
Temporal lobe epilepsy	27	15	56
West syndrome	24	11	46
Lennox–Gastaut syndrome	30	6	20
Childhood absence epilepsy	12	0	0
Juvenile myoclonic epilepsy	3	0	0

showed no difference in the numbers of neurons in any sector, compared with the age matched controls. This was in contrast to the group with temporal lobe epilepsy, where there was a significant reduction in the neuron density in sector CA4. There was a clear correlation between the number of neurons in sector CA4 and the total number of generalised tonic-clonic seizures (GTCS).

The total number of GTCS in the CAE group ranged between 10 and 700, with an average of 425, compared with an average of 1070 in the temporal lobe group. This indicates that the neuron loss in sector CA4 might be a consequence of seizures, related to the total number of GTCS during life.

DEVELOPMENTAL DISTURBANCES

Microdysgenesis was the predominant finding in CAE. In contrast, microdysgenesis was found in 50 per cent of cases of Lennox–Gastaut and West syndromes and in only 7 per cent of patients who had temporal lobe epilepsy. These three syndromes had much more severe developmental disturbances in 11–16 per cent of cases, which were not seen in CAE (Table 15.4).

Table 15.4. Frequency of migration disturbances in different epilepsy syndromes

Syndrome	N	Migration disturbances			
		Severe		Microdysgenesis	
		N	%	N	%
Temporal lobe epilepsy	27	3	11	2	7
West syndrome	24	3	13	12	50
Lennox–Gastaut syndrome	30	5	16	15	50
Childhood absence epilepsy	12	0	0	12	100
Juvenile myoclonic epilepsy	3	0	0	3	100

Microdysgenesis is a summarising term, which includes a large variety of architectural disturbances (Fig. 15.1). We have described diffuse or focal increase of dystopic neurons in the stratum moleculare, protrusions of nerve cells from deep cortical layers up to the stratum moleculare, pits and hollows, sub-pial clustering of nerve cells, architectural disturbances of deeper cortical

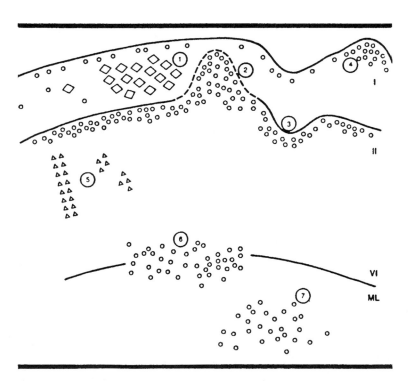

Fig. 15.1 Heteromorphism of microdysgenesis. 1) Diffuse or focal increase of dystopic neurons. 2) Protrusions of nerve cells. 3) Pits and hollows. 4) Subpial groups of nerve cells. 5) Architectural disturbances of deeper cortical layers. 6) Diffuse border zones. 7) Dystopic nerve cells in the white matter.

layers with disruption of the lamina organisation, including clustering of neurons, diffuse border zones between laminar VI and sub-cortical white matter and dystopic nerve cells in the white matter. In CAE the diffuse increase of dystopic neurons in the stratum moleculare and diffuse border zones between lamina VI and sub-cortical white matter, as well as dystopic neurons in the white matter, were the most common abnormalities.

The significance of microdysgenesis is controversial (Meencke & Janz, 1984; Meencke & Janz, 1985; Lyon & Gastaut, 1985) due, among other factors, to the fine and diffuse changes in cell density which are visually difficult to delineate (Figs 15.2, 15.3). Therefore, we started morphometric studies of neuron density in order to get valid data on these fine architectural changes. Neuron cell density was measured in the stratum moleculare of the frontal lobe (areas 9, 45 and 46), the temporal lobe (area 22) and the occipital lobe (area 18). Cell density was also measured in the sub-cortical white matter of the frontal lobe (areas 10, 45, 46). In the hippocampus cell density was defined in the stratum radiatum, lacunosum moleculare and oriens (Meencke, 1983; Meencke, 1985).

Neocortex

Neuron density is clearly related to brain development and also shows a distinct topographic pattern within the brain. Nerve cell density shortly after birth is about 15 000 cells/mm^3. During the first 2 years of life, the number of cells decreases markedly (Fig 15.4). After the second decade, there follows a

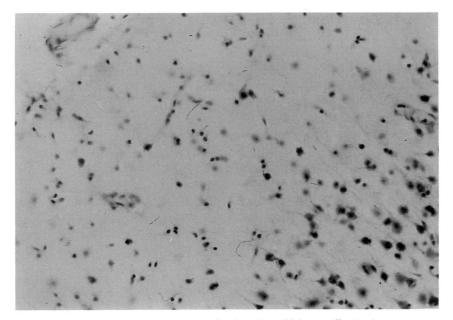

Fig. 15.2 Dystopic neurons in the stratum moleculare. Frontal lobe, paraffin Nissl stain.

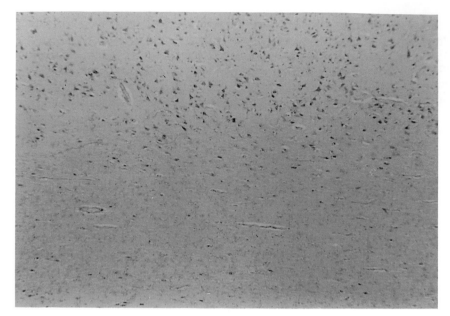

Fig. 15.3 Dystopic neurons in the subcortical white matter. Frontal lobe, paraffin Nissl strain.

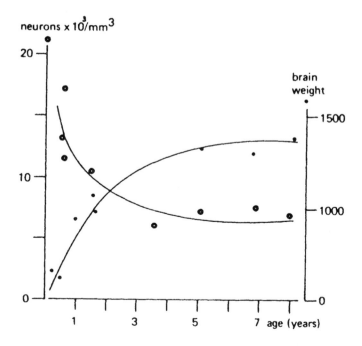

Fig. 15.4 Neuron density of stratum moleculare (open circles) and brain weight in control subjects. Brain weight units, gms.

period of constant cell density, with a mean of 5000 cells/ mm³, which decreases slightly in the seventh and eighth decades. The first marked decrease in cell density corresponds to a reciprocal increase in brain weight and cortical volume. The frontal lobe has a significantly higher neuron density than the temporal and occipital lobes, which have almost the same values (Fig. 15.5).

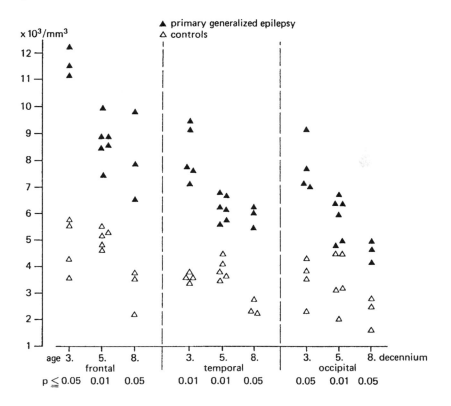

Fig. 15.5 Neuron density in stratum moleculare in patients with idiopathic generalised epilepsy (solid triangles), controls (open triangles). x-axis units, decades.

There are only two previous reports with counts of the cell density of lamina I, using the brains of middle-aged subjects. Schlote (1959) reported 5000 cells per mm³ in the frontal cortex, without indicating the area more precisely. Haug et al (1983) found 4000 cells per mm³ in area 11. These figures are in close agreement with our findings of neuron density in the steady state period.

The CAE group had a significantly higher cell count in the stratum moleculare than age-matched controls. The values in the third decade were twice as high as in controls of corresponding age. Moreover, the change of neuron density with age also differed between non-epileptic controls and cases with CAE. Cases with idiopathic generalised epilepsy had a decrease in density between the fourth and fifth decades but not, as in the controls, between the fifth and eighth decades. This phenomenon could be due to the greater vulnerability of dystopic neurons (and could thus be an expression of an earlier ageing process) or it could be an expression of a delayed post-maturing effect.

Subcortical white matter

The neuron density in the sub-cortical white matter of the frontal lobe in generalised epilepsies was also significantly higher than in age-matched controls.

Hippocampus

Neuron density in stratum radiatum, lacunosum and moleculare and in stratum oriens of the hippocampus differed from that in controls only in the younger age group, between 20–50 years of age (Fig. 15.6). After 50 years of

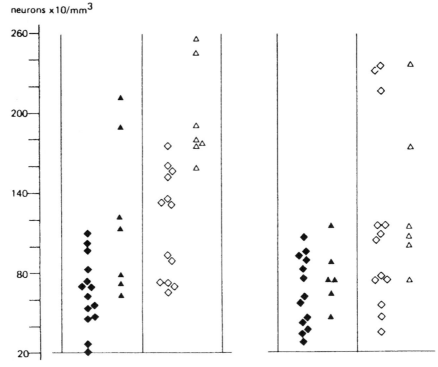

Fig. 15.6 Neuron density in stratum radiatum, lacunosum and moleculare of the hippocampus (CA1) in subjects aged 20–50 (left) and in subjects aged over 50 (right). Solid diamonds, large neurons (3 µm), controls; open diamonds, small neurons (1.6 µm), controls; solid triangles, large neurons (3 µm), idiopathic generalised epilepsy; open triangles, small neurons (1.6 µm), idiopathic generalised epilepsy

age, patients with epilepsy and non-epileptic controls had no significant differences. In the stratum radiatum, lacunosum and moleculare the densities were different for two cell types: for large neurons with a nucleolus diameter of 3.0 μm and also for small neurons with an average nucleolus diameter of 1.6 μm. In the stratum oriens the differences were significant only for the small neurons.

The finding of no significant differences in neuron densities in the older age group could be an expression of the increased vulnerability of dystopic neurons.

CONCLUSIONS

Our studies have demonstrated microdysgenesis in CAE. Increased numbers of dystopic neurons were found in the neocortex, in the sub-cortical white matter of the frontal lobe and in different laminae of the hippocampus outside of the stratum pyramidale. The dystopic neurons had a different age-related behaviour showing either a delayed maturation effect or an earlier onset of the ageing process.

Dystopic neurons in the stratum moleculare and in the sub-cortical white matter have been described by several authors. Ranke (1910), Oppermann (1929), Scholz (1955) and Veith and Wicke (1968) all described on a qualitative basis dystopic neurons in various cortical and sub-cortical structures. Jakob (1914) stated that neurons in the stratum moleculare also occur in brains of non-epileptic patients (up to then it was thought that neurons in the stratum moleculare were a phenomenon only of the fetal period) and he emphasised the differences between the brains of normal and epileptic individuals to prove the pathological significance in epilepsy.

Veith (1973) noted that 86 per cent of patients with peripheral malformations have microdysgenesis, as did only 10 per cent of patients without, and concluded that microdysgenesis could have a certain pathological significance. Hardiman et al (1988) found an increase of dystopic neurons in the sub-cortical white matter in 42 per cent of resected specimens from patients undergoing surgery for temporal lobe epilepsy. Nordborg et al (1987) and Andermann et al (1987) described dystopic neurons in the stratum moleculare of resected temporal lobe specimens. Neither group made a morphometric analysis. Our morphometric analysis of neuron density in the stratum moleculare in temporal lobe patients showed no significant differences in neuron density between controls and patients with temporal lobe epilepsy.

Roberts et al (1985) found increased numbers of small neurons in the inferior colliculus of the genetic epilepsy-prone rat. This increase occurred before the onset of seizures and it was suggested that the increase in cell numbers is not compensatory to the seizure activity, but is genetically programmed. This is the first finding from an animal model of idiopathic generalised epilepsy and supports our finding of slight developmental disturbances in human idiopathic generalised epilepsy.

The question arises whether these dislocated neurons represent disorders from the migrational period. The increased density of dystopic neurons could be the result of: disturbed migration; neuronal defect; glial defect; disturbed programmed cell death; or disturbed outgrowing neuropil. If disturbed migration were the cause of dystopic neurons, the relevant period of brain development for these disturbances would be months 5–7 of fetal life. The defect could either be of neuronal or glial origin. The relationship of developmental disturbances to vascular territories could support the idea that vascular-related disturbances of glial fibres might be responsible for this type of architectural abnormality.

Another aetiological aspect of increased neuron density could be a disturbed programme of cell death. Programmed cell death includes the phenomenon of necrosis, atrophy and apoptosis. An over-population of neurons during development is necessary in order to build up interneuronal connections. After establishing interneuronal contacts, 20–85 per cent of the primary nerve cells die. This physiological cell death is programmed genetically (Rorke, 1994). In some non-vertebrate animals genes responsible for this programmed cell death have been identified. In human CAE there could be a link between the genes responsible for this architectural disturbance and for the epileptic syndrome.

The functional correlation between microdysgenesis and CAE is still unclear. Microdysgenesis could be associated with general epileptogenesis. This would be supported by the finding that microdysgenesis is found in several distinct epileptic syndromes (Meencke, 1989). Our finding of increased numbers of dystopic neurons in patients with post traumatic epilepsy compared to non-epileptic patients with the same brain trauma, indicates some correlation between microdysgenesis and general epileptogenesis (Meencke, 1983). On the other hand there is also some evidence that microdysgenesis could be more specific for distinct syndromes. This is supported by our findings of a significant increase of dystopic neurons in the stratum moleculare of patients with CAE, something not found in patients with temporal lobe epilepsy. If these findings were not specific for distinct syndromes, it is less likely that they are causative.

REFERENCES

Andermann F, Olivier A, Melanson D, Robitaille Y 1987 Epilepsy due to focal cortical dysplasia with macrogyria and the forme fruste of tuberous sclerosis: a study of 15 patients. Advances in Epileptology 16: 35–38
Bridge EM 1949 Epilepsy and convulsive disorders in children. McGraw Hill, New York
Cohen R 1968 A neuropathological study of a case with petit mal epilepsy. Electroencephalography and Clinical Neurophysiology 24: 282
Hardiman O, Burke T, Philips J, et al 1988 Microdysgenesis in resected temporal neocortex: incidence and clinical significance in focal epilepsy. Neurology 38: 1041–1047
Haug H, Barmwater U, Eggers R, Fischer D, Kuhl S, Sass NL 1983 Anatomical changes in aging brain: morphometric analysis of the human prosencephalon. In: Cervos-Navarro J, Sarkander HJ (eds) Brain aging: Neuropathology and neuropharmacology (Aging Vol. 21) Raven Press, New York

Jakob A 1914 Zur Pathologie der Epilepsie. Z. Neurol 23: 1–65
Lyon G, Gastaut H 1985 Considerations of the significance attributed to unusual cerebral
   histological findings recently described in eight patients with primary generalized epilepsy.
   Epilepsia 26: 365–367
Meencke HJ 1983 The density of dystopic neurons in the white matter of the gyrus frontalis
   inferior in epilepsies. Journal of Neurology 230: 171–181
Meencke HJ 1985 Neuron density in the molecular layer of the frontal cortex in primary
   generalized epilepsy. Epilepsia 26: 450–454
Meencke HJ 1989 Pathology of childhood epilepsies. Cleveland Journal of Medicine 56:
   111–120
Meencke HJ, Janz D 1984 Neuropathological findings in primary generalized epilepsy: a study
   of eight cases. Epilepsia 25: 8–21
Meencke HJ, Janz D 1985 The significance of microdysgenesis in primary generalized
   epilepsy: an answer to the considerations of Lyon and Gastaut. Epilepsia 26: 368–371
Meencke HJ, Veith G 1985 Neuropathologische Aspekte des myoklonisch-astatischen Petit mal
   (Lennox-Syndrom). In: Kruse R (ed) Epilepsie 84 Einhorn-Presse, Reinbek pp 305–313
Nordborg C, Sourander P, Silfvenius H, Blom S, Zetterlund B 1987 Mild cortical dysplasia in
   patients with intractable partial seizures: a histological study. Advances in Epileptology 16:
   29-33
Oppermann K 1929 Cajal'sche Horizontalzellen in Ganglienzellen des Marks. Z Neurol 120:
   121-137
Ranke O 1910 Beiträge Zur Kenntnis der normalen und pathologischen Hirnrindenbildung.
   Beitr. Pathol. Anat. 47: 51
Roberts RC, Kim HL, Ribak CE 1985 Increased numbers of neurons occur in inferior
   colliculus of the young genetically epilepsy-prone rat. Developments in Brain Research 23:
   227–281
Rorke LB 1994 A perspective: the role of disordered genetic control of neurogenesis in the
   pathogenesis of migration disorders. Journal of Neuropathology and Experimental Neurology
   53: 105–117
Schlote 1959 W Zur Gliaarchitektonik der menschlichen Großhirnrinde im Nissl-Bild Archiv
   fur Psychiatrie und Nervenkrankheiten 199:573–595
Scholz W 1955 Die Krampfschadingungen des Gehirns. In: Monograph. Ges. Neurol.
   Psychiatr. Gruhle, Spatz, Vogel (eds) Springer, Berlin
Veith G, Wicke R 1968 Cerebrale Differenzierungsstorungen bei Epilepsie. Jahrbuch 1968.
   Westdeutscher Verlag, Koln-Oplanden
Veith G 1973 Der angeborene Hirnschaden. Anat. Grund. Kinderkrankheilkd. 121: 152–139

DISCUSSION

Gloor: Did those patients with idiopathic generalised epilepsy who were examined also have generalised tonic-clonic seizures?

Meencke: Yes.

Gloor: Did they have neuronal loss in the CA4 region of the hippocampus?

Meencke: No, they did not and this was probably related to the lower average number of generalised tonic-clonic seizures.

Panayiotopoulos: I have some anxiety regarding the finding of structural changes in the brain in a disease, typical absence epilepsy, which is age-related and generally self-limiting. Did they have pure childhood absence epilepsy?

Meencke: Yes. They had absences from 6–7 years to 20 or 25 years. Some of these cases developed generalised tonic-clonic seizures.

Panayiotopoulos: If they continued having absences and had generalised tonic-clonic seizures, they did not have the benign form of childhood absence epilepsy.

Janz: No. That would be a pure and benign form, without generalised tonic-clonic seizures. These patients did not die of their epilepsy. They had rather a normal epilepsy with generalised tonic-clonic seizures at intervals of months.

Meencke: Of the three patients who died in their seventies, for example, the severity of their epilepsy waxed and waned. They had long seizure-free periods.

Panayiotopoulos: I do not dispute what you said and I have great respect for this. It is just my anxiety relating structural abnormalities with a condition which I believe is usually benign.

Meencke: I agree, we have to be precise in the definition of the clinical features. Also, we have to be very clear in our definition of dysplasias and not mix up our findings in localisation-related epilepsies with those in generalised epilepsies.

Panayiotopoulos: Are abnormalities like this seen in the normal population, and is age an important factor?

Meencke: Yes. This was the reason for having our measurements age-related. We have age-matched controls and age-matched epilepsy groups, so we can get an estimate of the development of neuron density.

Fish: Was the distribution of the microdysgenesis within the brain more posterior or more anterior?

Meencke: Frontal. The frontal basal predominance of neuron density probably reflects neuronal migration in the cortex. The migration starts in the rolandic area and then moves down to the basal frontal lobe. It is the last populated area and also the last area where the remigration of the outer granular layer starts. The predominance of this area probably has some relationship to the physiological processes of development.

16. Investigations in humans – consensus statement

David Fish

Professor Gloor bridged the gap between animal and human investigations. He presented a variety of data from both animals and humans and drew the personal conclusion that cortical abnormalities were more likely to underlie the physiology of idiopathic generalised epilepsy than thalamic abnormalities, although clearly demonstrated the need for a cortico-thalamic loop in the production of generalised spike and wave.

Dr Prevett presented data on positron emission tomography (PET) in patients with generalised epilepsies and demonstrated the involvement of the thalamus in typical absences. It was clear that there was some discordance in the published literature on the effect of absences on cerebral blood flow (CBF), particularly with regard to recent work from the Strasbourg group on middle cerebral artery blood flow during absences. It was difficult to reconcile these different reports other than to accept differences in methodology or patient material. One of the problems with PET is the limited temporal resolution. Functional MRI has a theoretical temporal resolution of 100 msec, but detection of changes remains limited by the 0.5–1 sec lag between electrographic activity and a change in CBF. Future research with PET would concentrate much more on work with new ligands to explore abnormalities of neuro-transmission rather than CBF.

Dr Smith presented an overview of neurophysiological changes in humans with idiopathic generalised epilepsies. She showed a continuum of the neurophysiological changes with increased excitability in those syndromes with associated myoclonus.

Dr Berkovic presented work on magnetic stimulation in the idiopathic generalised epilepsies. This appeared to be a useful research tool but has not yet entered the clinical domain. He reported that there was a reduced threshold for magnetic stimulation in untreated patients with idiopathic generalised epilepsies and that this was partially reversed by treatment with anti-epileptic drugs. However, there was no change in latency or amplitude of response and this discrepancy was unexplained.

Dr Mirsky presented data on attentional changes during absence seizures and also during the inter-ictal phase. He also explored abnormalities of attention in relatives of people with absence seizures. Questions were raised about the control data as there appeared to be a difference between males and females which may have influenced some of the findings. In addition there was uncertainty about the effect of anti-epileptic drugs on the results, although Dr Mirsky thought that anti-epileptic medication was unlikely to have been responsible for the differences he reported.

Professor Meencke presented the neuropathological findings in patients with childhood absence epilepsy. Microdysgenesis was found in all of these subjects, predominantly anteriorly. This was a much higher incidence than in control groups. Both Professor Meencke and Dr Panayiotopoulos stressed the need for careful clinical description of cases and use of agreed terminology. Some of the patients had continued to have seizures throughout life and died of old age. These interesting neuropathological findings, which were documented very clearly, received considerable discussion given the immense implications for the pathogenesis of this condition.

In summary, during this session a variety of data were presented covering different aspects of investigations in humans showing the range of investigative findings and relating these to possible pathogenic processes. It remains of much interest to determine whether or not there are clear pathological substrates for some different forms of idiopathic generalised epilepsies.

17. The epidemiology and prognosis of typical absence seizures

J. W. A. S. Sander

The interpretation of epidemiological data in the epilepsies is often complicated and unsatisfactory and this is largely due to methodological problems
(Sander & Shorvon, 1987). The epidemiology of epileptic syndromes with
typical absences is a good example in that there are problems with case
ascertainment, case definition and patient selection bias.

Typical absences predominantly affect children and adolescents, females
usually more than males (Dreifuss, 1991; Loiseau, 1992). There is a higher
than expected incidence of a positive family history of epilepsy in patients
with the condition; first-degree relatives also have a higher rate of EEG
abnormalities. Typical absence seizures may be associated with myoclonic
and generalised tonic-clonic seizures. The term absence seizure or absence
epilepsy, however, has been applied inappropriately to a number of different
epileptic conditions featuring impairment of consciousness.

In this paper, the incidence (the measure of the rate of new cases of a
condition per unit of time within a specified population), prevalence (the
proportion of a population with the condition at a specified time), cumulative incidence (the risk of developing the condition in a population at any
point in life), prognosis (the chance of terminal remission) and mortality
(the chance of dying from or in association with the condition) of typical
absence seizures in the general population are discussed. The published literature on the subject is reviewed and the impact of methodological problems on findings are appraised.

THE PROBLEMS

Under-reporting of absences by patients or carers

Typical absence seizures are characterised by the abrupt but brief suppression, or decrease, of awareness with little or no other associated motor manifestations. It can usually only be diagnosed historically, though occasionally
there may be the chance observation of a seizure. Some patients, particularly
those who have no other associated seizure type, may never come to medical
attention, either because they or their guardians ignore or misinterpret the

symptoms or may be unaware of them. Indeed, it is not rare for patients with absence seizures to come to medical attention only when generalised tonic-clonic or myoclonic seizures develop or when they are referred for another reason, for instance, investigation for lack of concentration at school. In some of these patients, a diagnosis of absences seizures going back a considerable amount of time can then be made.

It is plausible, therefore, that all population studies of epilepsy, both cross-sectional and longitudinal, miss patients with typical absence seizures unless sensitive screening techniques for the condition are included in the case ascertainment. It could be argued that patients not presenting to a medical agency should not be considered a problem. This may hold sway in clinical practice but in the field of epidemiology it is extremely important that all cases are included if meaningful measurements are to be obtained.

The diagnosis

Idiopathic generalised epilepsy with typical absences is defined by the occurrence of absence seizures with a concomitant characteristic EEG discharge that are triggered by hyperventilation in most patients and by photosensitivity in up to a quarter of patients. Contrary to most other epileptic syndromes in which the diagnosis is essentially clinical and the role of the EEG is mainly in classification, in this condition the EEG is essential as the diagnosis is only confirmed when the characteristic discharges are recorded.

Not all patients with absence-like seizures or with 3 Hz spike and wave discharges, however, have typical absences. Absences may be associated with localisation-related epilepsy or may occur in association with other generalised or undetermined epileptic syndromes. For instance, in 346 patients with 3 Hz spike and wave discharges studied by Dalby (1969), only 44% had typical absence seizures, 20% had localisation-related epilepsies and the remainder had other epileptic syndromes.

A problem with reliance on EEG for diagnosis is that occasionally individuals are identified with the characteristic 3 Hz spike and wave discharges on the EEG without a history of seizures. Sometimes these individuals are close relatives of patients with the condition. Whether these subjects should be considered cases or false positives remains a controversial issue. In epidemiological terms, the inclusion or otherwise of such individuals may alter the incidence and prevalence figure to a significant extent.

Case ascertainment

For epidemiological purposes, ideally all cases of a condition should be registered with a study at the time of onset. With epilepsy this is seldom the case. The most common method of case ascertainment is that of a retrospective review of medical notes. In the case of typical absences this usually involves the screening of EEG records or reports searching for the presence of 3 Hz spike and wave discharges. This is a major source of inaccuracy as some cases do not get investigated by EEG. The method is useful, however, to establish cohorts of patients with the condition to assess long-term prognosis.

An epidemiological approach that does not rely on prior diagnosis is to carry out a community or house to house survey using a screening questionnaire that is sensitive and specific. This strategy works for generalised tonic-clonic seizures and other seizure types with florid clinical symptomatology. For typical absences, however, this may not be accurate as a pragmatic screening instrument for this condition has not yet been designed. Indeed, a recent attempt to design such a questionnaire had to be abandoned due to the low specificity of questions relating to absence seizures that would render any field survey using it impractical (Placencia et al, 1992a).

The optimum method to obtain accurate prevalence rates for this condition would be to interview all persons and their close relatives or friends (witnesses) in the proband population or all persons in specific age groups to ascertain a history of absence seizures. This should be followed by recording an EEG with over-breathing in all persons in the population (or only in suspected cases). For an incidence study the whole population in question, particularly those in susceptible age groups, would have to be monitored closely for a specified period of time to identify all new cases at the time of onset. This approach, however, is highly unrealistic in view of the logistical difficulties.

Definitions

In epidemiological work, even if case ascertainment is excellent, problems may arise in the use of definitions and classification. The classification of a seizure as a typical absence depends primarily on a skilfully obtained seizure description and an EEG recording showing the distinguishing discharges. However, even when presented with an EEG recording and clinical data, specialists often fail to agree on seizure classification. EEG recording and the use of enhancing techniques vary from centre to centre and this may complicate the comparison of different studies. The use of EEG in field surveys or retrospective reviews of medical records is also very often impractical. Some published epidemiological studies, however, have quoted figures for generalised absence epilepsy without EEG data (Gomez et al, 1978; Cruz et al, 1986; Haerer et al, 1986; Marino et al, 1987; Osuntokun et al, 1987; Bharucha et al, 1988; Placencia et al, 1992b). The validity of this approach is dubious.

A source of difficulty, particularly in prevalence studies, is the patient with inactive epilepsy. In the majority of people with typical absences, seizures cease but there is no general agreement as to what length of time free of seizures should occur before a patient is no longer designated a case.

All epidemiological surveys reporting on absence seizures should have clear definitions and fixed EEG and clinical criteria on which to base the diagnosis of absences, although these have seldom been published.

Selection bias in study populations

Population selection bias may have an important influence on incidence and prevalence statistics, particularly in a condition like idiopathic generalised epilepsy that has a strong genetic predisposition. There are likely to be regional differences in the incidence of the condition, reflecting genetic factors, although to date this has not yet been clearly shown. Another important factor is that of the demographic characteristics of the population studied. Age is one of the most important variables as the great majority of patients have the onset of typical absences between the ages of 3 and 12 years. Preferential sampling outside the susceptible age group may therefore introduce considerable bias. Age-specific rates should be given where possible. Standardised rates are preferable if standardised data on the population is available. In practice standardised rates for idiopathic generalised epilepsy and typical absences have seldom been reported.

THE PREVALENCE AND INCIDENCE OF TYPICAL ABSENCE SEIZURES

For the reasons discussed above it is likely that there are substantial inaccuracies in all the published epidemiological data for idiopathic generalised epilepsy and typical absences. It is difficult to assess if these inaccuracies are over- or under-estimations of the problem but, on balance, they are more likely to be over-estimations.

Incidence

Estimations of incidence have been made in a number of studies and these range from 0.7–4.6 per 100 000 people in the general population and from 6–8 per 100 000 in children and adolescents up to the age of 15 years. In the Faroe Islands an annual rate of typical absences of 0.7 per 100 000 people in the general population was estimated from a retrospective review of all medical and EEG records covering a period of 11 years. In this study absences presumed to be typical accounted for 1.5% of all cases of epilepsy (Joensen, 1986). In Rochester, Minnesota, epilepsy with typical absences was diagnosed in 3% of all cases of epilepsy in the Mayo Clinic Linkage system and an annual rate of 1.3 per 100 000 population was estimated retrospectively (Hauser & Kurland, 1975). A study of new cases of epilepsy in the Italian district of Copparo over a 15-year observation period estimated an average annual incidence rate of typical absences of 1.9 per 100 000 (Granieri et al,

1983). An annual rate of 2.7 per 100 000 (based on two cases) was assessed retrospectively for the general population in Northern Ecuador (Placencia et al, 1992b); absence seizures were ascertained without recourse to EEG data in this study and were estimated to account for less than 2% of all cases of epilepsy (the minimum annual incidence rate for all types of epilepsy in this region was estimated to be 122 per 100 000). A review of medical records of schoolchildren covering a period of five years in Modena, Italy, estimated a rate of 4.6 per 100 000 for typical absences, although it is likely that other types of absence seizures were included in this group. In this study a rate of 82 per 100 000 for the epilepsies as a whole was given (Cavazzuti, 1980).

In France, an annual incidence rate of 6 per 100 000 children under the age of 16 and of 1.4 per 100 000 for the general population was calculated. This was based on 14 new cases attending specialised clinics in the Department of Gironde over a one-year period (Loiseau et al, 1990). A prospective study of children presenting to paediatric clinics in northern Sweden identified four patients with typical absences during the study year and an annual incidence rate of 8 per 100 000 children aged 0–16 years was derived (Blom et al, 1978). Another study based on a review of all EEG records for children under the age of 16 years carried out in south-west Sweden estimated an annual incidence rate of typical absence seizures of 6.3 per 100 000 children aged 0–15 years and a cumulative incidence at age 15 years of 98 per 100 000 (Olsson, 1988). This later figure compares with a cumulative incidence of 4 per 100 000 at age 14 years, obtained in a study in Tokyo. The case ascertainment in the latter study was based on the attendance of children at a health centre (Tsuboi, 1988; Hauser & Annegers, 1993). It is difficult to determine if this 24-fold difference is entirely due to differences in case ascertainment or to true variations among the populations studied. Typical absences seem, therefore, to be rare in the general population even among the susceptible age group.

Prevalence

Prevalence can be derived from cross-sectional studies in smaller populations than are needed for incidence studies. Although there are many more published studies of prevalence available than of incidence, these are usually of epilepsy as a whole and few quote prevalence figures for typical absences separately. Another compounding factor is that no EEG data is available in many prevalence studies, particularly those carried out in the field. The prevalence rates for typical absences, however, derived from the figures quoted in studies of the general population, are very small, usually in the order of 0.05–0.5 per 1000; typical absences usually account for less than 2% of the patients identified (Hauser & Kurland, 1975; Gomez et al, 1978; Granieri et al, 1983; Li et al, 1985; Marino et al, 1987; Koul et al, 1988;

Keranen et al, 1989; Tekle-Haimanot et al, 1990; Placencia et al, 1992b).

The proportion of patients with typical absences among people with epilepsy has also been given in a number of community- or hospital-based studies covering unselected populations. A figure of around 3% is usually given (Juul-Jensen & Foldspang, 1983; Goodridge & Shorvon, 1983; Keranen et al, 1988; Sander et al, 1990). In the susceptible age groups, figures of up to 10% of all cases of epilepsy have been quoted (Livingston et al, 1965; Sillanpaa, 1973; Hagberg & Hansson, 1976; Blom et al, 1978; Cavazzuti, 1980; Hauser, 1994), although some have suggested a higher figure (Dalby, 1969; Gastaut et al, 1975); the latter, however, may be due to patient selection bias.

THE PROGNOSIS OF IDIOPATHIC GENERALISED EPILEPSY WITH TYPICAL ABSENCE SEIZURES

All indications are that patients with typical absences have an overall good prognosis with regard to full seizure control, particularly if there are no associated complicating factors. In a study of 117 patients with typical absences followed from the onset of the condition, 79% were reported to be seizure-free at age 20 (Livingston et al, 1965). Similarly, Dalby (1969) reported that 79% of patients with typical absences with no other associated seizure types became seizure-free; when absences were associated with generalised tonic-clonic seizures, however, only 33% were seizure-free at the end of a six-year follow-up. Several other studies confirmed this observation (Gordon,1965; Barnhardt et al, 1969; Gibberd, 1972; Oller-Daurella, 1981; Loiseau et al, 1983; Wolf & Inoue, 1984). Other factors put forward as being associated with a worse prognosis include: mental retardation (Lugaresi et al, 1973); onset before the age of 4 years (Currier et al, 1963; Dalby, 1969; Livingston et al, 1965); a positive family history (Sato et al, 1983); abnormal neurological examination or the presence of brain damage; abnormal EEG background; delay in the initiation of treatment (Dalby, 1969); and a long history. There have also been suggestions that females have a slightly less favourable prognosis than males (Dalby, 1969; Sato et al, 1983).

Sato et al (1983), using multivariate analysis, reported a >90% chance of a patient becoming totally seizure-free if at least three of the following factors were present: a negative history of generalised tonic-clonic seizures; IQ of 90 or above; a negative family history; short history; male sex; a normal neurological examination; and normal EEG background activity.

There have, however, been dissenting voices. Gibberd (1972) and Wolf & Inoue (1984) have suggested that a long history of the condition does not rule out the chance of achieving a terminal remission. The presence of absence status epilepticus also does not seem to jeopardise this long-term outcome (Shorvon, 1994).

A major problem with all prognostic series of typical absences is that most studies have used different definitions, case ascertainment and duration of follow-up. Another problem is that more patients with well-controlled seizures tend to be lost to follow-up than those with uncontrolled epilepsy; this may artificially inflate the number of patients with an unfavourable outcome in prognostic series. Despite all these methodological problems, most studies show an excellent prognosis with regard to seizure control. Unlike other types of epilepsy which have been consistently associated with an increased mortality (Nashef et al, 1994), no study so far has suggested such an increase among patients with typical absences.

CONCLUSION

Little is known about the true epidemiology of typical absences in the general population as definitive studies are lacking. Available data, despite its shortcomings, suggests that typical absences are rare, occurring in no more than 3% of all cases of epilepsy in the general population. The condition may, however, be commoner in specific age groups, ie, children and adolescents. Individuals who develop the condition, if there are no complicating factors, have an overall good prognosis both concerning full seizure control and for life.

If future studies are to extend our knowledge in this area, these should be large scale, general population based incidence studies with enhanced standardised EEG recordings as part of case ascertainment. Cohorts of patients so identified should then be prospectively followed in the long term to determine overall prognosis accurately. However, this may not be a feasible proposition in view of the sample size required and the practical and logistical difficulties such studies would pose.

REFERENCES

Barnhardt DA, Newson T, Crawley JW, Zion TE 1969 Long term prognosis of petit mal epilepsy. Electroencephalography and Clinical Neurophysiology 27: 549–550
Bharucha NE, Bharucha EP, Bharucha AE et al 1988 Prevalence of epilepsy in the Parsi community of Bombay. Epilepsia 29: 111–115
Blom S, Heijbel J, Bergfors PG 1978 Incidence of epilepsy in children: a follow-up study three years after the first seizure. Epilepsia 19: 343–350
Cavazzuti GB 1980 Epidemiology of different types of epilepsy in school age children of Modena, Italy. Epilepsia 21: 57–62
Cruz ME, Barberia P, Schoenberg BS 1986 Epidemiology of epilepsy. In: Poeck K, Freund HJ, Ganshirt H (eds) Neurology: Proceedings of the XIII World Congress of Neurology, Springer-Verlag, Berlin pp229–239
Currier RD, Koi K, Saidmann LJ 1963 Prognosis of pure petit mal: a follow-up study. Neurology 13: 959–967
Dalby MA 1969 Epilepsy and 3 per second spike and wave rhythms. A clinical, electroencephalographic and prognostic analysis of 346 patients. Acta Neurologica Scandinavia 45 (Suppl.40)
Dreifuss F 1991 Absences epilepsies. In: Dam M, Gram L (eds) Comprehensive epileptology. Raven Press, New York pp145–153
Gastaut H, Gastaut JL, Goncalves-Silva G, Sanchez GEF 1975 Relative frequency of different

types of epilepsy: a study following the classification of the International League against epilepsy. Epilepsia 16: 457–467

Gibberd FB 1972 The prognosis of petit mal. Epilepsia 13: 171–175

Gomez JG, Arciniegas E, Torres J 1978 Prevalence of epilepsy in Bogota, Colombia. Neurology 28: 90–94

Goodridge DMG, Shorvon SD 1983 Epileptic seizures in a population of 6,000. I: demography, diagnosis and classification and role of the hospital services. British Medical Journal 287: 641–644

Gordon N 1965 The natural history of petit mal epilepsy. Developmental Medicine and Child Neurology 7: 537–542

Granieri E, Rosati G, Tola R et al 1983 A descriptive study of epilepsy in the district of Copparo, Italy, 1964-1978. Epilepsia 24: 502–514

Juul-Jensen P, Foldspang A 1983 Natural history of epileptic seizures. Epilepsia 24: 297–312

Haerer AF, Anderson DW, Schoenberg BS 1986 Prevalence and clinical features of epilepsy in a biracial US population. Epilepsia 27: 66–75

Hagberg G, Hansson O 1976 Childhood seizures. Lancet 2: 208

Hauser WA 1994 The prevalence and incidence of convulsive disorders in children. Epilepsia 35 (Suppl. 2): 1–6

Hauser WA, Annegers JF 1993 Epidemiology of epilepsy. In: Richens A, Chadwick D, Laidlaw J (eds) A textbook of epilepsy. Churchill Livingstone, Edinburgh pp23–45

Hauser WA, Hesdorffer DH 1990 Epilepsy: frequency, causes and consequences. Demos Press, New York

Hauser WA, Kurland LT 1975 The epidemiology of epilepsy in Rochester, Minnesota 1935-1967. Epilepsia 16: 1–66

Joensen P 1986 Prevalence, incidence and classification of epilepsy in the Faroes. Acta Neurologica Scandinavia 76: 150–155

Keranen T, Sillanpaa M, Riekkinen PJ 1988 Distribution of seizure types in an epileptic population. Epilepsia 29: 1–7

Keranen T, Riekkinen PJ, Sillanpaa M 1989 Incidence and prevalence of epilepsy in adults in Eastern Finland. Epilepsia 30: 413–421

Koul R, Razdan S, Motta A 1988 Prevalence and pattern of epilepsy in rural Kashmir, India. Epilepsia 29: 116–122

Li SC, Schoenber BS, Wang CC et al 1985 Epidemiology of epilepsy in urban areas of the People's Republic of China. Epilepsia 26: 391–394

Livingston S, Torres I, Pauli LL, Rider RV 1965 Petit mal epilepsy: results of a prolonged follow-up study in 117 patients. Journal of the American Medical Association 194: 113–118

Loiseau P, Pestre M, Dartigues J et al 1983 Long term prognosis in two forms of childhood epilepsy. Annals of Neurology 13: 642–648

Loiseau P 1992 Absence epilepsy. In: Roger J, Bureau M, Dravet C et al (eds) Epileptic Syndromes in infancy, childhood and adolescence. John Libbey, London pp135–150

Loiseau J, Loiseau P, Guyot M et al 1990 Survey of seizure disorders in the French Southwest: 1. Incidence of epileptic syndromes. Epilepsia 31: 391–396

Lugaresi E, Pazzaglia P, Franck L et al 1973 Evolution and prognosis of generalised epilepsy of the petit mal absence type. In: Lugaresi E, Pazzaglia P, Tassinari CA (eds) Evolution and prognosis of epilepsy. Aulo Gaggi, Bologna pp2–22

Marino Jr R, Cukiert A, Pinho E 1987 Epidemiological aspects of epilepsy in Sao Paulo, Brazil: a prevalence rate study. In: Wolf P, Dam M, Janz D, Dreifuss FE (eds) Advances in epileptology, Vol.16. Raven Press, New York pp759–764

Nashef L, Sander JWAS, Shorvon SD 1994 The mortality of epilepsy. In: Meldrum B, Pedley T (eds) Recent advances in epilepsy. Vol. 6, Churchill Livingstone, Edinburgh (in press)

Oller-Daurella L, Sanchez ME 1981 Evolucion de las ausencias tipicas. Revue Neurologique 9: 81–102

Olsson I 1988 Epidemiology of absence epilepsy: 1. Concepts and incidence. Acta Paediatrica Scandinavia 77: 860–865

Osuntokun BO, Adeuja AOG, Nottidge VA et al 1987 Prevalence of the epilepsies in Nigerian Africans: a community-based study. Epilepsia 28: 272–279

Placencia M, Sander JWAS, Shorvon SD, Ellison RH 1992a Validation of a screening questionnaire for the detection of epilepsy in epidemiological studies. Brain 115: 783–794

Placencia M, Shorvon SD, Paredes V, Sander JWAS, Suarez J, Cascante SM 1992b Epileptic seizures in an Andean region of Ecuador: prevalence, incidence and regional variation. Brain

115: 771–782

Placencia M, Sander JWAS Roman M et al 1994 The characteristics of epilepsy in a largely untreated population in rural Ecuador. Journal of Neurology Neurosurgery Psychiatry 57: 320–325

Sander JWAS, Shorvon SD 1987 Incidence and prevalence studies in epilepsy and their methodological problems: a review. Journal Neurology Neurosurgery Psychiatry 50: 829–839

Sander JWAS, Hart YM, Johnson AJ, Shorvon SD 1990 National general practice study of epilepsy: newly diagnosed epileptic seizures in a general population. Lancet 336: 1267–1271

Sato S, Dreifuss FE, Penry JK 1976 Prognostic factors in absence seizures. Neurology 26: 788–796

Shorvon SD 1994 Status epilepticus in adults and children. Cambridge University Press, Cambridge

Sillanpaa M 1973 Medico-social prognosis of children with epilepsy. Epidemiological study and analysis of 245 patients. Acta Neurologica Scandinavia, (Suppl.) 237: 1–104

Tekle-Haimanot R, Forsgren L, Abebe M, Gebre-Mariam A, Heijbel J, Holmgren G, Ekstedt J 1990 Clinical and electroencephalographic characteristics of epilepsy in rural Ethiopia: a community based study. Epilepsy Research 7: 230–239

Tsuboi T 1988 Prevalence and incidence of epilepsy in Tokio. Epilepsia 29: 103–110

Wolf P, Inoue Y 1984 Therapeutic response of absence seizures in patients of an epilepsy clinic for adolescent and adults. Journal of Neurology 231: 225–229

DISCUSSION

Stephenson: Sander did not separate epidemiology into separate epileptic syndromes. Was this because he does not believe in them or because he thinks it is too difficult?

Sander: I am a firm believer in the syndromes. I looked at typical absences or syndromes with typical absences.

Mirsky: Perhaps Dr Sander is too pessimistic about epidemiological studies. They could be done at various levels. For example, we are involved in a study in Ecuador. The study involves 6118 subjects and we are doing our stratified sample with 327 with extensive neuropsychological analysis. Working together with an epidemiologist, Dr Sander and his colleagues could come up with a sampling method that would give them better data and it may not be necessary to do everything on every subject in their cohort.

Sander: I agree with the problems, having been involved in another study in Ecuador with 72 000 people and knowing how rare this condition is (even in 72 000 people we did not find enough cases to do anything more sophisticated). Apart from screening the entire population with EEG I can see no way out.

Mirsky: It is important to mention behavioural assessment as part of screening. One of the things we did in Ecuador was to use a continuous performance test, as well as other neuro-psychological tasks. This can help to identify cases.

Stephenson: Get everybody to do deep breathing, which invariably reveals typical absences.

Brodie: Nowadays we see confidence intervals with this sort of data and they give us a better idea of the possible figures we can have from the smallish numbers of patients.

Sander: I could recommend quite a good literature on the discussion of the place of confidence intervals in population data. If we look in the general population, the population is what we get and it is one of the places where confidence intervals do not have that much weight. If we screen the whole population we will get our own confidence intervals within that population.

Berkovic: It might not be feasible to do a proper door-to-door epidemiological study, but would it be ethical? Is it proper to find out about the occasional absence?

Sander: I agree entirely. I said very clearly that it was probably not feasible in view of the other issues involved. From a medical point of view, someone with atypical or typical absence who does not come to attention is not a problem. If we are looking epidemiologically, if we are missing a case we have a problem. In epidemiology we should not miss anyone.

18. Definitions and ictal manifestations of typical absences

Joseph Roger   Pierre Genton

The concept of 'typical absences' (TA) was introduced in the 1970 Clinical and EEG Classification of Epileptic Seizures (Gastaut, 1970), but was properly defined only ten years later, in the 1981 International Classification of Epileptic Seizures (Commission, 1981). In both cases the definitions were made negatively, by contrasting clinical and electroencephalographic (EEG) patterns of TA against those of other types of absence seizures.

The 1970 classification only distinguishes between two types of absence seizures: 'simple' absences, with only altered consciousness, and 'complex' absences, which are associated with other clinical phenomena. However, EEG criteria separated 'typical' absences, associated with rhythmic, 3 Hz spike and wave (SW) discharges (and considered characteristic of petit mal), from 'atypical' absences, which are associated with another type of ictal pattern, either slow SW or fast activity, and which were correlated with a 'petit mal variant'. The 1970 classification thus used a two-tier classification of absences, either clinical (simple as opposed to complex) or EEG (typical as opposed to atypical).

The 1981 classification distinguished only between TAs, which are plain 'absence seizures' and are associated with the 3 Hz SW discharges, and atypical absences, which are associated with other ictal patterns. TAs are thus defined by their EEG pattern (whatever the clinical semiology), while all absence seizures associated with other ictal patterns are considered 'atypical'. This dichotomy is in accordance with the accepted rule by which a seizure should be defined both by its clinical and EEG characteristics, and it would be incorrect to classify within the same category seizures that are clinically similar but have different EEG patterns.

ABSENCES AND EPILEPTIC SYNDROMES

The terms 'typical' and 'atypical' are perhaps ill-chosen. What are these absences typical for? Typical absences are found in patients who have idiopathic generalised epilepsy (IGE), while atypical absences are found in patients who do not have IGE. Thus it may be more accurate to state that typical absences are those occurring in IGE and atypical absences are those occurring in other types of epilepsy.

ABSENCES IN EPILEPSIES THAT ARE NOT IGEs

Absences are generalised seizures. Ictal manifestations that resemble absences but are associated with a focal EEG discharge are not absences. These are complex partial seizures, mostly of temporal or frontal lobe origin. Such seizures have been described in the literature as 'pseudo-absences'.

The situation is not always this simple. A focal discharge (that is, mostly sub-clinical and may even not be seen on surface EEG, but only when depth electrodes are used, especially in frontal lobe epilepsies) can be followed by a diffuse or generalised 3 Hz SW discharge that is associated with a clinical symptomatology compatible with the diagnosis of absence. If such a discharge is clinically characterised by loss of contact, and on the EEG by diffuse SWs, why can't it be called a 'typical' absence? Such absences may occur in children with the uncommon but well-characterised syndrome of continuous spikes and waves during slow wave sleep (Tassinari et al, 1992a) or in frontal lobe epilepsies (Roger & Bureau, 1992). In these patients the seizure pattern can be ascribed to secondary bilateral synchrony. In other types of epilepsy, such as the Lennox–Gastaut syndrome, the absences will be considered atypical.

ABSENCES IN IGEs

The International Classification of Epilepsies and Epileptic Syndromes (Commission, 1989) recognised two syndromes of IGE in which absence seizures are the main seizure type: childhood absence epilepsy (CAE) and juvenile absence epilepsy (JAE). A third syndrome of 'epilepsy with myoclonic absences' (Tassinari et al, 1992b) has been classified among 'cryptogenic or symptomatic' generalised epilepsies (see Ch. 23). The 1989 classification does not contain much information about the precise symptomatology of absence seizures in IGEs but it gives important clues concerning their frequency: absences are pyknoleptic (occurring many times per day) in CAE but rather infrequent in JAE. Absences may also occur in other types of IGE (see Ch. 27).

THE SEMIOLOGY OF TYPICAL ABSENCES

The clinical and EEG correlates of absence seizures have been analysed carefully in a number of papers (Penry et al, 1975; Loiseau & Cohadon, 1971; Berkovic et al, 1987; Dreifuss, 1991; Loiseau, 1992; Wolf, 1992; Berkovic, 1993). The seven sub-forms recognised by the 1971 classification (simple absences plus six forms of 'complex' absences) and by the 1981 classification (absence seizures) are summarised in Table 18.1.

At the present stage of our knowledge, one can only agree with Berkovic (1993):

The frequency of the various features depends on how carefully they are sought and the referral base from which cases are drawn. On the basis of ordinary history taking, simple absences and absences with mild clonic components are by far the most common, followed by absences with automatisms and decreased postural tone. Study using videotape increases the frequency of the less commonly identified types and mixed forms. The categorization of typical absences into the seven subforms, although useful descriptively, has dubious clinical or neurobiologic significance.

The important point is that data established concerning the semiology of typical absence seizures depend entirely on the tools used to study the absences, from the simple clinical interview with the parents of the child with epilepsy to the detailed analysis of video-EEG tapes that can be replayed at slow speed.

In their landmark paper using simple video monitoring, Penry et al (1975) found only 9.4% of simple absences (34 out of 374 recorded absences)

Table 18.1 Clinical and ictal EEG definitions of absences

1971 Clinical and EEG classification of epileptic seizures
Simple absences (with impairment of consciousness only)
- with rhythmic 3-Hz SW discharges ('petit mal' or typical absences)
- without 3Hz (variant of 'petit mal' or atypical absence)
  - low-voltage fast activity or rhythmic discharge at 10 Hz or more
  - more or less rhythmic discharge of sharp and slow waves, sometimes asymmetrical

Complex absences, with other phenomena associated with impairment of consciousness
  - with mild clonic components (myoclonic absences)
  - with increase of postural tone (retropulsive absences)
  - with diminution or abolition of postural tone (atonic absences)
  - with automatisms (automatic absences)
  - with autonomic phenomena (e.g. enuretic absences)
  - as mixed forms

1981 Proposal for revised clinical and electroencephalographic classification of epileptic seizures
Absence seizures
    EEG: Usually regular and symmetrical 3 Hz but may be 2–4 Hz spike-and-slow wave complexes and may have multiple spike-and-slow wave complexes
        Bilateral abnormalities
  a.   impairment of consciousness only
  b.   with mild clonic components
  c.   with atonic components
  d.   with tonic components
  e.   with automatisms
  f.   with autonomic components
  b–f   may be used alone or in combination

Atypical absence
    EEG: More heterogenous; may include irregular spike-and-slow wave complexes, fast activity or other paroxysmal activity. Abnormalities are bilateral but often irregular and asymmetrical.

    may have:
  - changes in tone that are more pronounced than in absence seizures
  - gradual onset and/or cessation

Adapted from Epilepsia 1971;11:102–113, and Epilepsia, 1981;22:489–501 and close to 60% of absences were associated with automatisms. They failed, however, to report autonomic components (pallor, flushing, enuresis, pupillary dilation) that are thought to be frequent symptoms of typical absences. In this context, it must be noted also that the absence of polygraphic channels may lead to an under-estimation of myoclonic, atonic and myoclono-atonic components.

It has often been stated that absences always have the same symptomatology in any given patient. This has not been convincingly demonstrated, however, and it has been shown that the clinical expression can change when the environment is modified, leading, for instance, to the appearance of previously non-existent automatisms. Long-term EEG recordings using telemetry have also shown that the semiology of absences changes over the day. They are strongly dependent on environmental factors, to such a degree that one may wonder whether a patient can choose to have a clinically evident absence or not when he experiences a 3 Hz SW discharge (Beaumanoir, 1976).

THE PROGNOSTIC VALUE OF THE SYMPTOMATOLOGY OF TYPICAL ABSENCES

The literature indicates that the precise symptomatology of typical absence seizures is variable, even in a given patient, and does not give any clue as to the long-term outcome that is clouded by the possible resistance to drug therapy and by the later occurrence of generalised tonic-clonic seizures. It is even possible that the precise symptomatology does not give any clue on the precise syndrome of IGE the 'absence epilepsy' may be classified into.

However, these data are not satisfactory. There are several reasons for thinking that typical absences may be associated with different types of evolutions (benign or more severe), may have different consequences on the patient's cognitive function, social adjustment and overall long-term outcome. This points to the existence of different types of absence epilepsies, probably far beyond the two major types (CAE and JAE).

There are no precise data on the coherence of the ictal symptomatology. The only correlation that seems to be well established is the association between the duration of the absence and the occurrence of automatisms (the longer the absence, the more automatisms) (Penry et al, 1975). Another major element is represented by the degree of 'loss of consciousness', or the precise type of cognitive impairment, that occurs during a typical absence. This has not been studied, either in correlation with the duration of the absences, with the other symptoms or with the ictal EEG changes.

Another major blank in our knowledge concerns the precise EEG symptomatology. Although it is considered, by definition, to consist of generalised, symmetrical, rhythmic 3 Hz SW discharges, our clinical experience shows us that other, less 'typical' patterns may be found in patients with one of the clinical variants of typical absences. For example, it has been demonstrated that the EEG symptomatology of 'myoclonic absences', found in a more severe type of epilepsy (Tassinari et al, 1992), is not equivalent to that of 'simple' absences. The EEG symptomatology of 'eyelid myoclonias with absences' (Jeavons, 1977) is not at all comparable with that of the typical absence. In certain families there is a genetic, probably dominant trait that appears as typical absences that are specifically triggered by photic stimulation in the laboratory (Grinspan et al, 1992). The precise neurophysiological correlates of such 'photo-sensitive absences' remain largely unknown.

A more sophisticated approach to the neurophysiological characteristics of absence seizures, using modern electrophysiological tools, will probably yield interesting results. Such studies should be performed to compare the characteristics of absences in the various types of IGE, and in sub-groups of patients characterised by particular clinical traits, in correlation with the outcome of epilepsy, and they will probably cause many entrenched opinions to change.

CONCLUSIONS

In spite of an abundant literature, all has not been said about typical absences. Given the paucity of precise data on the neuropsychological and neurophysiological correlates of absences, it appears that there are different absence types and different clinical entities that do not fit into the major categories of the present classification systems. There is still no proof that absences are all part of a single continuum, varying mainly according to the patient's age and neurological background. In our opinion, absences are syndrome-related, and there are still syndromes characterised by absences that have to be defined more accurately.

REFERENCES

Beaumanoir A 1976 Les épilepsies infantiles. Problèmes de diagnostic et de traitement. Editions Roche, Basle, pp41–48
Berkovic SF 1993 Generalized absence seizures. In: Wyllie E (ed) The treatment of epilepsy. Principles and practice. Lea and Febiger, Philadelphia, pp401–410
Berkovic SF, Andermann F, Andermann E, Gloor P 1987 Concepts of absence epilepsy: discrete syndromes or biological continuum? Neurology 37: 993–1000
Commission on Classification and Terminology of the International League Against Epilepsy 1981 Proposal for revised clinical and electroencephalographic classification of epileptic seizures. Epilepsia 22: 489–501
Commission on Classification and Terminology of the International League Against Epilepsy 1989 Proposal for revised classification of epilepsies and epileptic syndromes. Epilepsia 30: 389–399
Dreifuss FE 1991 Absence epilepsies. In: Dam M, Gram L (eds) Comprehensive epileptology. Raven Press, New York, pp145–153
Gastaut H 1970 Clinical and EEG classification of epileptic seizures. Epilepsia 17: 102–13
Grinspan A, Hirsch E, Malafosse A, Marescaux C 1992 Epilepsie – absences photosensible familiale: un nouveau syndrome? Epilepsies 4: 245–250

Jeavons PM 1977 Nosological problems of myoclonic epilepsies of childhood and adolescence. Developmental Medicine and Child Neurology 19: 3–8

Loiseau P, Cohadon S 1971 Le petit mal et ses frontières. Masson, Paris

Loiseau P 1992 Childhood absence epilepsy. In: Roger J, Bureau M, Dravet C, Dreifuss FE, Wolf P, Perret A (eds) Epileptic syndromes in infancy, childhood and adolescence, 2nd edn. John Libbey Eurotext, London-Paris, pp135–150

Penry JK, Porter RJ, Dreifuss FE 1975 Simultaneous recording of absence seizures with video tape and electroencephalography. A study of 374 seizures in 48 patients. Brain 98: 427–440

Roger J, Bureau M 1992 Distinctive characteristics of frontal lobe epilepsy versus idiopathic generalized epilepsy. In: Cauvel P, Delgado-Escueta AV, Halgren E, Bancaud J (eds) Advances in Neurology, Vol. 57. Raven Press, New York, pp399–410

Tassinari CA, Bureau M, Dravet C, Dalla Bernardina B, Roger J 1992a Epilepsy with continuous spikes and waves during slow sleep – otherwise described as ESES (epilepsy with electrical status epilepticus during slow sleep). In: Roger J, Bureau M, Dravet C, Dreifuss FE, Wolf P, Perret A (eds) Epileptic syndromes in infancy, childhood and adolescence, 2nd edn. John Libbey Eurotext, London-Paris, pp245–256

Tassinari CA, Bureau M, Thomas P 1992b Epilepsy with myoclonic absences. In: Roger J, Bureau M, Dravet C, Dreifuss FE, Wolf P, Perret A (eds) Epileptic syndromes in infancy, childhood and adolescence, 2nd edn. John Libbey Eurotext, London-Paris, pp151–160

Wolf P 1992 Juvenile absence epilepsy. In: Roger J, Bureau M, Dravet C, Dreifuss FE, Wolf P, Perret A (eds) Epileptic syndromes in infancy, childhood and adolescence, 2nd edn. John Libbey Eurotext, London-Paris, pp307–312

DISCUSSION

Panayiotopoulos: I would like to comment on automatisms and typical absence seizures. There is a widely held view that automatisms are related to the length of absence seizures; this is true only if impairment of consciousness is severe. An automatism, by definition, is automatic behaviour released by clouding of consciousness, and therefore they do not occur when cognition is unimpaired or mildly impaired. This is why automatisms are extremely rare in adults with absences, who may have long generalised discharges with no apparent clinical manifestations.

Furthermore, automatisms cannot have a prognostic value, as the same patient may have both simple and complex absences. We have previously shown that a simple absence seizure can be transformed to a complex one through ictal activation of a group of muscles by appropriate passive movements, which often result in automatisms performed by the same group of muscles and related muscles.

Moreover, from the clinical point of view, automatisms are not stereotyped in typical absences, and this may serve in the differential diagnosis from complex partial seizures on the few occasions when difficulties may arise.

Genton: I would agree. By definition, automatisms occur in someone who is not aware of the movement. On the other hand, I read a paper the other day entitled 'Automatisms with preservation of consciousness', so not everybody agrees with this concept of automatisms.

Dreifuss: I want to emphasise that, if one follows up patients with video recording over years, one finds that patients who have been totally unaware and unresponsive in early childhood begin to retain awareness, and very often responsiveness, during absence attacks as they get older.

They recommence breathing long before the attack is over, and may even remember what is said to them during the period of absence. This seems to be a fairly regular occurrence with increasing age. The repertoire of the act changes.

19. Childhood absence epilepsy

Pierre Loiseau   Bernard Duché

Childhood absence epilepsy (CAE) is both a well-known and an ill-known epileptic syndrome. It was first described long ago, but a clear definition has been agreed upon only recently (Commission, 1989). Before that, children suffering from CAE were not considered apart from patients presenting with other types of minor seizures or, after the discovery of a suggestive EEG pattern, those with other forms of typical absences. All were diagnosed petit mal. When clustered under this heading, absence seizures (AS) are very heterogeneous. Benign and malignant progressive varieties of petit mal were described formerly. Patients included otherwise healthy children as well as children suffering from fixed or progressive encephalopathies. Onset of seizures ranged from infancy to adulthood. AS were not necessarily the first type of seizures. This explains why knowledge of the course and prognosis of CAE remains rather limited.

Three milestones mark the history of CAE. A benign paroxysmal disorder in children was characterised by German authors at the beginning of the century (Janz, 1969). In 1906, Friedmann published a paper entitled: 'Über die nichtepileptischen Absencen oder kurzen narkoleptischen Anfälle.' Immediately, Heilbronner denied a relationship between narcolepsy and these 'gehäufte kleine Anfälle'. In 1912 and 1915, Friedmann republished accounts of these frequent short attacks. The term pyknolepsy was given by Sauer in 1916: 'über gehaüfte kleine Anfälle by Kindern (pyknolepsy).' Sauer was of the opinion that it was an epileptic condition.

In 1924, Adie summarised pyknolepsy as follows: 'A disease with an explosive onset between the ages of 4 and 14 years, of frequent, short, very slight, monotonous minor epileptiform seizures of uniform severity which recur almost daily for weeks, months or years, are uninfluenced by antiepileptic remedies, do not impede normal mental and psychological development, and ultimately cease spontaneously never to return.' Adie concluded: 'The disease is only a variety of epilepsy but its clinical characters are so distinct that it seems worthy of a separate name.' One can say, therefore, that at that point a disorder very close to CAE had been recognised, on purely clinical grounds, with as main characters the age of the patients, the high number of absence seizures and a favourable outcome.

The next period came with Janz's contribution. The German epileptologist gave a penetrating description of the various forms of AS and asked for a distinction between petit mal, a term which should encompass all minor seizures, and pyknolepsy, which he held to be a distinct form of childhood epilepsy called pyknoleptic petit mal. For him, the frequency of AS was an important feature (pyknoleptic versus spanioleptic, or non-pyknoleptic absences).

The third period is the current conception, arrived upon as a consequence of an international classification of epileptic syndromes. Modern epileptologists have to determine what qualifies and what does not qualify as CAE. One of the aims of the concept of epileptic syndromes is to allow a prognosis in the presence of a cluster of signs and symptoms. Therefore, the characteristics and the limits of an epileptic syndrome must be precise.

DEFINITION

Childhood absence epilepsy is currently defined as follows:

1. A form of epilepsy with an onset at school age (or before puberty);
2. Occurring in a previously healthy child;
3. Absences as the initial type of seizures;
4. Very frequent AS of any type except myoclonic absences;
5. AS associated in the EEG with bilateral, symmmetrical and synchronous spike-waves, usually at 3 Hz on a normal background activity.

Obviously, CAE corresponds to 'pure petit mal' and to pyknolepsy in the literature.

EPIDEMIOLOGY

CAE is the most frequent syndrome of absence epilepsies, but is not a frequent form of epilepsy. Its annual incidence rate has been estimated between 6.3–8.0 per 100 000 in children aged 1–15 years (Loiseau et al, 1990). In the literature its prevalence rate among epileptic children ranged from 2.3–37.7% due to different case ascertainment and to different recruitment. It represented 8% in school-age epileptic children in one study (Cavazzuti, 1980). In population-based surveys, the prevalence rate of AS has been found to be 0.1–0.7 per 1000 in persons under 16 years of age. Of course, these data might be slightly biased by inclusion of some patients with other types of AS than CAE. CAE is clearly more frequent in girls than in boys (Loiseau, 1992).

AETIOLOGY

Genetics

The evidence for a genetic predisposition in CAE is clear. A positive family history of epilepsy is frequent, reported in 15–44% of cases, but the nature and relative importance of the genetic factors is debated.

Acquired factors

Many factors, such as perinatal anoxia, post-natal head trauma and cerebral inflammatory disease have been reported in the history of 7–30% of children with CAE. They have been proposed as potentially aetiologic. However, without a control group the relationship is only speculative. A population-based case-control study of risk factors failed to detect any significant association between AS and perinatal factors (Rocca et al, 1987).

AGE OF ONSET

Classically, CAE begins between 3 and 12 years of age, with a peak at 6–8 years. An earlier onset is rare but indisputable (Cavazzuti et al, 1989). A second peak has been documented at 11–12 years of age (Oller-Daurella & Sanchez, 1981). One might question its meaning, because it has also been estimated to be the usual age of onset of juvenile absence epilepsy.

SEIZURES

In CAE, AS have some particular electro-clinical features.

Duration

It ranges from 2–3 s to 1–2 min, but is in most cases from 5–10 s and rarely lasts longer than 45 s (Penry et al, 1975).

Signs

The International Classification of Epileptic Seizures (Commission, 1981) distinguishes six types of typical AS, according to their associated clinical features. These distinctions are mainly based on ancient clinical observations and might be considered as an over-simplification of this seizure type – for nosological purposes incomplete and meaningless. Intensive video-EEG monitoring has shown that, in almost 50% of cases, at least two components are present during a given AS and that several of these artificial types of AS may co-exist in a given patient despite a statistically significant tendency for individual patients to have seizures of the same sort (Penry et al, 1975). Janz (1969) observed that no single form of AS is characteristic of pyknoleptic petit mal. Significant clinical and EEG differences have been reported in the AS patterns of CAE, JAE, JME and myoclonic absence epilepsy (Panayiotopoulos et al, 1989).

Three signs are of value. The first one is the degree of impairment of consciousness: a complete abolition of awareness, responsiveness and memory is the rule. The second one is important because it may lead to a wrong diagnosis. Automatisms are quite often observed. They are related to the duration of the attack, their frequency increasing with increasing absence duration, ranging from 22% in a seizure lasting less than 3 s to 95% in a seizure lasting more than 16 s (Penry et al, 1975). They are no more specific for CAE than the other components of so-called complex AS. The third sign held to be a characteristic clinical manifestation of AS in CAE is an early eye-opening (Panayiotopoulos et al, 1989).

EEG

The classical inter-ictal and ictal EEG abnormality is the 3 Hz spike and wave, with a possible faster onset, at 3.5 Hz, gradually slowing to 2.5 Hz. In the past, more irregular spike-wave discharges were considered compatible with a diagnosis of CAE. Panayiotopoulos (1994) considers them as exclusion criteria. Endorsing this opinion are the results of an important study of absence seizures in children (Holmes et al, 1987). The authors operationally defined absence seizures as typical or atypical using EEG criteria alone, whatever the clinical picture. AS were considered as typical only when associated with regular 3 Hz spike-waves. Atypical absence seizures were defined either by slow spike-waves or by faster but irregular multiple spike-and-wave discharges. Even though the authors concluded that typical and atypical absence seizures form a continuum, a diagnosis of CAE is much more likely in patients with typical absences.

Some children exhibit an inter-ictal delta rhythm, usually as long bursts of high-voltage regular activity, at 3 Hz, in occipital and occipito-parietal areas. This is probably specific for CAE and is considered a favourable prognostic sign. A marked photo-sensitivity should be a criterion of exclusion.

Repetition

Attacks are very frequent throughout the day. Their true frequency is most often under-estimated by clinical observation, as demonstrated by prolonged EEG recordings.

OUTCOME

At the beginning of the century most authorities were of the opinion that the disorder had a good prognosis. It was Adie's pyknolepsy. It was Lennox's opinion, too. Later on, the prognosis of petit mal was considered to be poor. Most of the literature is inconclusive concerning the evolution and prognosis of CAE for two reasons. First, different forms of absence epilepsies have been mixed under the heading of petit mal or typical absences. Secondly, a prolonged follow-up is mandatory to ascertain the long-term outcome of the syndrome. Control of AS is not an absolute indication of good prognosis, since generalised tonic-clonic seizures may occur many years after the cessation of AS.

The short-term follow-up of treated patients shows that ethosuximide and valproate have a similar efficacy. Alone or in combination they control 70–80% of patients. In Europe, valproate is the first-line drug because of its efficacy in the control of GTCS. The importance of lamotrigine is still unknown.

The long-term follow-up of patients having experienced CAE indicates three outcomes:

- Patients become rapidly seizure-free and do not relapse after stopping medication. A wide range of remission rates has been given. It has been stated that the longer the follow-up, the smaller the percentage of controlled patients.
- Absence seizures persist. This is a rare occurrence. AS become less frequent and tend to be very short, not very troublesome to the patient.
- Tonic-clonic seizures develop. They begin in most cases between 10–15 years of age, but may appear in some patients beyond 20 and even 30 years of age. Onset of GTCS is most frequently 5–10 years after the onset of AS, but the time-lag may be shorter or longer. A distinction has been made between two groups of patients presenting with GTCS: (1) incidental seizures occuring above the age of 16 in association with precipitating factors like insufficient sleep, alcohol abuse, stress etc; and (2) GTCS beginning between 8–15 years of age without relation to precipitating factors. They may be frequent and difficult to treat (Dieterich et al, 1985). Predisposing factors for a favourable outcome are: female gender, onset before the age of 8, short duration of AS period, rapid response to therapy and posterior delta rhythms.

CONCLUSIONS

A precise diagnosis allows an accurate prognosis and a correct risk-benefit analysis of treatment for an individual patient. However, the syndromic approach implies that we do not squeeze patients into syndromes where they do not strictly fit. Not all patients are classifiable. A diagnosis may be compared to a jigsaw puzzle: the picture takes shape only when a sufficient number of pieces are in place. No single sign is characteristic of CAE.

Let us come back to the definition of CAE (Commission, 1989):

1. A form of epilepsy with an onset at school age (or before puberty). School age is not very precise. Puberty is not a safe item, because of marked chronological variations in sexual development. The simplest definition is one fixing an age range. In this case a period ranging from 1 to 9 or 10 years seems reasonable. However, all AS occurring in this age span do not belong to CAE. In JME with an early onset, AS are usually the presenting sign of this distinct syndrome. We do not believe that CAE can occasion-

ally evolve into JME. A misdiagnosis would have serious consequences because of the different outcome and therapy duration in the two syndromes. Juvenile absence epilepsy with spanioleptic absences may begin before puberty. Conversely, CAE may have a late onset.

2. Otherwise normal children. Individuals with idiopathic mental subnormality belong to a normal population.
3. Absences as the initial type of seizures. This is a mandatory criterion.
4. Very frequent AS. This sign, too, is a very important clue for a diagnosis of CAE. As Lennox wrote: 'If attacks do not recur daily, the diagnosis may be questioned.'
5. On EEG, bilateral, synchronous symmetrical spike-waves, usually 3 Hz, on a normal background activity. This pattern is necessary but is not sufficient. Other absence epilepsies share it with CAE.

The Commission on Classification and Terminology of the International League Against Epilepsy added: 'During adolescence, GTCS often develop. Otherwise, absences may remit or, more rarely, persist as the only seizure type.' Often means between 40 and 60%.

APPENDIX

We tried to challenge this pessimistic opinion with a retrospective study of 89 patients (55 girls) diagnosed as CAE. Inclusion criteria were as follows: consecutive patients with typical AS occurring between 3 and 10 years of age as a presenting sign in normal children, with no history except febrile seizures, daily and EEG-recorded AS, seen within the year of onset of AS or of treatment, and aged >20 years at follow-up. EEG with multiple or irregular spike-waves and or photo-sensitivity were excluded..

It was a difficult and disappointing task because 36 (40%) patients were lost to follow-up. The striking points in the remaining 53 patients were as follows:

- AS persisted beyond the age of 20 in five patients only, remaining the sole seizure type in two (now aged 27 and 47 years).
- GTCS were noted in 14 patients. Eleven had isolated or rare seizures, and only two had experienced seizures in the previous two years. An under-estimation of the frequency of GTCS in this series is unlikely. Of course, seizures can occur later in younger patients: one experienced a first seizure at 25 years. However, there is some evidence that lost patients would have come back if experiencing a seizure. A difference was noted according to the patient's age at onset of AS: only six of the 37 who were under 9 years at onset developed GTCS, compared with eight of the 16 with an onset at 9 or 10 years.
- Posterior delta rhythm was recorded in 11 patients. All of them are controlled. However, one experienced a single GTCS; another, now aged 29,

experienced numerous GTCS between the ages of 17 and 24.

- There is good evidence that AS may be rapidly controlled, resulting in a highly favourable outcome (Oller-Daurella & Sanchez, 1981). In this series, AS definitely disappeared in 12 patients within some weeks of starting medication. However, they persisted for several years in most cases: between 1 and 4 years in 29 patients and up to 8, 11 and 19 years in individual patients. Furthermore, relapses were observed 1–5 years after an early response to therapy in six patients. Such relapses in seizure-free patients were related to poor compliance and incidental factors (Dieterich et al, 1985). We were also surprised by the length of therapy in this series. For controlled patients having experienced AS only, it ranged from 2–20 years (mean 7 years). At follow-up, 10 patients were still on medication. A general rule is to taper patients off medication after two seizure-free years (Pearl & Holmes, 1993). Our data question this rule.

REFERENCES

Cavazzuti GB 1980 Epidemiology of different types of epilepsy in school age children of Modena, Italy. Epilepsia 21: 57–62
Cavazzuti GB, Ferrari F, Galli V, Benatti A 1989 Epilepsy with typical absence seizures with onset during the first year of life. Epilepsia 30: 802–806
Commission on Classification and Terminology of the International League Against Epilepsy 1981 Proposal for revised clinical and electroencephalographic classification of epileptic seizures. Epilepsia 22: 489–501
Commission on Classification and Terminology of the International League Against Epilepsy 1989 Proposal for revised classification of epilepsies and epileptic syndromes. Epilepsia 30: 389–399
Dieterich E, Baier WK, Doose H, Tuxhorn I, Fischel H 1985 Long-term follow-up of childhood epilepsy with absences. I. Epilepsies with absences at onset. Neuropediatrics 16: 149–154
Holmes GH, MacKeever M, Adamson M 1987 Absence seizures in children: clinical and electroencephalographic features. Annals of Neurology 21: 268–273
Janz D 1969 Die Epilepsien. Spezielle Pathologie und Therapie. Georg Thieme, Stuttgart
Loiseau P 1992 Childhood absence epilepsy. In: Roger J, Bureau M, Dravet Ch, Dreifuss FE, Perret A, Wolf P (eds) Epileptic syndromes in infancy, childhood and adolescence. John Libbey, London, pp135–150
Loiseau J, Loiseau P, Guyot M, Duché, B, Dartigues JF, Aublet B 1990 Survey of seizure disorders in the French Southwest. I. Incidence of epileptic syndromes. Epilepsia 31: 391–396
Oller-Daurella L, Sanchez ME 1981 Evolucion de las ausencias tipicas. Revista de Neurologia 9: 81–102
Panayiotopoulos CP The clinical spectrum of typical absence seizures and absence epilepsies. In: Malafasse A, Genton P, Hirsch E, Marescaux C, Broglin D, Bernasconi R (eds) Idiopathic generalised epilepsies: clinical, experimental and genetic aspects. John Libbey, London, pp 73–83
Panayiotopoulos CP, Obeid T, Waheed G 1989 Differentiation of typical absences in epileptic syndromes. A video EEG study of 224 seizures in 20 patients. Brain 112: 1039–1056
Pearl P L, Holmes GL 1993 Absence seizures. In: Dodson WE, Pellock JM (eds) Pediatric epilepsy: diagnosis and therapy. Demos, New York, pp 157–169
Penry JK, Porter RJ, Dreifuss FE 1975 Simultaneous recording of absence seizures with

videotape and electroencephalography: a study of 374 seizures in 48 patients. Brain 98: 427–440

Rocca WA, Sharbrough FW, Hauser WA, Annegers JF, Schoenberg BS 1987 Risk factors for absence seizures: a population-based case-control study in Rochester, Minnesota. Neurology 37: 1309–1314

DISCUSSION

Wolf: Photo-sensitivity was said to be rare in childhood absence epilepsy. In our study, childhood absence epilepsy had photo-sensitivity in about 15%, which means that this is one of three syndromes that are correlated significantly with photo-sensitivity.

Loiseau: We looked at it in terms of prognosis. We do not consider photo-sensitive patients as having childhood absence epilepsy. We discarded it.

Panayiotopoulos: Loiseau is considered very experienced and conservative. In his definition of childhood absence epilepsy he expects children to have severe impairment of consciousness. Therefore, patients who may have absences in childhood without severe impairment of consciousness he would not consider as having childhood absence epilepsy.

Secondly, he does not include in childhood absence epilepsy patients with photo-sensitivity because of the relatively bad prognosis. For example, eyelid myoclonia with absences is not and should not be included in childhood absence epilepsy. He also emphasised that he would exclude from CAE absences with marked myoclonic jerks and polyspikes.

The other point is that he does not agree with those who say that juvenile myoclonic epilepsy starts as childhood absence epilepsy or juvenile absence epilepsy. The fact is that JME may start with absences in childhood or adolescence but these absences of JME are different to CAE or JAE. Is that right?

Loiseau: Yes. It is not only a question of age. It was clearly written by Dieter Janz: childhood absence epilepsies, pyknoleptic absences. If at 13 or 14 years of age they begin absence seizures with severe impairment of consciousness and 50 absences a day, then even though they are older it is childhood absence epilepsy.

Berkovic: I am troubled by photo-sensitivity. The observation that children who have absences and photo-sensitivity and tonic-clonic seizures have a worse prognosis than those who do not is interesting and very important, and probably not in dispute. But it does not make sense to suddenly make up our minds that if they do have that they do not have childhood absence epilepsy.

The best genetic evidence as I understand it probably comes from Doose et al. Their view is that the trait of photo-sensitivity is probably inherited independently, or at least partially independently, from the otherwise generalised spike-wave. We do ourselves a disservice in trying to understand these diseases if we make up our minds that photo-sensitivity is not childhood absence epilepsy.

Loiseau: The conception of Sanome is not to pick one thing but to put this data into a general framework. What I have to do is to help the parents understand the likely outcome for their child: how s/he will be in ten years' time, whether s/he will get a driving licence and so on. Without photo-sensitivity the prognosis is good but with photo-sensitivity I am not quite sure, and so I prefer to discount them and consider them as a special sub-group.

Berkovic: But we are mixing up prognosis and classification of disease, which is usually based on mechanism.

Panayiotopoulos: We have to. Prognosis is by definition an important criterion that we apply when we are making the diagnosis.

Berkovic: No. We diagnose the syndromes to identify patients so that we can understand what its underlying biology is, and its natural history, and what the treatment is.

Marescaux: One comment on photo-sensitivity. We should try to be precise. We have to differentiate severe photo-sensitivity, where clinical absences are consistently induced by light stimulation. I believe then that the prognosis is bad. This kind of patient never achieves remission and usually has tonic-clonic seizures. These severe forms of photo-sensitive absences should be differentiated from these where mild EEG generalised abnormalities are induced by photic stimulation.

20. Juvenile absence epilepsy

Peter Wolf

According to the Revised International Classification of Epilepsies and Epileptic Syndromes (Commission, 1989), juvenile absence epilepsy (JAE) is one of the age-related idiopathic generalised epilepsies. The following description is given: 'The absences of JAE are the same as in pyknolepsy, but absences with retropulsive movements are less common. Manifestation occurs around puberty. Seizure frequency is lower than in pyknolepsy, with absences occurring less frequently than every day, mostly sporadically. Association with GTCS is frequent, and GTCS precede the absence manifestations more often than in childhood absence epilepsy, often occurring on awakening. Not infrequently, the patients also have myoclonic seizures. Response to therapy is excellent.'

A more detailed and updated description was given by Wolf (1992). It is still under discussion if JAE and childhood absence epilepsy are separate syndromes or, rather, sub-varieties of one syndrome. Twin findings are in favour of their genetic disparity (Berkovic, 1994) but the definitive answer has to await more precise genetic data.

DESCRIPTION

There are no epidemiological data on the syndrome, but it can be assumed that the condition is less frequent than childhood absence epilepsy (CAE), and it seems that the sex distribution is equal. A family history of epilepsy is frequent, and identical twins who both have the syndrome have been reported by Berkovic (1994) and by Panayiotopoulos et al (1989). The latter author reported that in a Saudi Arabian population where consanguineous marriages are frequent and can be found in 47 per cent of the families of patients with Juvenile Myoclonic Epilepsy (JME), this was only true for one of 14 JAE families. It seems therefore likely that a recessive gene is important in JME but not JAE.

Age of onset is mostly in the range of 7–17 years. The seizure frequency is lower than in pyknolepsy, with clinical absences occurring less frequently than every day and mostly sporadically. The same types of absence occur as in CAE, but absences with retropulsive movements are less common. In one video-based study (Panayiotopoulos et al, 1989), language functions in JAE absences were less rapidly abolished, consciousness was less severely impaired, and hyperventilation stopped later than in CAE. Spontaneous eye opening was rare, and simple absences were more common.

The majority of patients also have GTC seizures, but it may be that JAE absences are often overlooked if they are the only seizure type. If the patients also have GTC seizures, their manifestation precedes that of the absences more often than in CAE. Most frequently, they belong to the awakening type.

Association with myoclonic seizures of the type seen in JME is more common than in CAE, probably in the order of 15–20%.

In the EEG, the background activity is usually normal. The characteristic feature of the interictal and ictal EEG is generalised symmetric SW discharge with frontal accentuation. The SW frequency is usually faster than 3 Hz (3.5–4 Hz), the first complex of a group sometimes being even faster. Often the slow wave is preceded by two or three spikes. According to Panayiotopoulos et al (1989), the ictal discharges were longer in JAE (16.3 ± 7.1 s) than in CAE (12.4 ± 2.1 s) and in JME (6.6 ± 4.2 s). They were more regular than in JME but could show fragmentation unlike in CAE. In one study (Wolf & Goosses, 1986), photosensitivity was less common than in other idiopathic generalised epilepsies, but this was not confirmed in the only other study (Waltz et al, 1990).

The response to therapy is good in spite of the frequent combination with GTC seizures. According to Wolf and Inoue (1984) non-pyknoleptic absences (i.e., the type in JAE) respond better to therapy with succinimides or valproic acid, or both, and combination with myoclonic seizures does not affect the prognosis. (A more detailed description may be found in Wolf, 1992.)

TWO CASE HISTORIES OF JUVENILE ABSENCES

Case 1: Anja K was 10 years old when I saw her following her first seizure. Her mother is in my treatment for a rather benign type of focal epilepsy. In her third decade of life she started to have sporadic isolated auras consisting of an indescribable feeling of strangeness. This didn't impress her as something pathological until, at the age of 39, she suffered a series of three and a single GTC seizure starting with such an aura. Her EEG never presented any epileptiform discharge and the only noticeable findings were some occipital delta rhythms. With carbamazepine monotherapy (her highest serum level ever found was 7.9 µg/ml) control was reached immediately. After seven years' treatment with decreasing dosage, and a further year free of drugs, she has now been completely seizure free for eight years.

Anja's first GTC seizure was observed by her brother. It occurred in the evening after school and her riding lesson. She was brought to a hospital where all investigations were normal apart from her EEG which presented 'generalised irregular SW paroxysms of up to 3 s duration' and, during sleep, right rolandic sharp waves. Another EEG one week later demon-strated photo-sensitivity with SW at flash frequency 6 Hz (her mother was not photo-sensitive at the age when she was investigated).

A video-EEG at our centre displayed photo-sensitivity at 20 Hz where a generalised SW discharge was provoked which outlasted the stimulus by 3.6 s (Fig. 20.1, left). In the unprovoked recording, focal sharp waves were observed at P4, 02, and P3, but no generalised discharges. There also were some short occipital delta rhythms similar to her mother's.

In a series of patients with first seizures Anja is exceptional because no convincing precipitating cause for her seizure could be identified. The fam-ily decided against pharmacotherapy and was counselled about avoidance of precipitants such as sleep irregularities.

Three months after the first, Anja had a second seizure without any pre-cipitant, at noon after school. A new video-EEG investigation now revealed, at hyperventilation, three brief generalised SW discharges (Fig. 20.1, right). Tests of responsiveness to an acoustic stimulus during these revealed impaired consciousness along with initial slight eyelid myoclonia. She was, however, not completely unconscious, reporting that at one point she had heard the acoustic signal but 'could not remember what was expected as a response'; at another she gave a correct but delayed response. Treatment with valproic acid 300 mg per day was started (serum levels around 15 µg/ml) and Anja has now been free of seizures and absences for two years. Her EEG contains no SW discharges.

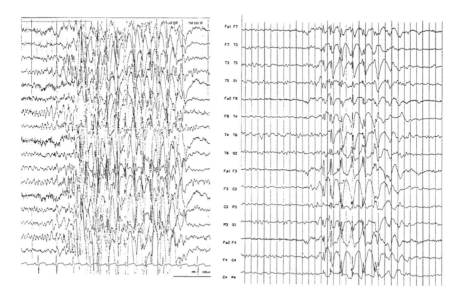

Fig. 20.1 Left: photo-sensitivity of Patient 1 with JAE; sub-clinical SW outlasting an intermittent light stimulus of 20 Hz. Right: absence in the same patient. There were some missing responses to an acoustic stimulus during the SW.

This was a rare case where, uninfluenced by drugs, the onset of JAE could be observed. Here the first manifestation was a GTC seizure which, according to Janz (1969), is slightly less common than onset with absences, although this mode of onset is more frequent in JAE than in childhood absence epilepsy (pyknolepsy). It is interesting to note, however, that this GTCS was unprovoked, unlike the usual first juvenile GTCS. It is noteworthy that Anja's mother also has a benign epilepsy but of a focal type, and the patient had, in her first EEG, some focal sharp waves. Nonetheless, this could be considered as a reasonably typical case of JAE.

Case 2: Heike K was 28 years old when first seen. Her history also starts with absences at the age of ten. According to a video-EEG investigation, she also has partly impaired consciousness. She is sometimes able to repeat a test word given to her during an SW discharge, sometimes not. Her EEG (Fig. 20.2) presents, on a slightly irregular background with a predominant 8 Hz alpha rhythm, more or less irregular 2.5–4.0 Hz SW preceded by a short run of generalised spikes. The most prominent clinical signs are myocloni, mostly of the axial and proximal limb muscles, which make the body shake or shudder, often accompanied by mild rhythmic cloni of the perioral musculature.

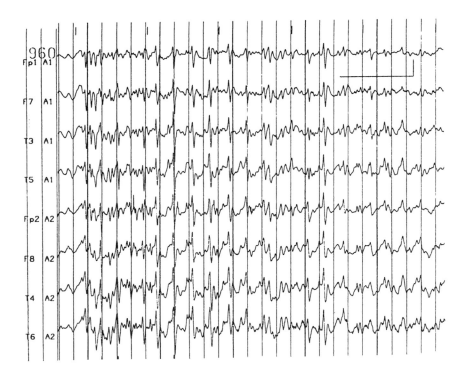

Fig. 20.2 Ictal EEG of Patient 2: absence with mild clonic components; onset with a run of generalised spikes (Gain 300 μV).

Heike has also had rare GTC seizures. Occasionally, tonic spasms of her right extremities were observed in an absence and, rarely, these could cause a fall. In her EEGs, focal spikes in variable loci of either hemisphere have rarely been described along with generalised SW and PSW discharge. This patient has no positive family history. She presents moderate to severe mental retardation, and some soft motor signs at neurological investigation. There is no indication of a specific aetiology but her birth was complicated by prolonged labour and severe postnatal blue asphyxia. Her cerebral CT presents mild symmetrical internal and external signs of atrophy and is considered consistent with mild perinatal brain damage.

Heike's epilepsy is very difficult to treat, having proved resistant to many anti-epileptic drugs in monotherapy and combinations. Classification is difficult. There are no clinical or EEG symptoms and signs which are not covered by the description in the International Classification of Epileptic Seizures (Commission, 1981) of absences with mild clonic (plus rare tonic) components, and there is no definite reason to classify them as 'atypical', apart perhaps from the fact that consciousness is not suddenly lost and regained. But the same is true for the highly 'typical' absences of Case 1, as indeed for many 'typical' absences if the patients are tested correctly, especially in JAE (Panayiotopoulos et al, 1989).

Why is this not a case of JAE? Because, at least periodically, Heike's absences are rather frequent? Maybe, but this is a rather soft symptom. Because they are highly pharmaco-resistant? It would be preferable to decide a diagnosis on better arguments than ex non juvantibus. Is it not JAE because she has obvious signs of exogenous brain damage? Perhaps, but are we sure that this is a case of symptomatic epilepsy? Why then should it produce a phenocopy of absences which do not qualify as 'atypical'? There is always the possibility that an idiopathic epilepsy syndrome happens to manifest in a person who also has some exogenous brain damage. Heike seems to suffer from the sequelae of some perinatal brain damage but may, in addition, have inherited a specific gene for JAE.

Should Heike's absences be considered atypical in a way which is not recognised by the International Classification (ICES)? I certainly believe they should, at least in the context of JAE, and mainly because of the unusual distribution of the myocloni, the pattern of which surely contains some clue regarding their pathophysiology and anatomy. Even if we are not yet able to read this message, some day we may understand why and how this deviates from JAE and other known syndromes, whether such absences are typical for some yet undefined syndrome, or if they are individual results of the random interplay of a variety of endogenous and exogenous pathogenetic factors.

DISCUSSION

The present classification of absence seizures was built on an incredibly small number of video-registered absences, and these had not yet been analysed in view of the syndrome classification which came later. Thus among the absence syndromes of the international classification there is one, epilepsy with myoclonic absences, the name-giving seizure type of which is not yet contained in the ICES, and is again different from the absences of our Case 2, which may also have tonic components. The absence sub-classes of the ICES are restricted to basic formal aspects regarding the movement types which can be observed. No attention is paid to their locali-sations and possible lateralisations.

This classification only separates 'absence seizures' from 'atypical absences'. The concept of 'typical' absences is thus implicit rather than explicit; it is neither discussed nor defined. All the recognised absence sub-classes, however, are included in this category.

This obviously is no definite solution but calls in fact for revision. It should more clearly differentiate seizures from syndromes and abstain from calling any seizure type 'atypical', which is a contradictio in adiectu anyway. The seizure classification is a classification of symptoms and should be strictly descriptive. Today, a much larger number of video-registered absences is available for analysis, and it could be tested whether their sub-classification in the 1981 ICES still stands as the best possibility, and what parameters or types should be added or changed. In addition, observed seizures can now be nosologically related to absence syndromes to find out the patterns which are typical for the various syndromes. A first such attempt was the study of Panayiotopoulos et al (1989), which indeed indi-cated the existence of typological differences between the various syn-dromes of idiopathic generalised epilepsy. In that study, however, only three patients with JAE could be included. Further investigations of this kind are highly desirable.

It is still not known exactly what happens when a genetically predeter-mined condition such as the idiopathic absence syndrome manifests in a patient whose brain has suffered some potentially epileptogenic exogenous insult. Will such a situation result in a singular individual pattern tainted by traces of the various pathogenetic influences? Should the genetic syn-drome prevail, how pure will the phenotype be? Therefore, such studies should also identify localising or lateralising clinical and electroencephalo-graphic symptoms and compare these with historical data and physical and ancillary findings to establish their possible relation to exogenous patho-genetic factors.

CONCLUSION

Far from being settled, the classification of absences calls for improvement in view of a better interlinkage of seizure and syndrome classification. The syndrome juvenile absence epilepsy like its counterpart, childhood absence epilepsy, still has to pass the test of genetic identification. Meanwhile, more clarification is needed concerning the semiology of the absences which are typical for the two conditions. At present it seems questionable whether the categorisation of the seizure classification is sufficient and adequate for such a syndromic analysis. Perhaps the most urgent question to be settled by future studies is: what do the typical absences of the various absence syndromes really look like?

REFERENCES

Berkovic S 1994 Lessons from twin studies. In: Wolf P (ed) Epileptic seizures and syndromes, with some of their theoretical implications. John Libbey, London, pp157–164
Commission on Classification and Terminology of the ILAE 1981 Proposal for revised clinical and electroencephalographic classification of epileptic seizures. Epilepsia 22: 489–501
Commission on Classification and Terminology of the ILAE 1989 Proposal for revised classification of epilepsies and epileptic syndromes. Epilepsia 30: 389–399
Janz D 1969 Die Epilepsien. Spezielle Pathologie und Therapie. Thieme, Stuttgart
Panayiotopoulos C P, Obeid T, Waheed G 1989 Differentiation of typical absence seizures in epileptic syndromes. Brain 112: 1039–1056
Waltz S, Beck Mannagetta G, Janz D 1990 Are there syndrome-related genetically determined spike and wave patterns? A comparison between syndromes of generalised epilepsy. Epilepsia 31: 919
Wolf P 1992 Juvenile absence epilepsy. In: Roger J, Bureau M, Dravet C, Dreifuss F, Perret A, Wolf P (eds) Epileptic syndromes in infancy, childhood and adolescence, 2nd edn. John Libbey, London, pp307–312
Wolf P, Inoue Y 1984 Therapeutic response of absence seizures in patients of an epilepsy clinic for adolescents. Journal of Neurology 231: 225–229
Wolf P, Goosses R 1986 Relation of photosensitivity to epileptic syndromes. Journal of Neurology, Neurosurgery and Psychiatry 49: 1386–1391

APPENDIX

Juvenile absence epilepsy: an alternative view

J. S. Duncan   C. P. Panayiotopoulos

The definition of juvenile absence epilepsy (JAE) is mainly based on the pioneer work of Doose et al (1965) and Janz (1969) (see for review Wolf, 1992; Porter, 1993). In accordance with this definition, the main criterion for the diagnosis of JAE is age of onset (after the age of ten years) and frequency of absences (non-pyknoleptic – ie, less frequent than in childhood absence epilepsy). Our belief is that the syndrome of JAE is expressed with many more additional clinical and EEG symptoms and signs which are clustered together in a non-fortuitous manner (Panayiotopoulos et al, 1989; 1992). There are also exclusion criteria which may be as important as inclusion criteria for JAE.

Juvenile absence epilepsy is an idiopathic generalised epileptic syndrome mainly characterised by typical absences which are manifested by abrupt and severe impairment of consciousness. In comparison with CAE the absences of JAe show less severe impairment of cognition (activity may be restored during the ictus), occur less fequently (1–10 per day) and are of longer duration (16±7 s). Random and infrequent myoclonic jerks as well as infrequent generalised tonic-clonic seizures occur in the majority of patients. Unlike in juvenile myoclonic epilepsy, absences are the predominant clinical feature. Age at onset of absences is between 7–16 years with a peak at 10–12 years. JAE is a lifelong disorder, although the absences tend to become less severe in terms of impairment of cognition, duration and frequency with age.

The ictal EEG shows generalised, spike or multiple spike and slow waves at 3 Hz. The frequency at the initial phase of the discharge should be >2.5 s. There is a gradual and smooth decline in frequency from the initial to the terminal phase. The discharge is regular, with well-formed spikes which retain a constant relation with the slow waves. The inter-actal EEG is normal or with mild abnormalities only.

Eyelid or perioral myoclonus, rhythmic limb jerking and single or arrhythmic myoclonic jerks of the head, trunk or limbs during the absence ictus are not compatible with JAE. Visual, photo-sensitive and other sensory precipitation of absences is against the diagnosis of JAE. Mild or no impairment of consciousness, which is common in JME, is not compatible with JAE.

A typical case of JAE is that of an 11-year-old child with frequent (1–10 per day) episodes of unresponsiveness lasting for 10–20 s. Witnesses described how 'The eyes glaze or stare and he is not with it.' There were frequent perioral and limb automatisms which varied in each absence. An EEG confirmed the 'absences' and the diagnosis of petit mal (unsatisfactory term) or 'childhood absence epilepsy' (erroneous diagnosis) was made. Absences responded only when sodium valproate was combined with ethosuximide.

Medication was slowly withdrawn after three years seizure-free but a generalised tonic-clonic seizure occurred half an hour after waking from a short sleep compounded by the excitement of a planned trip to celebrate the end of school examinations. Video-EEG revealed absences typical of JAE and the patient admitted occasional mild jerks of the hands, mainly at night. Retrospective evaluation of the first EEG revealed that the ictal EEG manifestations consisted of long (15–22 s) generalised discharges of multiple spike and wave at 3.5 Hz and that, although the child was usually unresponsive, he could occasionally remember numbers or phrases given to him and kept his eyes closed during the ictus. These are ictal manifestations favouring juvenile not childhood absence epilepsy.

Reviewed at 37 years of age, the patient still has occasional absences, particularly when excited, despite adequate doses of valproate and ethosuximide. He admitted occasional mild jerks occurring randomly in the day. Two GTCS had occurred at the ages of 18 and 19, after excessive and unaccustomed alcohol drinking and sleep deprivation in the first case and missing his tablets in the second.

Prevalence, genetics, precipitating factors and circadian distribution

The exact prevalence of JAE is unknown because the criteria and the definitions are not identical for all authors. JAE is probably less common than

CAE, two to three cases of which will be seen for every one of JAE (Wolf, 1992). The prevalence of JAE among adults with idiopathic generalised epilepsies and absences was 13.3% (see Ch. 14).

Sex and age

Although there is a clear female preponderance in other idiopathic epileptic syndromes with absence seizures, in JAE both sexes are equally affected (Wolf, 1992)

Absences start between 7–16 years with a peak at 10–12 years. Myoclonic jerks and GTCS usually begin 1–10 years from the onset of absences. However, reports of GTCS preceding absences have been published (Wolf, 1992).

Clinical and EEG manifestations

Typical absences are the characteristic and the predominant feature of JAE. Their onset varies from 7–16 years with a peak at 10–12 years and although less frequent (1–10 per day) than in childhood absence epilepsy, there are cases where absences occur several times per day, in a pyknoleptic frequency (Panayiotopoulos et al, 1989; 1992; Obeid, 1994). In JAE, absences show the following features:

- Ictal clinical manifestations demonstrate profound impairment of consciousness which is not as severe as in CAE. Awareness, perception, responsiveness, memory and recollection are deeply but not completely disturbed, with marked variation in severity from seizure to seizure even in the same patient. The patient may temporarily and inadequately maintain some mild awareness and responsiveness during the absence ictus. Even verbal responses may occur towards the end of the discharge. Automatisms (perioral more frequent than limb) are frequent and are proportional principally to the severity of the impairment of consciousness and secondarily to the length of the discharges. Breath counting during hyperventilation usually stops 3–6 s after the onset of the ictal discharge but may restart out of order in the middle or towards the end of the EEG paroxysms (Fig. 20.3). If the eyes are closed during the ictus they may remain closed or they may open spontaneously 3–7 s from its onset.
- The duration of the absences is long (Fig. 1), with a mean of 16±7 s (range 3–29 s).
- The ictal EEG discharges consist of a 3–4 Hz generalised spike and/or multiple spike and slow wave discharge which is regular and continuous.

The ictal clinical and EEG exclusion criteria are equally important as the inclusion criteria:

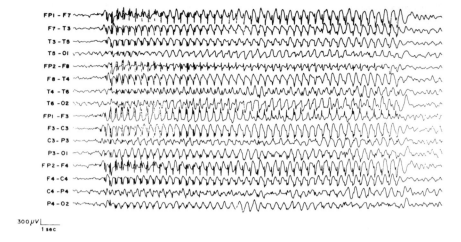

300 μV |____
       1 sec

Fig. 20.3 Video-EEG recording of a typical absence seizure from an 18-year-old patient who had frequent absences daily from age 12 years. His homozygotic twin brother also had JAE. Both brothers had infrequent GTCS together with their 'pyknoleptic' in frequency absences. During the discharge the patient had severe impairment of consciousness. Breath counting was discontinued at the initial phase of the discharge but was resumed, in wrong sequence, 6 seconds before termination. Automatisms occurred after 5 seconds from the onset. The EEG discharge is characterised by the multiple spike and slow wave complexes without fragmentations. The regularity of the discharge is also apparent.

Ictal clinical exclusion criteria
- Absences with marked eyelid or perioral myoclonus or marked single or rhythmic limb and trunk myoclonic jerks.
- Absences with exclusively mild or clinically undetectable impairment of consciousness.

Electroencephalographic exclusion criteria
- Irregular, arrhythmic spike/multiple spike and slow wave discharges with marked variations of the intradischarge frequency.
- Significant variations between the spike/multiple spike and slow wave relations.
- Predominantly brief discharges (less than 4–5 seconds).
- Markedly abnormal background. Focal abnormalities, particularly as the result of abortive discharges, are accepted.

Other types of seizures

Generalised tonic-clonic seizures occur in 80% of patients, mainly after awaking, although nocturnal or diurnal GTCS may also be experienced. GTCS are usually infrequent, occurring in non-compliant patients and often after sleep deprivation, alcohol consumption and fatigue. Myoclonic jerks occur in 15–25% of patients and they are usually mild, infrequent and of random distribution. These myoclonic jerks do not occur during the absence ictus. A patient may have all three types of generalised seizures but absences predominate.

Genetics

There is probably an increased incidence of epileptic disorders in families of patients with JAE (Janz, 1969; Janz et al, 1992) and there are reports of identical twins with JAE (Obeid et al, 1994). The exact mode of inheritance has not yet been established. A multivariant linkage analysis of 25 multiplex families of probands with idiopathic generalised epilepsies with absences (JME patients were not included) excluded EJM1 locus for contributing to the clinical expression of IGEs in these families (Sander et al, 1994).

Prognosis and treatment

JAE is a lifelong disorder which is not expected to remit although absences become less severe after the fourth decade. Therefore, the prognosis of JAE is not as good as in CAE, although more than 80% of patients become seizure-free with appropriate medication: sodium valproate alone or in combination with ethosuximide. In resistant cases, small doses of lamotrigine 25–50 mg added to sodium valproate resulted in complete cessation of absences in 50% of patients (Panayiotopoulos et al, 1993; Ferrie et al, 1994). Some authors have advocated the use of amantadine hydrochloride as an add-on drug in generalised epilepsies with absences (Drake et al, 1991). GTCS and myoclonic jerks occasionally persist even if absences are well controlled.

Differential diagnosis

JAE, an idiopathic generalised epilepsy, is easy to differentiate from syndromes with atypical absences which are mainly symptomatic or cryptogenic. However, the differentiation of JAE from other idiopathic generalised epilepsies with absences may impose considerable difficulties without appropriate video-EEG evaluation of the absences.

In children the differential diagnosis between CAE and JAE is often difficult because of overlapping features and similar manifestations. In JAE absences show less severe impairment of cognition, they are less frequent and of longer duration than in CAE. The eyes may remain closed during the ictus and the patient may restore counting or respond to commands in the last seconds before the end of the discharge (Panayiotopoulos et al, 1989). Automatisms are equally prominent in both CAE and JAE. Limb myoclonic jerks (not during the absences) and/or GTCS in the presence of severe absences indicate JAE.

JAE is different from eyelid myoclonia with absences (EMA). EMA is characterised by brief (3–6 s) absences with rapid eyelid myoclonia (fast, blinking-like jerks of the eyelids) together with tonic spasm and semi-opening of the eyelids and upwards deviation of the eyes. Patients with EMA are photo-sensitive and age at onset is earlier than in CAE and JAE (see Ch. 25).

Similarly, JAE is easily differentiated from perioral myoclonia with absences. This is a syndrome characterised by rhythmic perioral myoclonia during the absences which rarely show severe impairment of cognition and their duration is shorter than in JAE. Absence status and GTCS are common (see Ch. 26).

The rhythmic myoclonic movements of myoclonic absence epilepsy are characteristic and cannot be mistaken (see Ch. 23).

In adolescents, the differential diagnosis may be difficult between JAE and JME. However, absences are the major problem in JAE (more frequent and with severe impairment of consciousness) but not in JME, (where absences are often so mild as to be not easily discernible). Conversely, myoclonic jerks occurring mainly on awakening are the main seizure type in JME.

In adults absences are often misdiagnosed as complex partial seizures (Panayiotopoulos et al, 1992).

Comment

The significance of using stricter criteria for the definition of JAE than simply age at onset and frequency of absences is well illustrated in the two cases presented in the foregoing chapter. Both patients suffer from absences with juvenile onset, which, according to our thesis, is not the determining criterion of JAE. Neither of these cases meet the definition criteria for JAE. Absences in Case 1 were so mild and brief that neither the patient nor those around her were aware of them (Phantom absences? see Ch. 34); they were detected only by EEG and psychological testing. This is in contrast with the severe impairment of consciousness of absences in JAE. Case 2 had mental retardation and soft neurological signs which, by definition, is an exclusion criterion of idiopathic epilepsies. Furthermore, her absences with predominant myoclonic jerking do not show any similarities with those of JAE.

Conclusion

Juvenile absence epilepsy is a syndrome characterised mainly by absences, imitating those of CAE and infrequent myoclonic jerks and/or GTCS, imitating JME. The phenotypic manifestations of JAE are intermediate between CAE and JME. Whether this is also the case in their genotypes remains to be seen (Janz et al, 1992). Irrespective of this the clinical distinction of patients with JAE from CAE and JME is essential because of different prognosis and management.

REFERENCES

Drake ME Jr, Pakalnis A, Denio LS, Philips B 1991 Amantadine hydrochloride for refractory generalised epilepsy in adults. Acta Neurologica Belgica 91:159–164

Doose H, Volzke E, Scheffner D 1965 Verlaufsformen kindelicher Epilepsien mit Spike-Wave-Absencen. Arch Psychiatr Nervenkrh 207: 394–415.

Ferrie CD, Robinson RO, Panayiotopoulos CP, Knott C 1994 Lamotrigine in typical absence seizures. Acta Neurologica Scandinavica (in press)

Janz D 1969 Die Epilepsien. Spezielle Pathologie und Therapie. Thieme, Stuttgart

Janz D, Beck-Managetta G, Sander T 1992 Do idiopathic generalised epilepsies share a common susceptibility gene? Neurology 42 (Suppl. 5):48–55.

Obeid T 1994 Juvenile absence epilepsy. European Neurology (in press).

Panayiotopoulos C P, Chroni E, Daskalopoulos C, Baker A, Rowlinson S, Welsh P 1992 Typical absence seizures in adults: clinical, EEG, video-EEG findings and diagnostic/syndromic considerations. Journal of Neurology, Neurosurgery and Psychiatry 55: 1002–1008

Panayiotopoulos CP, Ferrie CD, Robinson RO, Knott C 1993 Interaction of lamotrigine with sodium valproate. Lancet 340: 1223

Panayiotopoulos CP, Obeid T, Waheed G 1989 Differentiation of typical absences in epileptic syndromes. A video EEG study of 224 seizures in 20 patients. Brain 112: 1039–1056

Porter RJ 1993 The absence epilepsies. A review. Epilepsia 34 (Suppl. 3): S42-S48

Sander T, Hildmann T, Beck-Managetta G, Neitzel H, Bianchi A, Janz D 1994 Exclusion of linkage between the EJM1 locus and idiopathic generalised epilepsies in absence families. In: Malafosse A, Genton P, Hirsch E, Marescaux C, Broglin D, Bernusconi R (eds) Idiopathic generalised epilepsies. John Libbey, London (in press)

Wolf P 1992 Juvenile absence epilepsy. In: Roger J, Bureau M, Dravet P, Dreifuss F E, Perret A, Wolf P (eds) Epileptic syndromes in infancy, childhood and adolescence. John Libbey, London, pp 307–312

21. Juvenile myoclonic epilepsy with absences

Dieter Janz   Stephan Waltz

Since its rediscovery by Delgado-Escueta & Enrile-Bacsal (1984) and Asconapé & Penry (1984), juvenile myoclonic epilepsy (JME) has become a prototype for a clinical and aetiologically homogeneous epileptic syndrome. The leading symptom is bilateral arrhythmical jerking of the arms and shoulders in full consciousness. An age of onset restricted to around puberty and characteristic fast spike-wave patterns on the EEG are also typical diagnostic criteria. Certainly there are other symptoms found also in other syndromes, such as generalised tonic-clonic seizures (GTCS) in about 90% and absences in about 30%. A review of the literature of 485 cases reveals 8% with myoclonic jerks as the only symptom and in 90% of cases a combination with GTCS (Table 21.1). A combination with absences was reported in 28%. Among these cases, 1% featured a combination of jerks with absences without GTCS, a finding which we have never observed.

Table 21.1 Type of seizure in JME

	Authors	Absences	Jerks and absences only	Jerks only	GTCS	Total
1984	Asconape & Penry	3	–	2	10	12
1984	Delgado-Escueta & Enrile-Bascal	17	–	1	42	43
1986	Numata et al	5	–	1	24	25
1988	Obeid & Panayiotopoulos	9	–	1	40	50
1989	Matsuoka	9	3	7	15	25
1989	Janz et al	19	–	13	168	181
1990	Sundqvist	51	1	3	70	74
1992	Canevini et al	18	1	7	52	60
1992	Grünewald et al	6	–	–	15	15
	N	137	5	35	435	485
	%	28	1	8	90	100

It is the presence of these absences with JME that is of interest in the overall theme of this symposium. We want to know if there is a difference between the absences of JME and the absences of childhood absence epilepsy (CAE) and also those of juvenile absence epilepsy (JAE). Likewise, we are concerned to know whether there is a difference between JME with absences and JME without absences.

DEVELOPMENT

Absences can be the first symptom, or they can develop with the first jerks or GTCS, or they can appear after the GTCS or jerks have developed (Sundqvist, 1990). The absences in JME are mild, relatively short and often unremarked by the patient. Their detection is probably the result of special attention or specialist examination (EEG, video-EEG, etc) after the first jerk or GTCS. Panayiotopoulos et al (1994) reported that 'absences pre-dated myoclonic jerks and GTCS in all but two of their 22 patients who had simultaneous onset of absences and myoclonic jerks'. According to their observations, 'absences pre-dated myoclonic jerks by 3.4 ± 2.5 years (range 0–9 years)'.

Unfortunately the syndrome diagnosis of absences in JME is seldom reported. Canevini et al (1992) reported that two out of 18 JME absence patients had 'classical childhood absence epilepsy. . . with the characteristics of pyknolepsy. In all other patients, absences appeared either contemporary with (5 patients) or after the myoclonic jerks.' According to the frequency of absences, one can note that in the five cases of Numata et al (1986) only three had pyknoleptic absences daily. Panayiotopoulos et al (1994) classified his 22 cases according to the age of onset. In eight cases this was under 10 years and in 14 it was over 10.

In our 51 JME patients who also had absences, 11 had pyknolepsy (i.e. in the first months of the illness at least once a day) (Fig. 21.1). Of 181 cases of JME, 6% developed from absences with pyknolepsy and 22% were combined with absences, which, according to the frequency, corresponds with the frequency of juvenile absence seizures (Durner, 1988; Janz & Durner, 1991). The illustration also shows clearly the age of onset and the overlap of seizure types in the quartet of the four idiopathic generalised epilepsies beginning in childhood and adolescence.

If one looks at the development of both childhood and juvenile absences into JME, there are, according to our experience, 8% of pyknolepsies, which emerged around puberty in combination with JME and 16% of cases of JAE (Fig. 21.2). The figures are provisional because not all patients with a CAE have reached the age which is critical for the onset of JME, and also because the patients with CAE who attend a neurological clinic already show biased selection.

They are, however, not the most unfavourable therapy-resistant cases of CAE which go on to become JME. Canevini et al (1992) and Janz (1969) reported on patients with pyknolepsy who were controlled on treatment for a

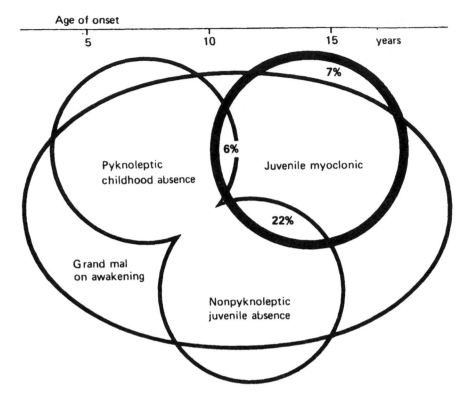

Fig. 21.1 Sub-types of idiopathic generalised epilepsy. Incidence of myoclonic jerks only, of pyknoleptic absences and of non-pyknoleptic absences in JME (Janz, 1990).

long time, when during the JME specific age onset the first myoclonic jerks and then soon after GTCS developed. This experience convinced us that drug treatment for absence epilepsy should be continued beyond puberty.

SEIZURE PATTERNS

As a rule the absences in JME are simple and brief (Janz, 1969; 1985; 1990; Delgado-Escueta & Enrile-Bacsal, 1984; Asconapé & Penry, 1984; Panayiotopoulos et al, 1989a; 1989b; Canevini et al, 1992). The absences are often unnoticed by others and they are experienced by the patients as short-lived disruptions of concentration, which are not reported unless prompted. Not uncommonly, the first absences are noticed during the EEG examination, which Panayiotopoulos et al (1989a) have convincingly demonstrated in three patients, who did not have discernible ictal clinical symptoms, despite numerous 2.5–4 Hz spike and slow-wave generalised discharges in the EEG which lasted up to 8 s.

There are, however, cases of absences with mild clonic jerks of the eyelids, the eyeballs, the head and arms and even with automatisms, as in one of the 19 patients described in more detail by Panayiotopoulos et al (1989a).

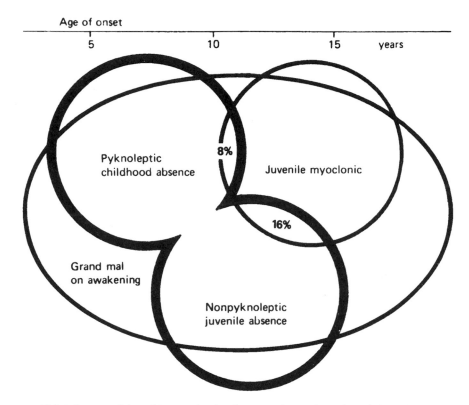

Fig. 21.2 Sub-types of idiopathic generalised epilepsy. Incidence of myoclonic jerks in childhood absence epilepsy and juvenile absence epilepsy (Janz et al, 1992)

In our experience of 51 cases with absences in JME, so far as this can be observed with the EEG, three-quarters of the cases had only simple absences until the time of investigation, and one-quarter had absences with mild rhythmic motor symptoms or with automatisms (Durner, 1988) (Table 21.2). These findings correspond with clinical experience that absences in CAE show more marked symptoms than in JAE. Both syndromes differ in the frequency of absences but especially in age of onset. According to our experiences, pyknolepsies begin at an average age of 8.3 ± 4.5 years and JAE at the age of 14.8 ± 8.3 (Wolf & Inoue, 1984). These facts emphasise that the development of absences depends largely upon the age of onset.

Table 21.2 Symptomatology of absences in JME (Durner, 1988)

Absences	Simple	Complex	Total
pyknoleptic	7	4	11 (22%)
non-pyknoleptic	20	10	40 (78%)
Total	37 (73%)	14 (27%)	51

Panayiotopoulos et al (1989a; 1989b; 1994) have confirmed these observations through systematic clinical and video-EEG investigations. They found that the absences of seven patients, which had begun before ten years of age, would occur more often and would be combined with 'severe impairment of consciousness and occasionally with automatisms'. Conversely, among nine patients with absences that began after the age of 10, in only two cases were these combined 'with sudden discontinuation of activities and staring', whereas in the other patients they were mild, short and without automatisms. They reported that these patients 'usually complain of brief impairment of concentration only without disturbance of cognition or daily activity.' The authors, however, dispute Panayiotopoulos' conclusions that the pyknoleptic absences of JME resemble the pyknoleptic absences of CAE only slightly and that the 'late onset absences of JME are different from those of juvenile absence epilepsy', because the absences of CAE improve in frequency and severity with age. Also, with JAE one can see short discharges with clinical symptoms and long ones without clinical manifestations, which are illustrated by two patients.

Figure 21.3 shows two 4.5 s discharges of fast spike-wave/multi-spike wave patterns in a 34-year-old man who had up to 15 short absences for several days during which rhythmic eye blinking was seen.

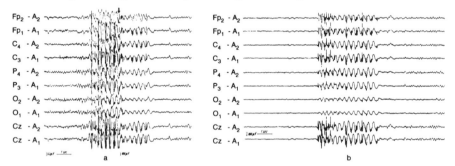

Fig. 21.3a, 3b Ictal EEG (provoked by hyperventilation) during absences with rhythmic fluttering of the eyelids (Janz, 1969).

The other patient was a 24-year-old man who from the age of 12 had suffered from GTCS on awakening. Absences were not reported despite EEG 3–5 Hz spike and wave discharges lasting for 24 s. His breathing remained quiet and he did not open his eyes (Fig. 21.4). He later commented that he had only felt slightly dizzy.

ELECTROENCEPHALOGRAPHY

Panayiotopoulos et al (1989b) reported that the spike multiple spike slow-wave complexes in JME absences were not rhythmic and frequently demonstrated variable spike slow-wave relationships. We can only partially confirm that these irregular multiple spike wave complexes do not apply for

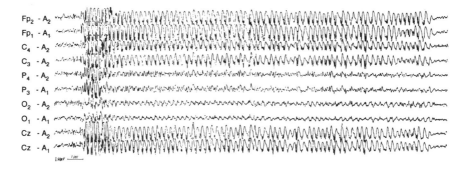

Fig. 21.4 Ictal EEG (provoked by hyperventilation) during an absence which was not noticed by the patient (Janz, 1969).

all absence types in JME and that the same pattern is also seen with JAE without JME.

Although the development of one syndrome into another is often observed, but rarely recorded. Figure 21.5 shows two EEGs of the same patient from Rabe's (1961) account of six cases of JME which developed from pyknolepsy. On the left side an absence is recorded in which the patient suddenly disrupts her ongoing activity, her eyes rhythmically jerking upwards and after which she continued with her activity. The patient was at the time 15 years old and had been having absences at least 10 times daily since the age of 11. She also had infrequent generalised tonic-clonic seizures on awakening from age 13 years. A year later, when treatment was discontinued because of adverse effects, the EEG showed, in addition to classical 3Hz spike wave complexes, for the first time multi-spike wave-

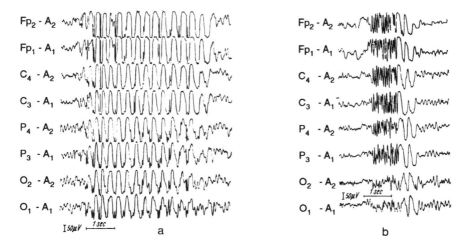

Fig. 21.5 Ictal EEG (a) in a 15-year-old girl during a short absence. Inter-ictal polyspike-wave pattern (b) one year later (Rabe, 1961).

complexes without clinical manifestations. She resumed treatment and again became seizure-free. However, six months later, on waking up in the morning, she experienced such violent jerking of both arms that she was unable to keep hold of any object in her hands. The EEG now showed both patterns: the one on the left as well as the one on right side.

The three epileptic syndromes in which typical absences are seen cannot be sharply divided clinically nor by means of the EEG. After a thorough analysis of over 2000 EEG records (76 patients with CAE, 66 with JAE and 165 with JME), Waltz et al (1990) came to the following conclusion: in CAE the classical 3 Hz spike-wave pattern is prevalent, in JAE the fast spike-wave pattern and in JME multi-spike-wave complexes but in all three forms, all patterns were seen (Table 21.3). However, the differences were not statistically significant.

Table 21.3 Incidence of spike-wave pattern in CAE, JAe and JME (Waltz et al, 1990)

Syndromes	Spike-wave discharges (%)			
	<2.5 Hz	2.5–3.5 Hz	>3.5 Hz	Poly-SW
childhood absence epilepsy N=76	18	75	64	47
juvenile absence epilepsy N=66	21	55	83	45
juvenile myoclonic epilepsy N=165	3	60	57	54

We have not found significant differences in the frequency of spike-wave patterns of JME with absences and of JME without absences (Pantazis, 1989). Also, no differences were found comparing the frequency of the spike-wave patterns between JME with CAE and JAE (Table 21.4). These results do not exclude the possibility that differences could arise if different criteria were applied. All three spike-wave patterns are seen significantly more often in female patients with JME than in male patients (Table 21.5). The sex dif-

Table 21.4 Incidence of spike-wave pattern in JME with and without absences (Pantazis, 1989)

Syndromes	Spike-wave discharges (%)			
	<2.5 Hz	2.5–3.5 Hz	>3.5 Hz	Poly-SW
JME with absences N=47	4	66	64	57
JME without absences N=118	3	84	54	53

Table 21.5 Sex-related incidence of spike-wave pattern in JME with and without absences (Pantazis, 1989)

Syndromes	Spike-wave discharges (%)			
	<2.5 Hz	2.5–3.5 Hz	>3.5 Hz	Poly-SW
JME with absences				
male N=24	4	42'	46"	38"
female N=23	4	91'	83"	78'''
JME without absences				
male N=45	4	73	46	44
female N=73	1	90	59	58

p' = 0.0003
p" = 0.008
p''' = 0.004

ference in patients with JME without absences is not significant. However, photo-sensitivity, which is less frequent in JME with absences (29%) than in JME without absences (42%), is more common in female patients with JME without absences (51%) than in male patients (27%).

GENETICS

To find out whether combinations of JME with absences have a different neurological basis to JME without absences, a genetic investigation would be most appropriate (genetic epidemiological investigation as well as a molecular genetic analysis). An epidemiological study is being carried out and it will soon become apparent whether the clinical types of epilepsy in close relatives differ in JME patients according to whether the subjects had absences or not. Together with a study group in Innsbruck we collected a total of 60 family trees of subjects with JME and/or absence epilepsies. We hope to report our results soon.

A second approach is derived from the hypothesis that a genetic heterogeneity between types with and without absences is present.

For questions concerning clinical characteristics indicating genetic heterogeneity the average lod scores may be compared (Table 21.6). JME-families with affected members with absence epilepsies show a remarkably higher lod score than families without absences, either as an additional symptom in the proband or in affected members (Janz et al, 1993). The interpretation of these findings is limited by the fact that higher lod scores correspond to a larger family size. The result is additionally confusing since we know that, for families of probands with absence epilepsies without any combination with JME, linkage to the HLA region is missing (Sander et al, 1993). According to our study (Sander et al, 1993) as well as that of Serratosa (1993), linkage between families of probands with absence epilepsies and RFLP-markers of the HRA-DQ locus on chromosones 6p could be

Table 21.6 Lod scores of 23 multiplex affected JME families. Index cases and/or affected family members

With absences		Without absences	
Family (n=11)	lod score	Family (n=12)	lod score
2	0.998	1	-0.027
3	0.205	5	0.002
6	0.523	7	-0.013
9	0.071	13	0.194
10	-0.134	15	-0.531
11	0.427	22	0.000
12	-0.172	30	-0.001
14	0.264	31	0.273
16	-0.044	34	0.001
23	0.012	35	0.017
32	0.013	38	0.017
		41	0.163
Σ	2.163	Σ	0.078

Family size: with absences, 7.9; without absences, 5.3. Analysis done under a dominant mode of inheritance, a male/female recombination fraction of $\Theta=0.01$, and a penetrance of 70%.

excluded. This was somewhat surprising because of the clinical evidence for a common genetic predisposition of JME and absence epilepsies (Janz et al, 1992).

It could be that other criteria are of importance to the understanding of the biological basis which we define through genetic factors, aside from the symptomatology. If it were the case that the age of onset has more importance for the genetic basis than symptomatology, then we would have to give up a separation based on symptomatological criteria, which would lead to more and more subtle entries, in favour of a separation according to biological criteria.

REFERENCES

Asconapé J, Penry JK 1984 Some clinical and EEG aspects of benign juvenile myoclonic epilepsy. Epilepsia 25: 108–114
Canevini MP, Mai R, Di Marco C, et al 1992 Juvenile myoclonic epilepsy of Janz: clinical observations in 60 patients. Seizure 1: 291–298
Delgado-Escueta AV, Enrile-Bacsal F 1984 Juvenile myoclonic epilepsy of Janz. Neurology 34: 285–294
Durner M 1988 HLA und Epilepsie mit Impulsiv-Petit mal-EineAssoziationsstudie. Inaugural dissertation. Freie Universität Berlin, Berlin
Grunewald R, Chroni E, Panayiotopoulos CP 1992 Delayed diagnosis of juvenile myoclonic epilepsy. Journal of Neurology, Neurosurgery and Psychiatry 55: 497–499
Janz D 1969 Die Epilepsien. Spezielle Pathologie und Therapie. Thieme, Stuttgart
Janz D 1985 Epilepsy with impulsive petit mal (juvenile myoclonic epilepsy). Acta Neurologica Scandinavia 72: 449–459

Janz F 1990 Juvenile myoclonic epilepsy. In: Dam M, Gram L (eds) Comprehensive epileptology. Raven Press, New York, pp171–185

Janz D, Beck-Mannagetta G, Sander T 1992 Do idiopathic generalized epilepsies share a common susceptibility gene? Neurology 42 (Suppl. 5): 48–55

Janz D, Beck Mannagetta G, Sander T, Hildman T 1993 Phenotypic variability of idiopathic generalized epilepsies in JME families. International Workshop on Idiopathic Generalized Epilepsies, Alsace, April 22–25 (Abstract)

Janz D, Durner M 1991 Verlauf und Genetik der Juvenilen Myoklonischen Epilepsie. In: Jacobi G, Meier-Ewert K (eds) Epilepsien im Kindesalter. Therapie und Prognose. Fischer, Stuttgart, pp67–82

Janz D, Durner M, Beck-Mannagetta G, Pantazis G 1989 Family studies on the genetics of juvenile myoclonic epilepsy (epilepsy with impulsive petit mal). In: Beck-Mannagetta G, Andersson VE, Doose H, Janz D (eds) Genetics of the epilepsies. Springer, Berlin, pp43–52

Matsuoka H 1989 A clinical and electroencephalographic study of juvenile myoclonic epilepsy: its pathophysiological considerations based on the findings obtained from neuropsychological EEG activation. Psychiatria Neurologia Japonica 91: 318–346

Numata Y, Inoue Y, Hamada K, Yagi K, Seino M 1986 Clinical characteristics of 25 patients with juvenile myoclonic epilepsy. The Japanese Journal of Psychiatry and Neurology 40: 421–422

Obeid T, Panayiotopoulos CP 1988 Juvenile myoclonic epilepsy: a study in Saudi Arabia. Epilepsia 29: 280–282

Panayiotopoulos CP, Obeid T, Tahan AR 1994 Juvenile myoclonic epilepsy: a 5-year prospective study. Epilepsia 135: 285–296

Panayiotopoulos CP, Obeid T, Waheed G 1989a Absences in juvenile myoclonic epilepsy: a clinical and video-electroencephalographic study. Annals of Neurology 25: 391–397

Panayiotopoulos CP, Obeid T, Waheed G 1989b Differentiation of typical absence seizures in epileptic syndromes. A video EEG study of 224 seizures in 20 patients. Brain 112: 1039–1056

Pantazis G 1989 Elektroencephalografische Befunde bei Epilepsie mit Impulsiv-Petit mal (IPM). Inaugural dissertation, Freie Universität Berlin, Berlin.

Rabe F 1961 Zum Wechsel des Anfallcharakters epileptischer Anfälle. Deutsche Zeitschrift für Nervenheilkunde 182: 201

Sander T, Hildmann T, Beck-Managetta G et al 1994 Exclusion of linkage between the EJM1 locus and idiopathic generalised epilepsies in absence families. In: Malufosse A, Genton P, Hirsch E et al (eds) Idiopathic generalised epilepsies. John Libbey, London

Serratosa JM, Pelgado-Escueta AV, Liu WYA et al 1993 Exclusion of linkage between DNA markers in JME locus of chromosome 6p and childhood absence epilepsy. Epilepsia 4 (Suppl. 2): 149

Sundqvist A 1990 Juvenile myoclonic epilepsy: events before diagnosis. Journal of Epilepsy 3: 189–192

Waltz S, Beck-Mannagetta G, Janz D 1990 Are there syndrome-related genetically determined spike and wave patterns? A comparison between syndromes of generalized epilepsy. Epilepsia 31: 819 (Abstract)

Wolf P, Inoue Y 1984 Therapeutic response of absence seizures in patients of an epilepsy clinic for adolescence and adults. Journal of Neurology 231: 225–229

DISCUSSION

Stephenson: The paper shows that syndromification is both separately in the direction of genetic analysis and in prediction. Do we then still need to have a prospective study of absences appearing, typical absences in childhood, to see if we can predict whether they are likely to have the prognosis of childhood absence epilepsy or juvenile myoclonic epilepsy?

Janz: We do.

22. Clinical aspects of typical absences and related syndromes – consensus statement I

John Stephenson

I have to admit that this is not a consensus statement but a brief personal view which is inevitably influenced by the proceedings of the remainder of the meeting. I have to preface what I say with a comment about assumptions regarding the underlying mechanisms of typical absences. Karl Popper has taught us that one exception will demolish the grandest hypothesis. I have perhaps two, in the form of children with what I call anoxic-epileptic seizures (Stephenson, 1990).

There is substantial acceptance that generalised epileptic seizures, of which typical absences are a special example, depend upon the integrity of a cortical-thalamic circuit. I doubt the universality of this proposition for the following reasons. Generalised epileptic seizures may be induced by syncopes (Stephenson, 1983) and such anoxic-epileptic seizures may be typical absence in the form of absence status (Battaglia et al, 1989), but observation of the EEG in such a case does not assist in the understanding of the mechanisms since there is no way of recognising such a provoked absence before generalised 3 Hz spike and wave appears in the scalp record.

Such a difficulty does not obtain with the closely related 'generalised' clonic seizure. When this type of epileptic seizure is triggered by vagal-mediated cardiac standstill, the rhythmic and apparently 3 Hz motor manifestations of the cloni (such as EMG and movement artefacts) appear on the trace several seconds before the end of the isoelectric phase of the EEG and the onset of visible rhythmic discharges (3 Hz) (Stephenson, 1990). This evidence seems to show that, although the cerebral cortex is necessary for the generation of 3 Hz spike and wave, functional neocortex is not required for the genesis of deep 3 Hz bilaterally diffusing (but of course not generalised) epileptic activity. I think that I have seen the same phenomenon in a case of myoclonic absences induced by syncopes (Stephenson, 1990), but there are no convincing records.

Ignoring such questions of mechanism, let us turn to the clinical definition of typical absence. It is evident that the definition used by the epidemiologist might not be precisely the same as that used by the classifier of syndromes, bearing in mind that the purpose of classification – to unravel the genetics, to optimise therapy, or to improve prediction and prognosis – may influence which definition is found more useful. The definition of typical absence may vary from one epidemiological study to another or be assumed to be self-evident, whereas one physician's common- sense understanding of what is a typical absence may be quite different from that of another. Attempts have been made, of course, to unify and harmonise definitions by international commissions and so forth but it may be that Franco-Italian epileptologists find this easier than Anglo-Saxons.

Leaving definitions of typical absences without total consensus, let us turn to definitions of typical absence syndromes and their usefulness. I will attempt to concentrate on the middle ground. In typical childhood absence epilepsy (CAE) typical absences are expected to be the first and only type of epileptic seizure. Actually in a substantial proportion, maybe 20 or 30%, there is a previous history of febrile seizures of presumably epileptic mechanism although available published data is inadequate. The typical absences are supposed to be very frequent and to be unaccompanied by myoclonus. Some would have it that photosensitivity, meaning in this context the reproducible induction of absences by photostimulation, implies a separate syndrome whereas others would maintain only that photosensitivity implies a worse prognosis. This is an example of the importance of recognising the purpose of a definition of classification. If one is looking for genetic or biological insights it might be reasonable to lump together those with absences with and without photosensitivity, but if one is classifying for prognosis it would seem better to split off the photo-responders.

I am not going to say anything about juvenile absence epilepsy, except to admit that I am not sure if I understand it, and that if I do, I am not sure how helpful it is to know about it. I will therefore pass promptly to juvenile myoclonic epilepsy with absence (JMEA) and discuss the importance and validity of distinguishing these typical absences from those of CAE. The general consensus is that there is a distinct electro-clinical syndrome of juvenile myoclonic epilepsy (JME). I do not recollect any good data related to the relative incidence of typical absences in childhood in those who will eventually be classified as CAE and those who will eventually be classified as JMEA. Information on this balance would be important because the significance of a diagnostic test depends on the expected likelihood of the disorder in the population studied. Differentiating diagnostic criteria have indeed been proposed by Panayiotopoulos (1989).

In summary, my interpretation of the alleged characteristics is as follows. The absences of CAE are associated with severe loss of awareness (or loss of responsiveness) accompanying 3 Hz spike and wave in which there is one spike and only one spike for each wave. The absences of JMEA are associated with less complete unresponsiveness, double spikes (Ws) or even polyspikes between some of the waves, complete interruptions in the spike and waves so that it stops and starts and more subtle interruptions in so far as there is not a spike for every wave. This is a distinction disputed by Janz at this meeting. I do not think that there are adequate prospective studies predicting the type of epilepsy from the first presenting absence and then following the children long enough to determine whether or not morning myoclonus develops. Such studies need to be undertaken by young, committed epilepsy investigators – preferably those with a good expectation of life themselves.

REFERENCES

Battaglia A, Guerrini R, Gastaut H 1989 Epileptic seizures induced by syncopal attacks. Journal of Epilepsy 2: 137–146
Panayiotopoulos CP, Obeid T, Waheed G 1989 Differentiation of typical absence seizures in epileptic syndromes. Brain 112: 1039–1056
Stephenson J 1983 Febrile convulsions and reflex anoxic seizures in epileptic syndromes. In: Rose FC (ed) Research progress in epilepsy.
Stephenson J 1990 Fits and faints. MacKeith Press, London

23. Myoclonic absence epilepsy

C. A. Tassinari   R. Michelucci   G. Rubboli   D. Passarelli
P. Riguzzi   L. Parmeggiani   L. Volpi   M. Bureau

Since 1969 we have repeatedly described myoclonic absences (MA) as an individual seizure type and proposed the existence of a specific epileptic syndrome (MA epilepsy) in which MA constitute the only or predominant seizure type (Tassinari et al, 1969,1992; Lugaresi et al, 1973; Tassinari & Bureau, 1985). Recently many general reviews have been devoted to this subject (Tassinari et al, 1994; Tassinari & Michelucci, 1994; Manonmani & Wallace, 1994).

The international classification of epilepsies and epileptic syndromes (Commission on Classification and Terminology of the ILAE, 1989) includes MA epilepsy among the cryptogenic or symptomatic forms of generalised epilepsy and gives the following definition of this syndrome:

The syndrome of epilepsy with myoclonic absences is clinically characterised by absences accompanied by severe bilateral rhythmical clonic jerks, often associated with a tonic contraction. On the EEG, these clinical features are always accompanied by bilateral, synchronous, and symmetrical discharge of rhythmical spike-waves at 3 Hz, similar to childhood absence. Seizures occur many times a day. Awareness of the jerks may be maintained. Associated seizures are rare. Age of onset is 7 years, and there is a male preponderance. Prognosis is less favourable than in pyknolepsy owing to resistance to therapy of the seizures, mental deterioration, and possible evolution to other types of epilepsy such as Lennox-Gastaut syndrome.

MYOCLONIC ABSENCES: AN INDIVIDUAL SEIZURE TYPE

Clinical symptomatology

MA are characterised by:

1. Impairment of consciousness, which is quite variable in intensity, ranging from a mild disruption of contact to a complete loss of consciousness. Sometimes patients are aware of the jerks and may recall the words pronounced by the examiner during the seizures.
2. Motor manifestations, which consist of bilateral myoclonic jerks, often associated with a discrete tonic contraction. The myoclonias mainly involve the muscles of shoulders, arms and legs. When facial myoclonias occur, they are more evident around the chin and mouth, whereas eyelid twitching is typically absent or rare. Due to concomitant tonic contrac-

tion the jerking of the arms is accompanied by a progressive elevation of the upper extremities, giving rise to a quite constant and recognisable pattern. When the patient is standing, falling is uncommon while backward or forward staggering occurs more often. Head and body deviation can be a clinically relevant feature in some patients (Fig. 23.1).

3. Autonomic manifestations, which consist of an arrest or change of respiration and sometimes incontinence of urine.

MA have an abrupt onset without any warning, last for 10–60 s and recur at a high frequency (many seizures per day). They are often precipitated by hyperventilation or awakening. MA may be also observed during the early stages of sleep, sometimes awakening the subject. Episodes of MA status, although distinctly rare, have been described (Tassinari et al, 1992; Manonmani & Wallace, 1994).

EEG and polygraphic symptomatology

The ictal EEG consists of a rhythmic spike and wave (SWs) discharge at 3 Hz: bilateral, synchronous and symmetrical, as observed in typical absences (Fig.23.2). The onset and end of SWs are abrupt except in rare cases in which the discharge ends progressively with delta waves in frontal areas, sometimes asymmetrical (Tassinari et al, 1992; Seino M, 1990, personal communication). In individual seizures, the typical SW discharges may be intermingled occasionally with polyspikes.

Polygraphic recording discloses the appearance of bilateral rhythmic

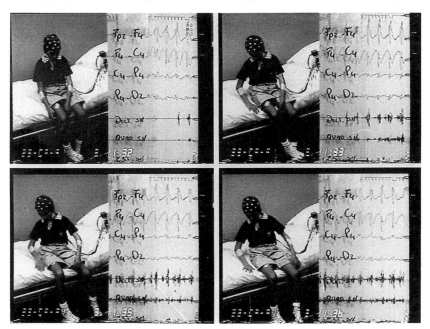

Fig. 23.1 MA: split-screen video-polygraphic recording. Note the elevation and abduction of both arms and the deviation of head and body to the right (delt sin: left deltoid; quad sin: left quadriceps).

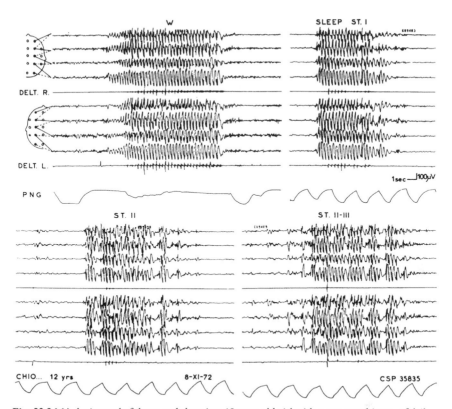

Fig. 23.2 MA during wakefulness and sleep in a 12-year-old girl with a one-year history of daily MA. Top left: spontaneous MA during wakefulness. Rhythmic SWs discharge at 3 Hz, bilateral and symmetrical, accompanied by rhythmic myoclonias, at the same frequency of the SWs, over both deltoid muscles. Note the associated tonic contraction and arrrest of respiration. Top right: MA during sleep stage 1, of shorter duration than during wakefulness. Bottom left and right: generalised SW discharges during sleep stage II and III. The SWs are irregular, fragmented and associated with mild and variable myoclonias.

myoclonias, at the same frequency as the SWs, which begin one second after the onset of EEG paroxysmal discharges and are followed by a tonic contraction, maximal in the shoulder and deltoid muscles (Fig. 23.2). Sometimes myoclonias and tonic contraction are unilateral or clearly asymmetrical despite a generalised EEG pattern (Figs 23.3,4).

Tassinari et al (1969,1971) provided a detailed analysis of the relationships between the SWs and motor events by means of high-speed oscilloscopic recording. They found a strict and constant relationship between the spike of the SW complex and the myoclonia. In detail the spike, morphologically related to a positive transient (Weir, 1965) of high amplitude, is followed on the EMG by a myoclonia with a latency of 15–40 msec for the more proximal muscles and of 50–70 msec for the more distal muscles. This myoclonia is itself followed by a brief silent period (60–120 msec) which breaks the tonic contraction.

The inter-ictal EEG shows a normal background activity in all cases, with superimposed generalised SWs (in one third of cases) or, more rarely

(14%), focal or multifocal SWs (Fig. 23.3). Photo-sensitivity is uncommon (14% of cases).

The sleep EEG shows a normal organisation and symmetrical physiological patterns. During sleep the evolution of the SW discharges is similar, on the whole, to that observed in childhood absence epilepsy (Tassinari et al, 1974). Clinically evident MA may occur during stage I. Generalised SW discharges of brief or long duration, sometimes associated with bursts of myoclonias, may also be observed during stages II and III (Figs 23.2–4). Irregular and fragmented SWs, predominant over one or the other anterior regions, are common during sleep (Fig. 23.3).

Differential diagnosis

The polygraphic recording (EEG + EMG of various muscles, particularly the deltoid muscles bilaterally) is mandatory when the clinical suspicion of MA is raised. Indeed, the diagnosis of MA rests on the polygraphic demonstration of SW discharges at 3 Hz accompanied by severe and diffuse rhythmic myoclonias. Therefore, MA can be differentiated easily from a variety of seizures which may be 'similar', on anamnestic description, to MA:

1. 'Generalised myoclonic seizures', which are accompanied by poly SW discharges and not by rhythmic 3 Hz SWs, do not occur in rhythmic clusters and are not associated with impairment of consciousness.
2. 'Absence seizures with mild clonic components' (as defined by the Commission on Classification and Terminology of the ILAE, 1981), in which myoclonias involve only the eyelids or the face.

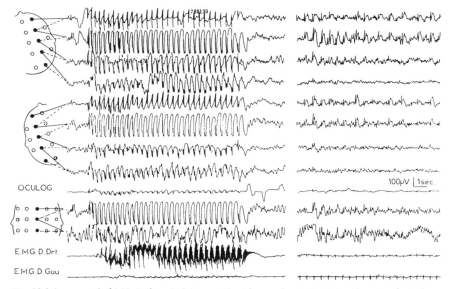

Fig. 23.3 Asymmetrical MA. Left: wakefulness; MA with myoclonias involving almost exclusively the right deltoid muscle, in spite of a generalised SW discharge. Right: sleep; inter-ictal bilateral and irregular SWs predominant over the right anterior regions (D Drt: right deltoid; D Gau: left deltoid).

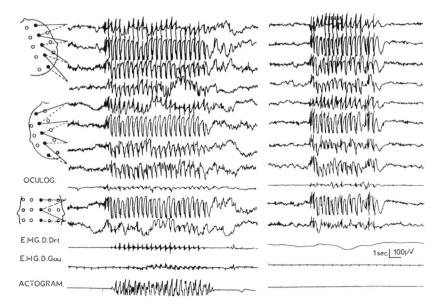

OCULOG.

E.M.G.D.Drt.

E.M.G.D.Gau.

ACTOGRAM.

1sec. 100μV

Fig. 23.4 Same patient and recording as in Fig. 23.3. Left: wakefulness; MA with bilateral myoclonias involving both deltoid muscles. Slight right predominance of the myoclonias. Right: sleep: inter-ictal generalised SW discharge. Legends: see **Fig. 23.3**. Actogram: channel recording global body movement.

3. 'Partial motor seizures', which may be considered in the differential diagnosis when the motor manifestations of MA are asymmetrical (with head and body turning) (Fig.23.1) or predominant on one side.

On anamnestic investigation the rhythmic myoclonic movements of MA may be overlooked due to predominant tonic contraction or when the myoclonias are of reduced intensity under the effect of treatment. In these cases, the polygraphic demonstration of MA and not of simple absences may be a surprise. Finally, MA-like seizures have been observed in a variety of epileptic encephalopathies. In these cases, however, polygraphic recording shows atypical features, consisting of more irregular SWs, a less abrupt onset and end of the discharge or the combination of myoclonic and atonic motor phenomena (Tassinari, 1992, unpublished data).

MYOCLONIC ABSENCE EPILEPSY: AN INDIVIDUAL EPILEPTIC SYNDROME

In MA epilepsy, other factors besides seizure type may justify the recognition of a specific syndrome distinct from other forms of generalised epilepsy. From the review of 49 cases (36 observed at the Centre St Paul in Marseille, 13 at the University Neurology Department, Bologna), the following features may be considered distinctive of MA epilepsy:

a. Incidence: this syndrome is rare, being found in 0.5–1% of patients referred to the St Paul Epilepsy Centre.
b. Sex ratio: there is a male preponderance (69%), which is at variance with

the female preponderance in childhood absence epilepsy.

c. Aetiological factors: these are of the same nature and frequency as in childhood absence epilepsy.

d. Genetic factors: a family history of epilepsy is found in 19% of the cases.

e. Age of onset: mean 7 years (range 11 months–12.2 years). Rare cases of MA beginning during the first year of life have been reported (Tassinari et al, 1992; Manonmani &Wallace, 1994; Aicardi, 1994; Giovanardi Rossi,1990, personal communication; Seino, 1990, personal communication; Panayiotopoulos, 1994, personal communication).

f. Seizures: in about one-third of cases MA represent the only seizure type. In the remaining patients, other seizures occur either before the onset of MA or in association with it. They consist of rare generalised tonic-clonic seizures (GTCS), absences or falling seizures.

g. Neurological and neuropsychological examination: neurological examination is normal in all cases. Mental retardation is present in about 45% of cases before the onset of MA. During the course of MA epilepsy, mental retardation occurs in a further 25% of cases, so that a total of 70% of patients present mental impairment at some time. These data constitute a very significant difference in comparison with the mental status observed in childhood absence epilepsy.

h. Evolution: MA were still present in half the patients followed up for a mean period of 20 years, whereas they had disappeared in the remaining patients after a mean period of 5.5 years from onset (Tassinari et al, 1992).

The two groups of patients differed for the frequency and type of associated seizures: patients with 'refractory' MA had a high incidence (85%) of associated seizures, mainly GTCS and atonic. Patients with remitting MA had a lower incidence (50%) of associated seizures, mainly of absence type.

Another factor which seems to influence the evolution is medical therapy. Recent observations indicate that a combination of valproic acid and ethosuximide at high doses with appropriate control of plasma levels leads to rapid remission of MA in most cases (Tassinari & Michelucci, 1994). On the other hand, the therapeutic history of patients with 'refractory' MA often discloses lower doses of these drugs or the use of different medical therapies.

The long duration of MA is likely to be an important factor for the appearance of mental retardation, since intellectual functions are constantly preserved in children with rapid remission of MA.

A particular evolution of epilepsy was described in five of the 36 cases observed at the St Paul Centre in Marseille. In these patients, absences with atypical SW discharges and clinical or sub-clinical tonic seizures occurred during the course of MA epilepsy, giving rise to a clinical picture similar to the Lennox-Gastaut syndrome (Figs 23.2,5,6).

MA epilepsy requires specific medical therapy which consists of the associated use of valproic acid and ethosuximide at high doses, with serum plasma levels ranging from 550–900 μmol/l and 500–770 μmol/l respectively.

Lamotrigine has been reported to be effective in suppressing MA in 'refractory' cases (Manonmani & Wallace, 1994).

CONCLUSIONS

We believe that MA represent a specific seizure type whose recognition rests on direct clinical observation and polygraphic recording of the seizures. The EEG-EMG pattern of MA is specific and allows differential diagnosis with other generalised seizure types. MA should therefore be included in the International Classification of epileptic seizures.

The diagnosis of MA is per se sufficient for the identification of a syndrome, namely myoclonic absence epilepsy, which stands in the international classification of the epilepsies and epileptic syndromes (Commission on Classification and Terminology of the ILAE, 1989) among generalised epilepsies of cryptogenic or symptomatic nature. The reasons which have allowed the identification of a specific syndrome, distinct from other forms of generalised epilepsy, include the distinctive electro-clinical features of MA and a less favourable prognosis than in childhood absence epilepsy due to resistance to therapy, mental retardation and possible evolution towards other types of epilepsy, such as Lennox-Gastaut syndrome.

Further research will be required to define better the long-term follow-up of MA once correct medical treatment is instituted, with special regard to the evolution of the epilepsy and neuropsychological assessment.

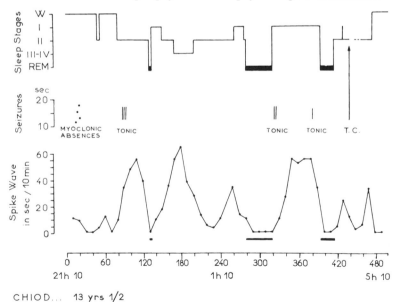

CHIOD... 13 yrs 1/2

Fig. 23.5 Evolution of MA epilepsy towards Lennox-Gastaut syndrome. Same patient as in Fig. 23.2. At the age of 13, she was admitted after the appearance of tonic seizures during sleep. The hypnogram of a full night's polygraphic recording is correlated with the SWs frequency and seizure number and type. Note the activation of the SWs during light sleep and the disappearance of the paroxysmal abnormalities furing REM sleep. Three types of seizures were recorded: MA (during wakefulness), tonic seizures and one tonic-clonic seizure (during sleep stages I-II).

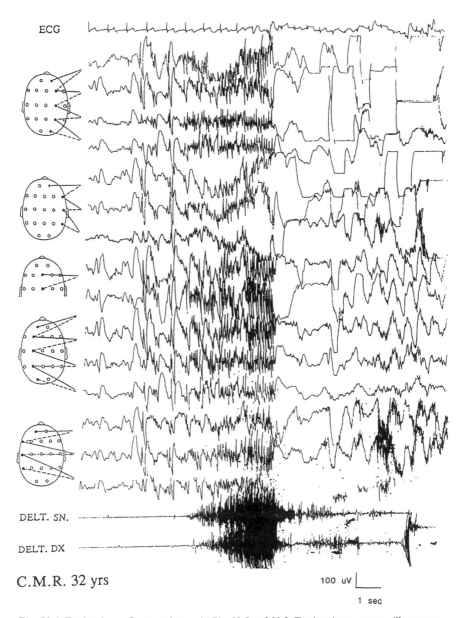

Fig. 23.6 Tonic seizure. Same patient as in Fig. 23.2 and 23.5. Tonic seizures were still present during sleep at the age of 32 years. At this time, falling seizures, absence-like episodes, tonic-clonic seizures and rare MA were also observed (delt sin: left deltoid; delt dx: right deltoid).

ACKNOWLEDGEMENTS

Supported by the 40% funds distributed by the Italian Ministry of Education and CNR. The financial support of Telethon (Grant E-109) is gratefully acknowledged.

REFERENCES

Aicardi J 1994 Typical absences in the first 2 years of life. In: Duncan JS, Panayiotopoulos CP (eds) Typical absences and related epileptic syndromes. Churchill Livingstone, London pp294-298

Commission on Classification and Terminology of the International League Against Epilepsy 1981 Proposal for revised clinical and electroencephalographic classification of epileptic seizures. Epilepsia 22: 489-501

Commission on Classification and Terminology of the International League Against Epilepsy 1989 Proposal for revised classification of epilepsies and epileptic syndromes. Epilepsia 30: 389–399

Lugaresi E, Pazzaglia P, Franck L et al 1973 Evolution and prognosis of primary generalized epilepsies of the petit mal absence type. In: Lugaresi E, Pazzaglia P, Tassinari CA (eds) Evolution and prognosis of epilepsy. Aulo Gaggi, Bologna, pp2–22

Manonmani V, Wallace SJ 1994 Epilepsy with myoclonic absences. Archives of Disease in Childhood 70: 288–290

Tassinari CA, Bureau M 1985 Epilepsy with myoclonic absences. In: Roger J, Dravet C, Bureau M, Dreifuss FE, Wolf P (eds) Epileptic syndromes in infancy, childhood and adolescence. John Libbey, London, pp123-131

Tassinari CA, Michelucci R 1994 Epilepsy with myoclonic absences: a reappraisal. In: Wolf P (ed) Epileptic seizures and syndromes. John Libbey, London, pp 137-161

Tassinari CA, Lyagoubi S, Santos V et al 1969 Etude des decharges de pointes ondes chez l'homme. II. Les aspects cliniques et electroencephalographiques des absences myocloniques. Revue Neurologique 121: 379-383

Tassinari CA, Lyagoubi S, Gambarelli F, Roger J, Gastaut H 1971 Relationships between EEG discharge and neuromuscular phenomena. Electroencephalography and Clinical Neurophysiology 31: 176

Tassinari CA, Bureau-Paillas M, Dalla Bernardina B et al 1974 Generalized epilepsies and seizures during sleep: a polygraphic study. In: Van Praag HM, Meinardi H (eds) Brain and sleep. De Erven Bhon, Amsterdam, pp 154-166

Tassinari CA, Bureau M, Thomas P 1992 Epilepsy with myoclonic absences. In: Roger J, Bureau M, Dravet C, Dreifuss FE, Perret A, Wolf P (eds) Epileptic syndromes in infancy, childhood and adolescence, 2nd edn. John Libbey, London, pp151-160

Tassinari CA, Rubboli G, Michelucci R 1995 Epilepsy with myoclonic absences. In: Wallace S (ed) Childhood epilepsy. Chapman & Hall, London (in press)

Weir B 1965 The morphology of the spike-wave complex. Electroencephalography and Clinical Neurophysiology 19: 284-290

DISCUSSION

Stephenson: As Professor Tassinari says, there are varieties of this syndrome. I saw a patient with typical myoclonic absences who now has a bright unilateral frontal abnormality on SPECT with normal brain imaging. One need not have a bad prognosis. One patient with myoclonic absences remitted completely and then relapsed again at seven years of age; he was controlled by a very small amount of clonazepam.

Hirsch: The case with the bad evolution I do not understand. Was the treatment at the beginning phenytoin? If it was phenytoin, could treatment modify the evolution and could the patient now be treated with different drugs (ethosuximide, valproic acid, lamotrigine) and have a different prognosis? Can treatment modify the phenotype of epileptic syndromes?

Tassinari: It could well be the natural course or the situation could be modified by treatment. Myoclonic absences tell us that we are facing absences that need more treatment and are more difficult. It is not a new syndrome or a new situation. It is useful semiological information.

Ethosuximide or valproate alone usually are not effective. A combination of these drugs at high levels is often successful. Lamotrigine has been tried by Wallace.

24. Towards an understanding of reflex epilepsy and the absence

Arnold Wilkins

'A simple reflex is probably a purely abstract conception because all parts of the nervous system are connected together and no part of it is ever capable of reaction without affecting and being affected by various other parts' (Sherrington, 1947).

The abstractness of the reflex concept is nowhere more apparent than in the case of the reflex epilepsies. These are epilepsies where there is clear evidence that seizures are precipitated by some identifiable factor. They include epilepsy induced by sensory stimulation (a pure tone, Zagury et al, 1989; a tap on the back, Deonna & Despland, 1989) and also epilepsy where there is no obvious stimulation and the seizures are the result of decision-making or other types of thinking (Wilkins et al, 1982; Andermann et al, 1989). Seizures due to less specific factors, such as stress or loss of sleep, are not usually referred to as reflex. There are a large number of these less specific factors and it is important to consider them, particularly when treating refractory epilepsy (Aird, 1983).

For a review of reflex epilepsies and their categorisation, Beaumanoir et al (1989) offer a compendium of fascinating cases. The only reflex seizures omitted from this review are those from video-games. This is a recent and somewhat puzzling group of epilepsies, not all of which are photo-sensitive (Ferrie et al, 1994; Harding et al, 1994). The purpose of this chapter is to describe some of the concepts necessary to understand the reflex epilepsies.

LOCALISED VERSUS DISTRIBUTED FUNCTION

A concept central to the understanding of reflex epilepsy is that of localisation of function within the brain. Historically, views on the extent to which function is localised have vacillated between two extremes. The phrenologists and the 19th-century neurologists who followed them sought to localise function by placing labels on a picture of the head or the brain. This approach was rightly criticised by Lashley who argued that deficits from brain lesions depended less upon which particular structures were removed than upon the extent of removal. Lashley's notion of equipotentiality was countermanded by neuropsychologists and single unit physiologists in the 1960s, particularly Brenda Milner and Hubel & Weisel, with their clear demonstrations of particular functions associated with particular brain structures. Later, the work of Sperry on callosal section once again emphasised the functional importance of connections between brain structures rather than the structures as such.

Sperry's work is linked to two current traditions of investigation: one on lateralisation of function and the other on distributed processing. The latter is the result of the recent development of neural network computing. This has provided a theoretical justification for notions of distributed representation. These notions receive empirical support from work on functional imaging, particularly positron emission tomography (PET). The current view is that there exists a localisation of sensation and motor output, language reception and production, spatial thinking and memory, but that the localisation is only partial. PET studies usually reveal a picture of brain metabolism consonant with that expected from dysfunction after lesions, but invariably with surprises. When the subject performs a sensory task the primary sensory areas show an increase in metabolic activity, but there are almost invariably other, more labile areas of activity, even in tasks that appear to be exclusively sensory or exclusively motor. For example, Petersen et al (1988, 1989) asked normal adult subjects to say a noun that was seen or heard and found an increase in blood flow in the bilateral primary motor and sylvian-insular cortices and supplementary motor area, but also increases in the paramedian cerebellum. When the task was made more complex by requiring the subject to say an appropriate verb in response to the noun, additional changes in local blood flow were observed in the left prefrontal and anterior cingulate cortices and in the right cerebellar hemisphere.

If the task is unfamiliar, the activation may be more generalised and frontal areas may be involved. Raichle et al (1994) examined regional blood flow using PET during naive and practised performance of the complex task above and showed that areas most active during naive performance (anterior cingulate, left prefrontal and left posterior temporal cortices) were all significantly less active during practised performance. These changes were accompanied by reciprocal changes in the sylvian-insular cortex bilaterally and left medial pre-striate cortex, making the distribution of activation similar to that for the simpler task of word repetition. Perhaps stressful conditions tend to result in a greater general activation; if so, this might explain why emotion and stress are some of the most powerful precipitants of seizures.

It has to be borne in mind that PET studies generally use techniques that subtract the spatial distribution of metabolic activity in one task from that in another. By concentrating on localisation in this way they tend to obscure one very important aspect of the relationship between thinking and brain function: the effects of a task on overall metabolism.

FOCAL CORTICAL TRIGGER FOR A GENERALISED DISCHARGE

Since the discovery by Hubel & Wiesel of neurones responding selectively to lines of a particular orientation in the visual field, there has been a rapid acquisition of knowledge about localisation of function in the visual cortex of the macaque, complemented by psychophysical evidence from human beings. This evidence has been combined with a detailed study of the stimulus characteristics of pattern-sensitive epilepsy. Some patients are sensitive only to a limited range of pattern orientations, confirming that orientationally selective units are involved. These units are cortical, and so the selective effects of pattern orientation point to a cortical locus for the seizure trigger. Many other characteristics of pattern-sensitivity are consistent with a cortical trigger (Wilkins et al, 1990). The trigger in pattern-sensitive epilepsy is, therefore, well localised despite the generalised nature of the discharge. This is a feature of other forms of reflex epilepsy. For example, in one case of seizures induced by thinking, tasks that presumably activated parietal areas were responsible for generalised discharges (Wilkins et al, 1982).

NON-UNIFORM HYPER-EXCITABILITY

How can there be a generalised seizure discharge from such a localised trigger? One explanation might be that, although the cortex is diffusely hyper-excitable, it is not uniformly so. The excitability may be greater in those brain areas that appear to be responsible for triggering the discharge. This might at first appear to be difficult to reconcile with the occurrence of bilaterally symmetric generalised discharges. However, close inspection of these discharges often reveals small asymmetries in amplitude. For example, asymmetries in the discharge obtained from diffuse intermittent photic stimulation are related to the lateral visual field in which patterns most readily elicit paroxysmal EEG activity. The amplitude of the discharge is greater over the hemisphere contralateral to the visual field showing the lowest pattern-sensitivity thresholds. Evidently the cortex is not necessarily uniformly hyper-excitable, even when a discharge is generalised, and close inspection can reveal asymmetries in the discharge that are consistent with other independent evidence of a non-uniform hyper-excitability (Wilkins et al, 1990).

CRITICAL MASS AND THE MASS ACTION OF INDEPENDENT NEURONAL AGGREGATES

There are further clues as to the nature of the seizure trigger mechanism to be gleaned from pattern sensitivity. The probability of paroxysmal activity is critically dependent on the size of pattern producing the discharge. Moreover, patterns that project to the same total area of visual cortex have the same epileptogenic effect. A small pattern projected to the centre of the visual field has the same effect as a large pattern presented in the periphery, for example. Even though the patterns are stimulating completely different cortical units, when the same 'amount' of brain receives stimulation the probability of the discharge is the same. This demonstrates that, although the trigger can be quite focal in one sense, it does not have to involve the same aggregate of neurones. The effects of pattern size indicate that a 'critical mass' of excitation is necessary; the greater the physiological activation, the greater the likelihood of seizures. Is this why emotion and stress are such common precipitants of seizures? Is this one of the mechanisms underlying startle epilepsy, in which there are presumably widespread afferents from the movement of the entire body? These afferents must be quite well synchronised by the nature of the startle reflex, and as we shall see, synchronisation is important at the inception of the discharge.

SYNCHRONISATION

Synchronisation may be an essential part of normal neural function. Singer (1990) has shown that there is synchronised activity over widespread areas of the visual cortex that may serve as a functional code. Synchronisation may also be assumed to occur as a result of normal sensory afferents. For example, when the eyes make a rapid jerk (saccade), there are doubtless consequential changes in activity in the visual cortex that are synchronised with that saccade. There is even a little indirect evidence that this is necessary for epileptogenesis in pattern-sensitive epilepsy.

When a patient looks at a pattern of stripes the likelihood of paroxysmal EEG activity is strongly dependent on the way the stripes move. If a pattern is divided into two halves, and in the left half the stripes drift towards the right and in the right half toward the left (ie, both halves towards the centre of gaze), then there is no optokinetic nystagmus. This drifting pattern is very unlikely to evoke paroxysmal activity. Presumably the contours of the pattern pass into and out of the overlapping receptive fields of visual neurones. But, because these receptive fields overlap, there is no synchronised pattern of activation in the network as a whole. However, when the pattern repeatedly changes its direction of motion it becomes highly epileptogenic. Under these circumstances the nerve network as a whole does show synchronisation because there are neurones that are selectively sensitive to one direction of motion and not the other. The large difference in the epileptogenic potential of patterns that drift in one direction and those that reverse direction suggests that synchronisation of activity in the neural network as a whole is necessary for epileptogenesis.

When a pattern is stationary it is more epileptogenic than a drifting pattern and less so than an oscillating pattern, presumably due to the synchronisation that results from microsaccades during fixation (Wilkins et al, 1990).

THE ABSENCE SEIZURE

Aarts et al (1984) have shown that isolated temporal spikes can be associated with an impairment of function. If the abnormality is right-sided, then the impairment is one of spatial memory; if it is left-sided, verbal memory is affected. This double dissociation indicates that the brain areas involved in a small focal discharge can show impaired function, provided the psychological testing is sufficiently sensitive to reveal it. In view of this finding, the impairment of consciousness during bilateral spike and wave is unsurprising. The poor synchronisation between the onset and offset of the discharge and the slowing of reaction time (Mirsky & van Buren, 1965) can be attributed to the failure of the surface EEG to show seizure activity in deep structures and the relative insensitivity of reaction time measures to cognitive deficits, or both of these.

Beginnings of an explanation

It is now possible to begin an explanation of reflex epilepsies and absences. The cortex is diffusely but not uniformly hyper-excitable. Physiological excitation of a hyper-excitable region, by thinking, by sensation, or by motor output, gives rise to a spread of activity. If a critical mass of excitation is achieved, a discharge is initiated which involves cortico-thalamic relays, increasing the degree of synchronisation in the cortex as a whole and further increasing the spread. This simple view provides a way of interpreting the complex clinical picture in many forms of reflex epilepsy. For example, in certain forms of reading epilepsy the trigger appears to involve the processing of language and by implication the language areas of the brain (Forster, 1977). In others, the pattern provided by text is a component of the trigger mechanism and presumably involves more posterior areas (Wilkins & Lindsay, 1985). When seizures are evoked by chess playing the trigger may seem behaviourally quite specific. In one such patient, however, tasks other than chess evoked paroxysmal EEG activity. The tasks were those that are generally impaired after lesions of the parietal lobe (Wilkins et al, 1982).

Vague and insufficient

It might justifiably be objected that any explanation couched in terms of the simple concepts of a non-uniform hyper-excitability, a critical mass and synchronisation, is necessarily so vague as to be unable to provide a testable theory. Vague though these concepts may be, they are insufficiently flexible to be able to account for the contrast between two simple forms of reflex epilepsy: photo-sensitive epilepsy and fixation-off sensitivity (FOS). Panayiotopoulos (1989) is responsible for elaborating the latter syndrome and drawing attention to some of its more intriguing aspects. In brief, patients with fixation-off sensitivity show spontaneous occipital spikes when they are in darkness, when their eyes are closed or when they are wearing diffusing goggles and deprived of contoured vision. Nevertheless, even the smallest visual signal (a small red light, for example) is sufficient to prevent the occurrence of the occipital spikes. These patients are not usually photo-sensitive.

In patients with FOS the occipital cortex exhibits spontaneous bursts of spikes. The visual cortex is evidently hyper-excitable but there is no response to intermittent photic stimulation. Why? It is conceivable that some visual neurones are Group 1 neurones (Wyler & Ward, 1980) that provide an epileptogenic critical mass but are damaged in such a way as to reduce the physiological effects of intermittent light. This seems unlikely given that there is no evidence of impaired visual function in these patients. The concepts developed so far seem insufficient to provide an explanation of the absence of photo-sensitivity in FOS, but perhaps an explanation can be sought by further consideration of the localisation of function that takes place in the visual pathways, specifically the division of magnocellular and parvocellular pathways.

More localisation of function

The characteristics of pattern-sensitive epilepsy are strongly reminiscent of the magnocellular division of the visual system.

1. The magnocellular system does not generally code for colour, and pattern-sensitive patients are not sensitive to gratings where the stripes differ in colour and not in brightness.
2. Neurones in the magno system are directionally coded, and, as we have seen, pattern-sensitive patients are sensitive to moving patterns in a way that is clearly dependent upon the direction of pattern motion.
3. Magnocellular neurones are tuned for binocular disparity. Patterns that fail to fuse in binocular vision are less epileptogenic than those that fuse.
4. The magnocellular system has a lower spatial resolution than the parvocellular system. The patterns to which patients are sensitive tend to have a fairly low spatial frequency.
5. Magnocellular neurones have a higher temporal resolution than parvocellular neurones. The upper frequency limit of sensitivity to diffuse intermittent photic stimulation can be as high as 60 Hz.
6. The magnocellular system is thought to project to parietal regions as part of the 'where' as opposed to the 'what' divisions of the visual system (Mishkin & Ungerleider, 1982). The isolated spikes in pattern-sensitive patients tend to be most marked over parietal electrodes (Darby et al, 1986).

The magnocellular system forms only a small proportion of the visual system as a whole. The parvocellular division is by far the larger. Perhaps patients who are sensitive to intermittent light have a hyper-excitability concentrated mainly within the magnocellular division. It is, after all, magno cells that might be expected to respond most effectively to intermittent light at frequencies of 20 Hz and above. Perhaps in FOS the sensitivity is more widespread and the relative involvement of the parvocellular system is greater. If parvocellular cortical networks are responsible for the occipital spikes, this might explain why patients with FOS are not photo-sensitive.

The separation of visual pathways might help explain why patients with FOS are not photosensitive. To explain why visual stimulation prevents the occurrence of occipital spikes, however, we need to supplement the concepts outlined earlier in this chapter to include another principle.

Competitive recruitment

Hughlings Jackson described a patient who could sometimes prevent the 'march' of a seizure from the extremities of a limb to the remainder of his body by vigorously rubbing the affected limb above the part involved in the seizure (Jackson, 1931). There are many other case studies suggesting that when parts of the neural network are recruited to subserve normal sensation and cognition this normal activity can interfere with the spread of an epileptic discharge. In the case of FOS, a small, steady, centrally fixated light appears sufficient to prevent the occipital spikes.

Presumably competitive recruitment occurs in relatively normal brain areas to which the hyper-excitable areas project. Presumably the functions normally subserved by these areas are responsible for preventing seizures. Perhaps the normal activity in these areas reduces synchronisation.

We have sought an explanation of some of the phenomena of reflex epilepsy in terms of four basic concepts: non-uniform hyper-excitability, critical mass, synchronisation and competitive recruitment. It is now time to turn these concepts to use in the treatment of reflex epilepsy.

TREATMENT TECHNIQUES

There are many different techniques that can be used in the non-pharmacological treatment of reflex epilepsy and they may be considered under three main headings.

Reduce the critical mass

It is sometimes possible to forestall the stimulus responsible for seizures or to reduce its intensity. Television epilepsy, for example, can sometimes be prevented by a selective and cosmetic form of monocular occlusion using polarisers. Unfortunately, there are other cases of television epilepsy where the television is used for self-induction (Wilkins & Lindsay, 1985). Cases of reading epilepsy where the trigger is not linguistic but due to the pattern provided by text can be helped by using a simple reading mask that reduces the number of lines of text that are visible (Wilkins & Lindsay, 1985).

Provide competitive recruitment

Cognitive therapy for depression or anxiety states is now well established and can be highly successful. The patient is taught to redirect the pathological train of thoughts. Baxter et al (1992) used PET in a study of patients with obsessive compulsive disorder. Patients were tested before and after treatment with either fluoxetine hydrochloride or behaviour therapy and results indicated that glucose metabolic rates in the right head of the caudate nuclear changed with successful treatment regardless of the modality used. Pardo et al (1993) report a study along similar lines in which PET was used to detect changes in cerebral blood flow associated with two self-induced states of mind. Given that PET studies have shown that cognitive therapy can result in a redistribution of neuronal activation, it might be possible in an analogous way to train patients to interrupt the train of thoughts that precipitates a seizure. Training of this kind is similar to the conditioning therapy discussed by Forster (1977).

Redistribute physiological excitation from the epileptogenic stimulus

We have seen that some triggers are exquisitely focal (eg, in pattern-sensitive epilepsy some patients respond only to patterns in certain orientations). Small changes in distribution of excitation within the nerve network may, therefore, be enough to reduce seizures in some patients. It is reasonable to infer that in the visual cortex the excitation resulting from normal visual input can be redistributed by changing the colour of the illuminating light. Although few of the cortical neurones code for colour, these neurones nevertheless have a non-uniform spectral sensitivity. We have preliminary evidence that changing the colour of illumination can offer effective treatment in some cases. Patients use an intuitive colorimeter (Wilkins et al, 1992) to select a coloured light that makes the eyes 'feel comfortable'. A pair of coloured glasses is then provided so that they experience this colour of light under normal conditions of illumination. Coloured glasses have been used to control seizures in photo-sensitive epilepsy since the work of Carterette & Symmes (1952), but it is only recently that it has become possible to tailor the colour of the lenses to suit the individual patient.

REFERENCES

Aarts JHP, Binnie CD, Smit AM, Wilkins AJ 1984 Selective cognitive impairment during focal and generalised epileptiform EEG activity. Brain 107: 293–308
Aird RB 1983 The importance of seizure-inducing factors in the control of refractory forms of epilepsy. Epilepsia 24: 567–583

Andermann F, Goossens L, Andermann E 1989 Clinical features and diagnosis of epilepsy induced by thinking. In: Beaumanoir A, Gastaut H, Naquet R (eds) Reflex seizures and reflex epilepsies. Editions Médecine et Hygiéne, Geneva, pp317–322

Baxter LR, Schwartz JM, Bergman KS et al 1992 Caudate glucose metabolic rate changes with both drug and behaviour therapy for obsessive-compulsive disorder. Archives of General Psychiatry 49: 681–689

Beaumanoir A, Gastaut H, Naquet R (eds) 1989 Reflex seizures and reflex epilepsies. Editions Médecine et Hygiéne, Geneva

Binnie CD, Darby CE, de Korte RA, Wilkins AJ 1981 Interhemispheric differences in photosensitivity thresholds. In: Dam M, Gram L, Penry JK (eds) Advances in epileptology: XIIth Epilepsy International Symposium. Raven Press, New York, pp403–412

Carterette EC, Symmes D 1952 Colour as an experimental variable in photic stimulation. Electroencephalography and Clinical Neurophysiology 4: 289–296

Darby CE, Park DM, Wilkins AJ 1986 EEG characteristics of epileptic pattern sensitivity and their relation to the nature of pattern stimulation and the effects of sodium valproate. Electroencephalography and Clinical Neurophysiology 63: 517–525

Deonna T, Despland PA 1989 Sensory-evoked (touch) idiopathic myoclonic epilepsy of infancy. In: Beaumanoir A, Gastaut H, Naquet R (eds) Reflex seizures and reflex epilepsies. Editions Médecine et Hygiéne, Geneva, pp99–102

Ferrie CD, de Marco P, Grünewald S, Giannakodimos S, Panayiotopoulos CP 1994 Video game induced seizures. Journal of Neurology, Neurosurgery and Psychiatry 57: 925–931

Forster FM 1977 Reflex epilepsy, behavioural therapy and conditional reflexes. Thomas, Springfield, Ill.

Harding GFA, Jeavons PM, Edson AS 1994 Video material and epilepsy (submitted for publication)

Hubel DH 1988 Eye, brain and vision. Scientific American Library, New York

Jackson JH 1931 Selected writings on epilepsy and epileptiform convulsions. Hodder and Stoughton, London

Livingstone MS, Hubel D 1988 Segregation of form, colour, movement and depth: anatomy, physiology and perception. Science 240: 740–749

Mirsky AF, van Buren JM 1965 On the nature of the 'absence' in centrencephalic epilepsy: a study of some behavioural, electroencephalographic and autonomic factors. Electroencephalography and Clinical Neurophysiology 18: 334–348

Mishkin M, Ungerleider LG 1982 Object vision and spatial vision: two cortical pathways. Trends in Neurosciences 6 (10): 414–417

Panayiotopoulos CP 1989 Fixation-off sensitive epilepsies. In: Beaumanoir A, Gastaut H, Naquet R (eds) Reflex seizures and reflex epilepsies. Editions Médecine et Hygiéne, Geneva, pp203–217

Pardo JV, Pardo PJ, Raichle ME 1993 Neural correlates of self-induced dysphoria. American Journal of Psychiatry 150: 713–719

Petersen SE, Fox PT, Posner MI, Mintun MA, Raichle ME 1988 Positron emission tomographic studies of cortical anatomy of single word processing. Nature 331: 585–589

Petersen SE, Fox PT, Posner MI, Mintun MA, Raichle ME 1989 Positron emission tomographic studies of the processing of single words. Journal of Cognitive Neuroscience 1: 153–170

Raichle ME, Fiez JA, Viden TO, MacLeod AK, Pardo JV, Fox PT, Petersen SE 1994 Practice-related changes in human brain functional anatomy during non-motor learning. Cerebral Cortex 4: 8–26

Sherrington C 1947 The integrative action of the nervous system. Yale University Press, New Hampshire

Singer W 1990 The formation of co-operative cell assemblies in the visual cortex. Journal of Experimental Biology 153: 177–197

Wilkins AJ, Zifkin B, Andermann F, McGovern E 1982 Seizures induced by thinking. Annals of Neurology 11: 608–612

Wilkins AJ, Lindsay J 1985 Common forms of reflex epilepsy: physiological mechanisms and techniques for treatment. In: Pedley TA, Meldrum BS (eds) Recent advances in epilepsy II. Churchill Livingstone, Edinburgh

Wilkins AJ, Binnie CD, Darby, CE, Kasteleijn-Nolst Trenité D 1990 Inferences regarding the visual precipitation of seizures, eye-strain and headaches. In: Avoli A, Gloor P, Kostopoulos

G, Naquet R (eds) Generalised epilepsy: neurological approaches. Birkhauser, Boston, pp314–326

Wilkins AJ et al 1992 Preliminary observations concerning treatment of visual discomfort and associated perceptual distortion. Ophthalmic and Physiological Optics 12: 257–263

Wyler AR, Ward AA Jr 1980 Epileptic neurones. In: Lockard JS, Ward AA Jr (eds) Epilepsy: a window to brain mechanisms. Raven Press, New York, pp51–68

Zagury S, Maury JA, Jomini-Jalanti RM 1989 Partial sensitive epilepsy triggered by a pure sound. A case report. In: Beaumanoir A, Gastaut H, Naquet R (eds) Reflex seizures and reflex epilepsies. Editions Médecine et Hygiéne, Geneva, pp251–254

DISCUSSION

Duncan: I am still not clear whether one can get typical absences as a reflex.

Wilkins: I find the discussions on clinical typologies difficult to follow, as I am not a clinician. I do not see these patients and so I do not have a good feel for their typology. There was one case I saw that had absences with stereotypical spike-wave. The patient was clearly pattern-sensitive, only had these discharges in response to patterns and only had absence seizures with stereotypical 3 per s spike and wave and no major attacks. So yes, I think it is possible.

Panayiotopoulos: Typical absences may be consistently induced by photic stimulation, patterns, emotions or mathematical calculations or thinking and somatosensory stimulation. These modalities of reflex absences are well documented in the literature. Let us also not forget self-induced photo-sensitive and pattern-sensitive epilepsy with absences. [See appendix pp 206–212.]

Mirsky: In that ingenious method for the patient to select the most comfortable colour, what is to prevent them from picking a colour that will make more seizures likely for those patients with self-induction?

Wilkins: An interesting question. Nothing as yet. Obviously at the moment I am doing all the work with concurrent EEG as a control. There are one or two patients where there is an EEG response which concurs with what they report to be the most uncomfortable colours. But in those cases where there is a clear history of self-induction and finding pleasurable sensations, I would not rely simply on the subjective report; one would have to do it with much more electrophysiological control. That is what I would like to do but I have not done it yet. Double-blind trials have only been based on the subjective reports.

Mirsky: It seems very intriguing.

Wilkins: Yes. It does seem to work. Not in everybody and certainly not in severe cases, but there are one or two where it does have a dramatic effect and it does not have the disadvantages of pharmacological treatment.

Robinson: If their absences got worse with a colour they liked, it would be equally interesting.

APPENDIX

J. S. Duncan   C. P. Panayiotopoulos

TYPICAL ABSENCES WITH SPECIFIC MODES OF PRECIPITATION (REFLEX ABSENCES): CLINICAL ASPECTS

Typical absences, like other epileptic seizures, generally arise in a 'spontaneous', unpredictable fashion without detectable precipitants. Less commonly they can be provoked by certain recognisable stimuli. Epileptic seizures which are consistently elicited by a specific stimulus are described as stimulus-sensitive (SSE), reflex, triggered or sensory-evoked; prevalence among patients with epilepsies is 4–7 per cent. The Commission of the International League Against Epilepsy (ILAE) describes them as 'Epilepsies characterised by seizures with specific modes of precipitation (reflex epilepsies)' (Commission, 1989). Wilkins (see pp. 206–215) has given an excellent account of the factors and brain mechanisms responsible for the precipitation of reflex seizures and absences. This brief review focuses on some clinical aspects related to reflex typical absences.

Stimulus-sensitive typical absences

Typical absences may be induced by flickering lights (photo-sensitivity), patterns (pattern-sensitivity), elimination of central vision and fixation (fixation-off sensitivity), somatosensory and probably other stimuli. It is recognised that absences are also common in self-induction. Stimuli may be extrinsic, as in the above examples, or proprioceptive (i.e. movements), or they may involve higher brain function, emotions and cognition (thinking, music, arithmetic).

Other types of generalised seizures may also be evoked by the same stimuli or they may be spontaneous. Generalised tonic-clonic seizures (GTCS) may occur de novo or follow a cluster of absences or myoclonic jerks. Myoclonic jerks may be manifested in the limbs or trunk or they may be localised in specific muscles such as those of the eyelids (eyelid myoclonia with absences).

These stimulus-sensitive typical absences are seen either independently or within the broad framework of certain epileptic syndromes.

Photo-sensitive epilepsies with typical absences

It should be emphasised that 'photo-sensitive epilepsy' (PE) is a broad term comprising all forms of epilepsies in which seizures are triggered by photic stimulation and does not correspond to a particular epileptic syndrome. For example, 30 per cent of patients with juvenile myoclonic epilepsy are photo-sensitive with or without absences (Figs 24.1, 24.2). Video-EEG and close questioning of photo-sensitive patients reveal that clinical manifestations (mild localised or generalised jerks and/or impairment of cognition or sub-

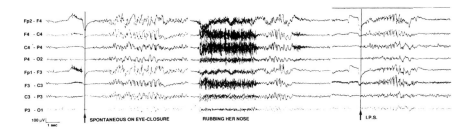

Fig. 24.1 EEG of a 26-year-old female patient with JME. Generalised spike and occasionally multiple spike and slow wave discharges occur after eye closure (left) and are also elicited by somatosensory stimulation such as rubbing the nose (centre) or intermittent photic stimulation (right). (From Panayiotopoulos et al, 1992, with the permission of the editor of the Journal of Neurology, Neurosurgery and Psychiatry).

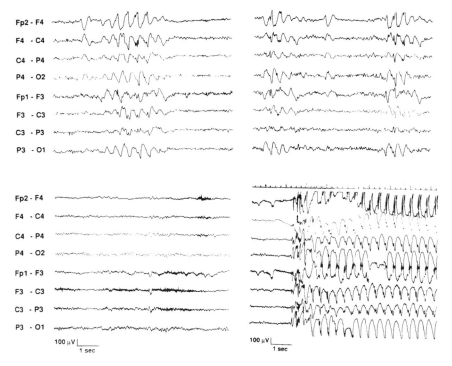

Fig. 24.2 EEG of a patient with JME who also had seizures induced by television viewing and video-games. (Case 1 reported by Ferrie et al, 1994.) A typical absence seizure is induced by intermittent photic stimulation (lower right). Spontaneous discharges and focal paroxysmal abnormalities were frequently recorded. (From Alberti et al, 1994, with the permission of the editor of Epilepsia.)

jective sensations) occur in more than 60 per cent of the photo-convulsive responses (Kasteleijn-Nolst Trenite, 1989). Thus the prevalence of absences in photo-sensitivity may be grossly under-estimated. Absences may be revealed with appropriate testing of cognition.

Generalised tonic-clonic seizures are reported far more commonly (87 per cent) than absences (6 per cent), partial seizures (2.5 per cent) and myoclonic jerks (1.5 per cent) (Jeavons & Harding, 1975; Newmark & Perry, 1979; Binnie & Jeavons, 1992). However, our experience with video-EEG recordings is that many patients categorised as having only GTCS frequently have mild spontaneous or photically-induced myoclonic jerks or absences either independently or preceding GTCS. The common problem in epilepsies is that minor phenomena like jerks and absences often go unreported.

Precipitants of seizures

Television, video-games, visual display units of computers, discotheques and natural flickering light (shining through trees or reflecting from the sea) are, in that order, common precipitants of seizures (Jeavons & Harding, 1975; Newmark & Penry, 1979). Video-game-induced seizures are increasingly common but should not always be equated with photo-sensitivity, from which only 70 per cent of patients suffer (Ferrie et al, 1994).

Eyelid myoclonia with absences (EMA)

EMA is probably the only well-defined syndrome of a form of photo-sensitive epilepsy, although it is not yet recognised by the ILAE (see Ch. 25). EMA is an idiopathic form of generalised epilepsy which persists in adult life. Photo-sensitivity and severity of absences may decline but eyelid myoclonia, mainly induced by eye closure, persists (Giannakodimos & Panayiotopoulos, 1995). Eyelid myoclonia with absences may be seen in patients with learning and behavioural problems which, though not belonging in the idiopathic generalised epilepsies, are difficult to categorise (see Ch. 29). We have been unable to confirm self-induction in eyelid myoclonia with absences (Appleton et al, 1993; Panayiotopoulos, 1994; Giannakodimos & Panayiotopoulos 1995) reported by other authors (Darby et al, 1980; Kasteleijn-Nolst Trenite et al, 1989).

Photically induced typical absences with onset in childhood or adolescence

Absences with onset in childhood are associated with a higher prevalence (18 per cent) of photo-sensitivity than those appearing in the second decade of life (7.5 per cent). Absences combined with photo-sensitivity have a worse prognosis than those of childhood absence epilepsy (see Ch. 19) and they should not be categorised as childhood absence epilepsy (CAE). Children with absences which are consistently elicited by photic stimuli (Fig. 24.3) may belong to syndromes other than CAE.

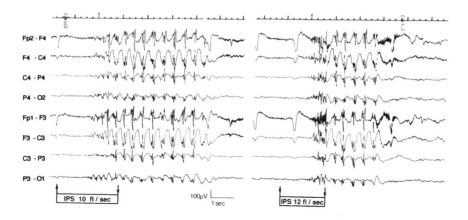

Fig. 24.3. Video-EEG-recorded typical absence seizures evoked in a photo-sensitive male aged 19 years. Patient is unresponsive and stares. He has suffered also since childhood from frequent absences, mainly in the morning after awakening, occasionally followed by generalised tonic-clonic seizures.

Self-induced seizures and absences

Self-induction has been well established as a mode of precipitation but prevalence is disputed from a small number to as high as 30 per cent of photo-sensitive patients (Andermann et al, 1962; Green, 1966; Jeavons & Harding, 1975; Darby et al, 1980; Kasteleijn-Nolst Trenite et al, 1989; Tassinari et al, 1989; Binnie & Jeavons, 1992). Self-induction of seizures, is practised not only by mentally handicapped patients, as was initially reported, but also by those of normal or above average intelligence. Techniques of self-induction vary from waving the abducted fingers in front of a bright light source to eyelid blinking, making the television screen roll or viewing geometric patterns

Absences and myoclonic jerks are the commoner types of self-induced seizures. A GTCS may be induced after a series of absences or jerks.

Video-game-induced seizures and absences

There is an increasing incidence of seizures induced by playing video-games (VGS) and recent media reports have highlighted the risk (Graf et al, 1994; Ferrie et al, 1994; Fish et al, 1994). This includes not only those games using an interlaced video-monitor (TV) but also small, hand-held liquid crystal displays and non-interlaced 70 Hz arcade games. Data analysed by Ferrie et al (1994) indicate that photo-sensitivity is a major precipitating factor (70 per cent) but VGS may also occur in non-photo-sensitive patients with idiopathic generalised epilepsies where sleep deprivation, fatigue, cognitive activities, decision-making and praxis may alone or in combination elicit an epileptic seizure. Occipital lobe epilepsy, mainly without photo-sensitivity, is the second most frequent (29 per cent) type of epilepsy. This is more often the case in arcade games.

VGS may be absences, jerks and GTCS or visual partial seizures with symptoms such as eye fatigue, headache and visual illusions, alone or pre-ceding a GTCS (Graf et al, 1994; Ferrie et al, 1994).

Pattern-sensitive epilepsy and absences

Pattern-sensitive epilepsy is a term used for epileptic seizures and/or EEG abnormalities induced by patterns. Pattern-sensitive epilepsy is closely related to photo-sensitivity; nearly all pattern-sensitive patients are also photo-sensitive. Pattern-sensitivity without photo-sensitivity has been reported (Brinciotti et al, 1994). Patients sensitive to non-geometric patterns are rare and probably not photo-sensitive. Self-induced pattern sensitivity with absences (Fig. 24.4) has been described (Panayiotopoulos, 1979; Matricardi et al, 1989).

Fixation-off-sensitive epilepsies

Fixation-off sensitivity (FOS) denotes the form/forms of epilepsy and/or EEG abnormalities which are elicited by elimination of central vision and fixation (Panayiotopoulos 1987). In routine EEG, performed in an illumi-nated room and conditions allowing preservation of fixation and central vision, FOS may be suspected if the EEG abnormalities appear and persist as long as the eyes remain closed and disappear when the eyes are opened – that is, they show a similar reactivity to that of the α-rhythm. FOS is mainly present in benign childhood epilepsy with occipital paroxysms; absences with FOS have been reported (Panayiotopoulos, 1987).

Thinking epilepsy and absences

Typical absences are probably the commonest type of seizures provoked by mental activity involved in calculations, studying mathematics, playing games such as cards, making complex decisions or emotions and excitement (Andermann et al, 1989; Martin da Silva et al, 1989; Danielle et al, 1989; Oller, 1989; Goossens et al, 1990; Panayiotopoulos et al, 1994; Ferrie et al, 1994; see also Ch. 14).

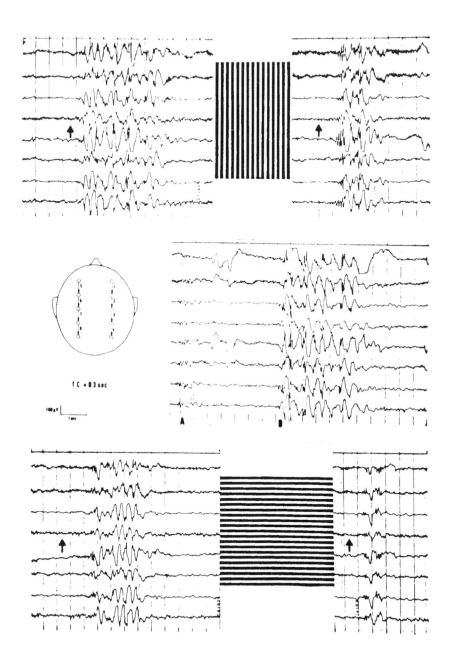

Fig. 24.4 Self-induced pattern-sensitive epilepsy. High-amplitude discharges of multiple/spike and slow wave are induced within 1 s of onset (arrow) of vertical (top) and horizontal pattern stimulation (bottom). Similar responses were induced when the patient looked (B) or glanced at a radiator with linear vertical patterns (middle). The patient was also photo-sensitive. (From Panayiotopoulos, 1979; with the permission of the editor of the Archives of Neurology).

REFERENCES

Alberti V, Grünewald RA, Panayiotopoulos CP, Chroni E 1994 Focal electroencephalographic abnormalities in juvenile myoclonic epilepsy. Epilepsia 32: 297–301

Andermann F, Goossens L, Andermann E 1989 Clinical features and diagnosis of epilepsy induced by thinking. In: Beaumanoir A, Gastaut H, Naquet R (eds) Reflex seizures and reflex epilepsies. Editions Médicine and Hygiéne, Geneva, pp317–322

Andermann K et al 1962 Self-induced epilepsy. Archives of Neuroogy 6: 49–79

Appleton R, Panayiotopoulos C P, Acomb A B, Beirne M 1993 Eyelid myoclonia with absences: an epilepsy syndrome. Journal of Neurology, Neurosurgery and Psychiatry 56: 1312–1316

Binnie C D, Darby C E, de Corte R A, Wilkins A J 1980 Self induction of epileptic seizures by eye closure: incidence and recognition. Journal of Neurology, Neurosurgery and Psychiatry 43: 386–389

Binnie C D, Jeavons P M 1992 Photo-sensitive epilepsies. In: Roger J, Bureau M, Dravet C, Dreifuss F E, Perret A, Wolf P (eds) Epileptic syndromes of infancy, childhood and adolescence, 2nd edn. John Libbey Eurotext, London, pp299-305

Brinciotti M, Matricardi M, Pellicia A, Trasatti G 1994 Pattern sensitivity and photosensitivity in epileptic children with visually induced seizures. Epilepsia 35: 842-849

Commission on Classification and Terminology of the International League against Epilepsy 1989 Proposal for classification of epilepsies and epileptic syndromes. Epilepsia 30: 389-399

Daniele O, Raieli V, Mataliano A, Natale E 1989 Seizures precipitated by unusual epileptogenic tasks. In: Beaumanoir A, Gastaut H, Naquet R (eds) Reflex seizures and reflex epilepsies. Editions Médicine and Hygiéne, Geneva, pp333–336

Darby C E, de Corte R A, Binnie C D, Wilkins A J 1980 The self-induction of epileptic seizures by eye-closure. Epilepsia 21: 31-41

Ferrie C D, de Marco P, Grunewald R A, Giannakodimos S, Panayiotopoulos C P 1994 Video game-induced seizures. Journal of Neurology, Neurosurgery and Psychiatry 57: 925-931

Fish D R, Quirk J A, Smith S J M, Sander J WAS, Shorvon S D, Allen P J 1994 National survey of photosensitivity and seizures induced by electronic screen games (video games, console games, computer games). Interim report and findings. HMSO, London

Giannakodimos S, Panayiotopoulos C P 1995 Eyelid myoclonia with absences in adults: a clinical and video-EEG study. Neurology (submitted)

Graf W D, Chatrian G E, Glass S T, Knauss TA 1994 Video game-related seizures: a report on 10 patients and a review of the literature. Pediatrics 93: 551-556

Green J B 1966 Self-induced seizures: clinical and electroencephalographic studies. Archives of Neurology 15: 579–586

Jayakar P, Chiappa K H 1990 Clinical correlations of photoparoxysmal responses. Electroencephalography and Clinical Neurophysiology 75: 251-254

Jeavons P M, Harding G F A 1975 Photo-sensitive epilepsy. Heinemann, London

Kasteleijn-Nolst Trenite D G A 1989 Photosensitivity in epilepsy: electrophysiological and clinical correlates. Acta Neurologica Scandinavica (Suppl.125): 3-149

Kasteleijn-Nolst Trenite D G A, Binnie C D, Meinardi H 1987 Photo-sensitive patients: symptoms and signs during intermittent photic stimulation and their relation to seizures in daily life. Journal of Neurology, Neurosurgery and Psychiatry 50:1546-1549

Martin da Silva A, Pinto R, Coutinho P 1989 Thinking epilepsy: Cognitive processes and cortical structures involved. In: Beaumanoir A, Gastaut H, Naquet R (eds) Reflex seizures and reflex epilepsies. Editions Médicine and Hygiéne, Geneva, pp323-331

Matricardi M, Brinciotti M, Trasatti G, Pellicia A 1989 Self-induced seizures by spatially structured visual stimuli. In: Beaumanoir A, Gastaut H, Naquet R (eds) Reflex seizures and reflex epilepsies. Editions Médicine and Hygiéne, Geneva, pp393-395

Newmark M E, Penry J K 1979 Photo-sensitive epilepsy: a review. Raven Press, New York

Oller F-V 1989 Absences provoked by mental activity. In: Beaumanoir A, Gastaut H, Naquet R (eds) Reflex seizures and reflex epilepsies. Editions Médicine and Hygiéne, Geneva, pp341-345

Panayiotopoulos C P 1979 Self-induced pattern-sensitive epilepsy. Archives of Neurology 36: 48-50

Panayiotopoulos C P 1987 Fixation-off sensitive epilepsy in eye-lid myoclonia with absence seizures. Annals of Neurology 22: 87–89

Panayiotopoulos C P 1994 Fixation-off sensitive epilepsies. In: Wolf P (ed) Epileptic seizures and epilepsies. John Libbey, London (in press)

Tassinari C A et al 1989 Self-induced seizures. In: Beaumanoir A, Gastaut H, Naquet R (eds) Reflex seizures and reflex epilepsies. Editions Médicine et Hygiène, Geneva, pp363–368

25. Eyelid myoclonia with absences

R. E. Appleton

Eyelid myoclonia with absences (EMA) has yet to be recognised by the International League Against Epilepsy (ILAE) as a separate syndrome within the classification of the epilepsies. It was first observed as a specific entity in 1977 (Jeavons 1977) and has recently been defined in detail (Appleton et al 1993). EMA satisfies the criteria for definition as a syndrome on the basis of uniform clinical and electro-encephalographic (EEG) features and a consistent prognosis. The main differential diagnosis includes typical absence and a self-induced epilepsy. The aim of this chapter is to describe the characteristic electro-clinical features of eyelid myoclonia with absences and to recommend its inclusion as a specific epilepsy syndrome in the future classifications of the epilepsies.

CLINICAL FEATURES

Seizure types

The clinical hallmarks of the syndrome are the eyelid myoclonia, typical absences and photo-sensitivity. The age of onset is always within the first decade, and usually within the first five years of life. Either the eyelid myoclonia or the absences maybe the first observed seizure type. However, the eyelid myoclonia may not be recognised as a seizure but as a tic or mannerism (Appleton et al, 1993). Eyelid myoclonia must be differentiated from eyelid flickering or fluttering (which may also resemble spontaneous eye-blinking); eyelid flicker/flutter may occur in childhood and juvenile-onset absence epilepsy (Commission, 1989; Panayiotopoulos et al, 1989), symptomatic absence epilepsy (Panayiotopoulos et al, 1992) and benign myoclonic epilepsy of infancy (Dravet & Bureau, 1981).

It may be difficult on clinical grounds alone to differentiate eyelid myoclonia from eyelid flutter. During the EEG eyelid myoclonia occurs simultaneously with spike-wave or polyspike discharges – the electro-encephalographic hallmark of EMA. The fast myoclonic jerks of the eyelids are frequently accompanied by upward deviation of the eyes and occasionally the head, and even shoulders, but rarely the limbs. However, limb myoclonus may rarely occur, independently from the eyelid myoclonia and absences. The episodes of eyelid myoclonia are brief, lasting from under 1 s to 2–3 s, and are frequently accompanied by a brief typical absence of the same duration.

At other times absences may occur both spontaneously and on awakening and also on hyper-ventilation. They seem to occur less frequently, and are of shorter duration (< 5 s) than in typical childhood/juvenile absence epilepsy. The precise age of onset of the absences in EMA is difficult to determine (due to under-recognition) but in the vast majority of patients it appears to be between 4–5 years of age. When occurring independently from eyelid myoclonia, the absences in EMA are not associated with other motor phenomena, such as lip-smacking or chewing movements or semi-purposeful hand movements, and are more likely to occur on waking.

Tonic-clonic seizures may occasionally develop after the age of 11–12 years but are infrequent and occur usually after provoking factors such as menstruation, sleep deprivation or photic stimulation.

The majority of patients with EMA reported thus far are photo-sensitive – both clinically and on EEG. In at least two of the patients described by Appleton et al (1993), clinical photo-sensitivity was the presenting symptom. One girl presented at the age of 2.5 years with repeated episodes of looking up, eyelid (and occasionally head) jerks and brief lapses in concentration. These episodes were initially thought to be caused by the wind on the child's face as they usually occurred on leaving a building and going outside (into bright sunshine). It is possible that clinical photo-sensitivity is present from an early age in these patients, but may remain undetected until demonstrated on intermittent photic stimulation (IPS) during an EEG. This is unlike the photo-sensitivity seen in the (other) idiopathic generalised epilepsies, which tends to develop around puberty.

Neurological and intellectual findings

Limited data have indicated that patients with EMA show no neurological abnormality and are of average or even above average intellectual ability. Despite the very early onset of all seizure types in EMA, no decline or 'fall-off' in cognitive function has been noted. Children may achieve academic qualifications, and, as adults, can secure most types of employment, including accountancy, banking and secretarial work. EMA has not been known to develop following either a traumatic or non-traumatic cerebral insult. The birth and perinatal history and early development have been normal in all patients reported.

Finally, none of the patients reported by Appleton et al (1993) or others (Giannakodimos & Panayiotopoulos, 1994) have admitted to self-inducing the seizures themselves over many years of follow-up (either spontaneously or on direct questioning) and self-induction was not demonstrated following repeated and prolonged video-EEG recordings.

Family history

Patients have been reported in whom there is no, or a definite family history of febrile, or afebrile seizures. The inheritance of all the epilepsies is complicated and multifactorial. This fact and the small number of patients previously reported with EMA precludes any definite comment on any genetic predisposition in this epilepsy syndrome. However, see twin cases with EMA by De Marco (1989), Bianchi (Ch. 37) and EMA among siblings (Giannakodimos & Panayiotopoulos, 1994).

When more data become available, and with further advances in molecular genetics, it may become possible to identify either a specific, genetically-determined epilepsy or at least a familial trait in EMA.

The electroencephalogram

The EEG (ictal and inter-ictal) is one of the most important criteria in defining any epilepsy syndrome. In EMA the inter-ictal EEG shows a normal background; the ictal EEG demonstrates generalised spike-wave or polyspike-wave discharges which occur on eye closure and also on IPS (Figs 25.1,2). Photo-sensitivity appears to be a common finding in EMA, although it was not observed in the patients reported by De Marco (1989). Photo-sensitivity may be marked, with frequent photo-convulsive responses. The generalised spike-wave or polyspike-wave discharges occur at a frequency of 3–6 Hz; they are seen from 0.5–4 s after eye closure and are brief, lasting between

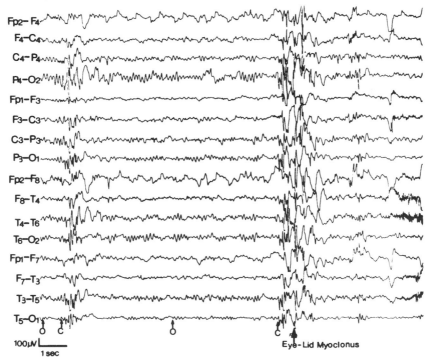

Fig. 25.1 Video-EEG in a child aged 13 years demonstrating normal background activity when eyes open (O), but, on eye closure (C), bursts of generalised, high-amplitude, irregular polyspike and spike slow-wave activity associated with eyelid myoclonus (from Appleton et al, 1993, with the permission of the editors of the Journal of Neurology, Neurosurgery and Psychiatry).

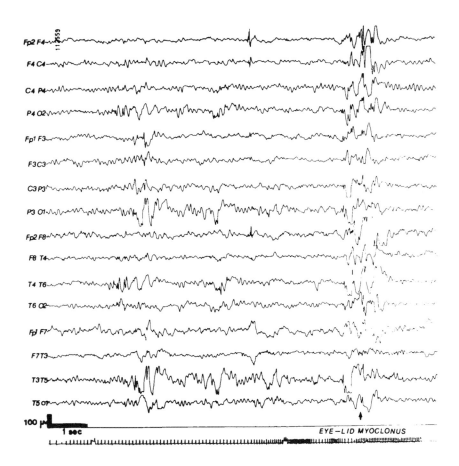

Fig. 25.2   EEG recording; response to intermittent photic stimulation (IPS) at 10–12 Hz with eyes closed – high amplitude spike and slow-wave and polyspike discharges with eyelid myoclonia and a very brief period of impaired consciousness.

1–4 s. In most patients the discharges are accompanied by simultaneous eyelid myoclonia and an absence. Generalised spike or polyspike and slow-wave discharges are also generated during hyper-ventilation on eye closure, but rarely with the eyes open.

Total darkness suppresses the eye closure-related abnormalities in all patients, both clinically and on EEG (Fig. 25.3). One patient (female) has shown fixation-off sensitivity (Panayiotopoulos, 1987). The electro-clinical features in EMA are easier to identify on awakening, particularly after sleep deprivation.

The demonstration of both the clinical events (which may be extremely brief) and abnormalities on the EEG may be difficult. Simultaneous split-screen video-EEG monitoring has proved extremely useful in establishing a diagnosis of EMA in most patients.

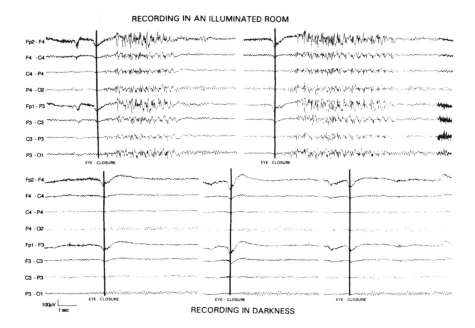

Fig. 25.3   Video-EEG recording of adult patient. Upper traces: EEG showing high amplitude spikes and multiple spikes and slow waves occurring on eye closure in normal light; the discharges were frequently associated with eyelid myoclonia and a very brief, mild impairment of consciousness. Lower traces: total darkness inhibited the abnormalities induced by eye closure (from Appleton et al, 1993, with the permission of the editors of the Journal of Neurology, Neurosurgery and Psychiatry).

EPIDEMIOLOGY

EMA appears to be rare. Whether this is real or reflects under-diagnosis, misdiagnosis or under-reporting is unclear. It may be a combination of all three factors. In the author's paediatric epilepsy clinic it represents approximately 1.2% of a total population of 380 patients; in a corresponding adult clinic the figure is 1.7% (Giannakodimos & Panayiotopoulos, 1994). There appears to be a sex bias, with 80% of patients being female (Appleton et al, 1993; De Marco, 1989; Giannakodimos & Panayiotopoulos, 1994).

DIFFERENTIAL DIAGNOSIS

As stated previously, it is important to differentiate eyelid myoclonia from eyelid flicker or flutter, which may be seen in a number of different epilepsy syndromes/epilepsies. Eyelid myoclonia, but not eyelid flicker, occurs simultaneously with spike-wave or polyspike and slow-wave activity on the EEG, and underlines the importance of obtaining a simultaneous split-screen video-EEG record in these patients. The absences in EMA are very brief (<5 s in duration), are not usually associated with additional motor phenomena and are not always accompanied by 3 Hz spike and slow-wave activity on the EEG, which may help to differentiate them from the absences seen in childhood and juvenile absence epilepsy. Four of 10 patients (Giannakodimos & Panayiotopoulos, 1994) and three of the five patients reported by Appleton et al (1993) were initially diagnosed as having childhood absence epilepsy. Early photo-sensitivity also appears to be a characteristic clinical and electroencephalographic feature of EMA and is not usually seen in the 'other' idiopathic generalised epilepsies, where the phenomenon tends to develop much later, usually between 10–18 years of age.

Finally, EMA must be differentiated from self-induced seizures whereby deliberate slow closure of the eyelids induces brief seizures characterised by an absence, with or without a myoclonic component (Binnie & Jeavons, 1992; Darby et al, 1980). This is clearly an important issue and, again, video-EEG may help to establish the correct diagnosis. In patients who self-induce their seizures the eye movements always precede the discharges and are much slower than in EMA, and the eye movements may persist in darkness (unassociated with any electrical discharges). Eye closure to command in these patients also fails to induce any discharges (Binnie, 1993, personal communication). It is also unlikely that self-induction can develop as young as two or three years of age, which was the age of onset in at least two of the patients reported by Appleton et al (1993). Most patients who self-induce admit to deriving some pleasure from the experience (Darby et al, 1980). In contrast, patients with EMA express considerable relief when seizure control is achieved, or even improved (Appleton et al, 1993; Giannakodimos & Panayiotopoulos, 1994). The majority of patients with EMA are of average or above average intelligence with no psycho-social or psychiatric problems, in contrast to most of the patients who self-induce (Binnie et al, 1980). The only reported exception to this were the twin girls reported by De Marco (1989), who demonstrated both learning difficulties and some behavioural disturbances. The possibility of self-induction was not discussed in that report, or in the patient described by Barclay et al (1993), who showed some of the features seen in EMA.

TREATMENT

Seizure control in EMA is usually more difficult than in typical absence and other generalised epilepsies (Appleton et al, 1993; De Marco, 1989), and it is thought that remission before adulthood is less likely. Generalised tonic-clonic seizures (if they occur) tend to be controlled easily, in contrast to the eyelid myoclonia, with or without absences, which may be reduced in frequency but still persist for years, despite treatment. Sodium valproate, with either ethosuximide (Appleton et al, 1993) or occasionally clobazam (De

Marco, 1989), appears to be more effective in treating this condition than if a single drug is used. Recently one of the author's patients has responded to a combination of lamotrigine and sodium valproate. It is possible that lamotrigine may prove to be effective in EMA, mirroring its early results in 'atypical' absences (Gibbs et al, 1991) and in myoclonic absence epilepsy (Manonmani & Wallace, 1994).

PROGNOSIS

None of the patients reported in the literature have achieved an obvious remission of seizures and only a few have shown complete seizure-control while receiving treatment. However, the patient population is clearly too small to allow a definitive comment on the long-term prognosis, at least in terms of the 'natural history' of the seizures. Nevertheless, preliminary data would suggest that anti-epileptic medication may need to be given for life and that less than total seizure control should be expected, with clear implications for driving and employment opportunities. In contrast, the information available suggests that there may be no significant adverse effect on intellectual status. In the first patient reported by Appleton et al (1993) there was a delay in diagnosis (and therefore in commencing treatment) of almost eight years with no obvious detrimental effect on development or academic progress. However, it is possible that continued, untreated absences could result in some subtle cognitive dysfunction as has been reported in adults who have had unrecognised/untreated absences throughout childhood (Loiseau et al, 1983).

CONCLUSION

Delineating epileptic syndromes permits a greater precision of diagnosis and, importantly, prognosis than simply classifying seizure types. When identifying a syndrome it is crucial to adhere to the criteria (clinical and EEG) which define the syndrome. Squeezing atypical cases into generally accepted syndromes must be avoided as this defeats the whole purpose of syndrome definition and precludes a consistent classification of the epilepsies.

Preliminary data would indicate that, on the basis of the clinical features, EEG findings, response to treatment and prognosis, EMA should be classified as a specific epilepsy syndrome within the generalised epilepsies. This hypothesis will no doubt be either confirmed or refuted with future DNA analysis.

REFERENCES

Appleton RE, Panayiotopoulos CP, Acomb BA, Beirne M 1993 Eyelid myoclonia with typical absences: an epilepsy syndrome. Journal of Neurology, Neurosurgery and Psychiatry 56:1312–1316

Barclay CL, Murphy WF, Lee MA, Darwish HZ 1993 Unusual form of seizures induced by eye closure. Epilepsia 34: 289–293

Binnie CD, Darby CE, de Korte RA, Wilkins AJ 1980 Self-induction of epileptic seizures by eye closure: incidence and recognition. Journal of Neurology, Neurosurgery and Psychiatry 43: 386–389

Commission on Classification and Terminology of the International League Against Epilepsy 1989 Proposal for classification of epilepsies and epileptic syndromes. Epilepsia 30: 389–399

Darby CE, de Korte RA, Binnie CD, Wilkins AJ 1980 The self-induction of epileptic seizures by eye closure. Epilepsia 21: 31–42

De Marco P 1989 Eyelid myoclonia with absences (EMA) in two monovular twins. Clinical Electroencephalography 20: 193–195

Dravet C, Bureau M 1981 L'epilepsie myoclonique benigne du nourrison. Revue Electroencephalographie Neurophysiologie Clinique 11: 438–444

Giannakodimos S, Panayiotopoulos CP 1994 Eyelid myoclonia with absences: a clinical and video-EEG study in adults. Electroencephalography and Clinical Neurophysiology: abstract in press

Gibbs JM, Appleton RE, Rosenbloom L, Yuen WC 1992 Lamotrigine for intractable childhood epilepsy: a preliminary communication. Developmental Medicine and Child Neurology 34: 368–371

Jeavons PM 1977 Nosological problems of myoclonic epilepsies in childhood and adolescence. Developmental Medicine and Child Neurology 19: 3–8

Loiseau P, Pestre M, Dartigues JF, Commenges D, Barbeger-Gateau C, Cohado S 1983 Long-term prognosis in two forms of childhood epilepsy: typical absences seizures and epilepsy with rolandic (centro-temporal) EEG foci. Annals of Neurology 13: 642–648

Manonmani V, Wallace SJ 1994 Epilepsy with myoclonic absences. Archives of Disease in Childhood 70: 288–290

Panayiotopoulos CP 1987 Fixation-off-sensitive epilepsy in eyelid myoclonia with absence seizures. Annals of Neurology 22: 87–89

Panayiotopoulos CP, Obeid T, Waheed G 1989 Differentiation of typical absence seizures in epileptic syndromes. Brain 112: 1039–1056

Panayiotopoulos CP, Chroni E, Daskalopoulos C, Baker A, Rowlinson S, Walsh P 1992 Typical absence seizures in adults: clinical, EEG, video-EEG findings and diagnostic/syndromic considerations. Journal of Neurology, Neurosurgery and Psychiatry 55: 1002–1008

26. Perioral myoclonia with absences

C. P. Panayiotopoulos   *C. D. Ferrie*   *S. Giannakodimos*
R. O. Robinson

Perioral myoclonia with absences is a syndrome of IGE with onset in child-hood or early adolescence, characterised by frequent typical absence seizures (TAS) with variable impairment of consciousness and ictal localised rhythmic myoclonus of the perioral facial muscles. Occasionally, the involvement of masticatory muscles may be more pronounced. The absences may be brief but absence status may also occur. GTCS always occur either early or many years after the onset of absences; they are usually heralded by absences or absence status and may be infrequent or rare. Absences and GTCS may be resistant to medication, unremitting and possibly lifelong. Family history is often positive for epilepsies. Ictal EEG shows high-amplitude generalised discharges of typical but often irregular, rhythmic spike, mainly multiple spike and slow waves at 3–4 Hz. There is no photo-sensitivity.

INTRODUCTION AND INVESTIGATIONAL APPROACH TO PATIENTS WITH TYPICAL ABSENCES

For many years it has been appreciated that patients with TAS do not behave uniformly, either in the association of absences with other seizure types, their response to treatment or their ultimate prognosis for remission of seizures. The Commission of the International League Against Epilepsy recognises that the current classification of epilepsies and epileptic syndromes is not wholly satisfactory (Commission, 1989). In particular, syndromes are often broadly defined. Tighter definitions have been proposed in which exclusion criteria are accorded equal prominence with the more usual inclusion criteria (Panayiotopoulos, 1994).

In order to improve our understanding of typical absence epilepsies the principal author has embarked on a long term study whose aim is both to define more closely current absence syndromes and to classify those patients with TAS who do not fit with existing syndromes. The approach is two-way: all patients seen in our epilepsy clinics are thoroughly investigated, including video-EEG recordings (Panayiotopoulos et al, 1989a; Panayiotopoulos 1992; 1993). All patients are prospectively followed. For those (mainly adults) with long-standing epilepsies, medical reports and records are carefully scrutinised retrospectively, while in newly diagnosed patients (mainly children) all possible clinical and video-EEG features are carefully collated. On the basis of combined clinico-EEG criteria we attempt to classify patients using the restricted definitions of the existing syndromes. Patients who do not fit are left unclassified and are periodically reviewed. With the aid of a computer data base, Epicare, we look for patients in whom clinico-EEG features appear to be clustering non-fortuitously. In so doing we may be in a position to propose classification of patients into new syndromes which can be tested prospectively in new patients. This method should enable more rapid identification of new syndromes than would be possible by a purely prospective study.

In a previously reported study of adults with TAS, two patients were identified who could not be classified satisfactorily (Panayiotopoulos et al, 1992) and in whom perioral myoclonus was a feature of absences. Using the method described above, four further patients were identified and the clinical and EEG features were described in detail (Panayiotopoulos et al, 1994). It was proposed that these patients be classified as perioral myoclonia with absences (PMA). This chapter gives details on two more patients with PMA, presents further epidemiological data and reviews the electro-clinical manifestations of the syndrome.

Case 7

This 22-year-old woman had a half-sister who died aged 19 from 'epilepsy'. At 10 years of age the patient had onset of TAS with a pyknolepsy frequency. These were brief, caused her to 'miss conversation' and were more frequent in the morning and after sleep deprivation. At 20 years of age she drank a lot of alcohol at an all-night party, slept for an hour and awoke to feel 'strange, dizzy in the head'. This episode of absence status lasted a few hours and terminated in a GTCS.

Video-EEG (Fig. 26.1) revealed one TAS with moderate impairment of consciousness in which rhythmic ictal myoclonus of the perioral muscles and muscles of mastication was noticed. Previously she had failed to respond to carbamazepine and ethosuximide. Valproate helped but compliance was poor.

Case 8

This 54-year-old man with no family history of seizures had onset at 10 years of age of frequent short episodes during which he would miss conversation and was aware of eyelid blinking. At 16 years GTCS began. These occurred once every few months and were consistently preceded by showers of the same brief episodes and occasionally by jerks of the upper limbs immediately prior to the GTCS. He was considered to have frequent com-

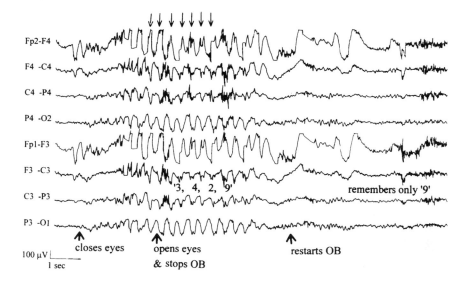

Fig. 26.1 Video-EEG recording from Case 7. During the discharge the patient was given a sequence of numbers to remember as shown. Arrows indicate perioral/jaw myoclonia. OB = over-breathing.

plex partial seizures with and without secondary generalisation and was treated with phenobarbitone, phenytoin and valproate. At 53 years of age he was admitted after being found by his family confused and with superficial burns caused by lying against a radiator. Later he recalled feeling 'slightly funny' on going to bed two days earlier and was amnesic for the following 48 h. During this time witnesses noted that he appeared very confused on the telephone. Neurological examination was normal except for residual signs of a mild cerebrovascular accident suffered a few years previously. Six weeks later an EEG revealed frequent brief generalised irregular polyspike and wave discharges with moderate impairment of consciousness accompanied by perioral myoclonus (Fig. 26.2).

EPIDEMIOLOGY

Six of our eight patients were female. Half had a family history of 'epilepsy'. We have recently reviewed all our adult patients with TAS (see Ch. 34) and the prevalence of PMA in this group of patients is 9.3%. The prevalence appears to be lower in children; we have seen only one case among over 50 children with video-EEG-documented typical absences.

CUMULATIVE DATA

Eight patients with PMA have been seen (Table 26.1).

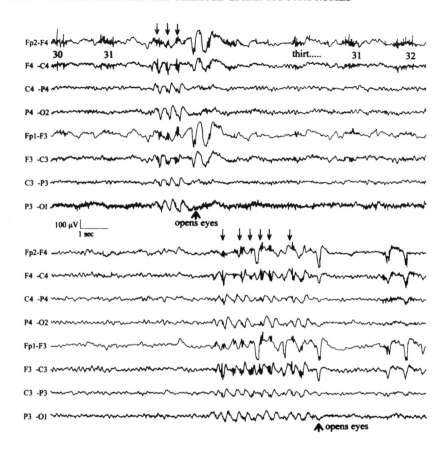

Fig. 26.2 Video-EEG recording from Case 8. The upper trace shows a TAS during over-breathing; the lower trace shows a spontaneous TAS. Arrows indicate perioral/jaw myoclonus. During both discharges arrhythmic eyelid blinking occurred.

CLINICAL AND EEG FEATURES

Patients with PMA may present from early childhood to early adolescence, usually following a GTCS, or less commonly with TAS or absence status (Fig. 26.3). Patients are of normal intelligence. Any neurological findings on examination are coincidental (Case 8) and neuro-imaging is normal.

Typical absences

Complex typical absences with perioral myoclonia are the defining feature of the syndrome. They have a wide range in their age of onset from 2–13 years (median 10) and vary both in their frequency (from 1–2 per week to pyknolepsy) and in the severity of impairment of consciousness. The absences, as revealed by video-EEG, are brief, lasting a mean of 3.7 s (range

Table 26.1 Summary data for patients with perioral myoclonia with absences

	Patient 1	Patient 2	Patient 3	Patient 4	Patient 5	Patient 6	Patient 7	Patient 8
Sex	female	female	female	female	male	female	female	male
Age last seen (years)	11	30	22	23	38	19	22	54
Onset of TAS (years)	3	11	7	13	2	11	10	10
Frequency of TAS	frequent	frequent	frequent	infrequent	unknown	1–2/week	frequent	frequent
PM noted by observers	yes	yes	yes	yes	yes	yes	no	no
IOC during TAS	severe	moderate	moderate	mild	very mild	moderate	moderate	moderate
Onset of GTCS (years)	33	11	7	22	2	11	22	16
Frequency of GTCS	1/month	0–12/year	0–3/year	1/life	3/life	3–6/year	1/life	1/few months
Last GTCS (years)	7	22	21	22	36	19	22	54
TAS leading to GTCS	not apparent	yes	yes	no	yes	yes	no	yes
Absence status	no	yes	possible	no	yes	possible	yes	yes
Other seizures	nil	nil	nil	nil	nil	yes***	no	no
Intellectual status	normal	normal	normal	normal	normal	normal	normal	normal
Family history	yes	no	yes	yes	no	no	yes	no
Neuroimaging (CT)	not done	normal	minor asymmetry	not done	normal	normal	not done	not done
Video-EEG	irregular PSW with PM	no ictal events	no ictal events	not done	irregular PSW with PM	irregular PSW with MP*,**	irregular PSW with PM*	irregular PSW with PM**

PM, perioral myoclonus; IOC impairment of consciousness; PSW, polyspike and wave discharge(s)

*, Including muscles of mastication;
**, Eyelid flickering also seen;
***, Infrequent, sporadic myoclonic limb jerks.

2.4–8.7 s). This is noticeably shorter than in CAE (mean 12.4±2.1 s) or JAE (16.3±-7.1 s) but is nearer to that in JME (6.6±4.2 s) (Panayiotopoulos, 1989a; Panayiotopoulos et al, 1989b). All discharges have multiple spikes and the number and amplitude of spikes show considerable inter- and intra-discharge variation. Often no regular relationship is seen between spikes and waves and abrupt frequency changes occur with discharge fragmentations.

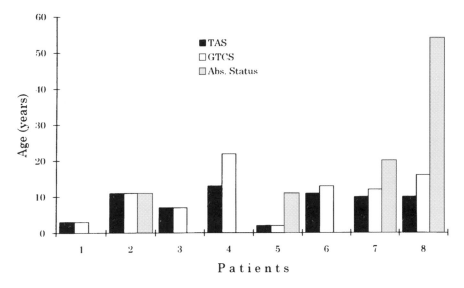

Fig. 26.3 Graph showing age of onset of seizure types in patients with PMA. Absence status was also suspected in Cases 3 and 6.

Perioral myoclonia occurred in all TAS and was confirmed by video-EEG in five patients. It consists of rhythmic contractions either of the orbicularis oris muscle, causing protrusion of the lips, contractions of the depressor anguli oris, causing twitching of the corners of the mouth, or more widespread involvement, including the muscles of mastication, causing jaw jerking. Each myoclonic jerk bears a close relationship to the polyspike component of the EEG discharge and myoclonia starts within the first second of the discharge and lasts for most of the ictus. Two patients, who also experienced eyelid flutter/blinking during TAS, described occasional longer absences in which spread of the myoclonus to the upper limbs preceded GTCS. No other symptoms are characteristic during TAS.

The inter-ictal EEG was normal or frequently showed focal abnormalities, including single spikes, spike wave complexes and theta waves with variable side emphasis. No patients were photo-sensitive, either clinically or on EEG.

Other seizure types

All patients develop GTCS. In four patients these had their onset in the months preceding recognition of absences. They are usually infrequent (range 1/life–12/year) and are often heralded by clusters of TAS or absence status. Absence status with perioral myoclonia is more common in PMA than in other syndromes of IGE with TAS. It was clearly described in four of our cases (Fig. 26.4) and was suspected in two others. It may end in a GTCS. Apart from these, other seizure types are not characteristic. Only one patient described random and infrequent myoclonic jerks of her upper limbs separate from TAS.

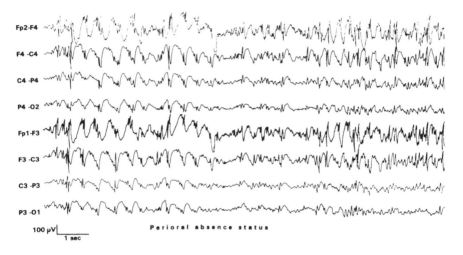

Fig. 26.4 Video-EEG of perioral absence status, which ended in a GTCS (Case 2).

Evolutionary aspects and treatment

The median age of our patients now is 22.5 years (range 11–54); all of them still require drug treatment. Persistence well into adult life appears to be a feature of the syndrome. Drug resistance is common; six of our patients required two or three drugs to achieve reasonable control. Valproate and ethosuximide were the drugs of choice; one patient responded to the addition of lamotrigine to valproate (Ferrie et al, 1993).

Differential diagnosis

Patients with PMA are frequently erroneously diagnosed as having partial seizures. This is a common mistake in adult patients with TAS (Panayiotopoulos et al, 1992) but is especially likely in PMA because of the prominent motor features of the absences. Perioral myoclonus is often reported/recorded as unilateral despite video-EEG evidence that it is bilateral. When it is accompanied by obvious impairment of consciousness the temptation to diagnose complex partial seizures is strong and is reinforced if, as commonly seen, clusters of absences or prolonged absences lead into GTCS. It is crucial that this mistake is avoided. This requires skill in the clinical art of diagnosing TAS (see Ch. 34). Doubt will frequently persist; the ictal EEG is, however, unmistakable and is exceptional in partial seizure disorders (see Ch. 34). A frequent mistake is to attach excessive weight to inter-ictal focal abnormalities, which are common in some syndromes of IGE (Aliberti et al, 1994). Where doubt persists sleep and awakening EEG are useful.

The importance of the syndromic classification of absence epilepsies is only now being appreciated. The majority of patients in this series might be classified as either childhood or juvenile absence epilepsy. In these a rapid response to treatment is expected and the former usually remits in childhood. Hence the recognition of PMA has important implications for therapy and prognosis. Onset of GTCS before or at the same age as TAS, the brief duration of TAS, the EEG irregularities and the occurrence of absence status are useful clinical indicators against either of these diagnoses. A clear history of marked perioral jerking, twitching, etc. is often obtained if a detailed history is taken. However, in most cases video-EEG is essential to confirm the diagnosis. We believe this investigation is a requirement for full evaluation of both children and adults with TAS.

CONCLUSIONS

Perioral myoclonia during TAS is a symptom which appears to be the hallmark for patients in whom absence status, GTCS, relative drug resistance and lack of remission can be expected. The clustering of clinical symptoms and EEG features warrants the designation of a separate syndrome of IGE. Some cases of myoclonic absence epilepsy, although classified as cryptogenic, may be idiopathic and those manifesting with perioral myoclonia may in fact belong to the syndrome of PMA. TAS in PMA are very different from those seen in either childhood or juvenile absence epilepsy and children or adolescents presenting with PMA have a completely different prognosis. The syndrome appears to be uncommon in children with TAS but, because it fails to remit, is relatively common in adults with TAS.

REFERENCES

Aliberti V, Grunewald RA, Panayiotopoulos CP, Chroni E 1994 Focal electroencephalographic abnormalities in juvenile myoclonic epilepsy. Epilepsia 32: 297–301
Commission on Classification and Terminology of the International League Against Epilepsy 1989 Proposal for revised classification of epilepsies and epileptic syndromes. Epilepsia 30: 389–399

Ferrie CD, Robinson RO, Panayiotopoulos CP, Knott C 1993 Lamotrigine in typical absence seizures. Neuropediatrics 24: 172

Panayiotopoulos CP, Obeid T, Waheed G 1989a Differentiation of typical absence seizures in epileptic syndromes. A video EEG study of 224 seizures in 20 patients. Brain 112: 1039–1056

Panayiotopoulos CP, Obeid T, Waheed 1989b Absences in juvenile myoclonic epilepsy: a clinical and video-electroencephalographic study. Annals of Neurology 25: 391–397

Panayiotopoulos CP, Chroni E, Daskalopoulos C, Baker A, Rowlinson S, Walsh P 1992 Typical absence seizures in adults: clinical, EEG, video EEG findings and diagnostic/syndromic considerations. Journal of Neurology, Neurosurgery and Psychiatry 55: 1002–1008

Panayiotopoulos CP 1993 The classification of epileptic syndromes and diseases: II Epileptic syndromes with typical absences. In: Epilepsy in children. Royal Society of Medicine, Paediatric and Neurology Sections, London

Panayiotopoulos CP, Baker A, Grunewald R, Rowlinson S, Walsh P 1993 Breath counting during 3 Hz generalised spike and wave discharges. Journal of Electrophysiological Technology 19: 15–23

Panayiotopoulos CP 1994 The clinical spectrum of typical absence seizures and absence epilepsies. In: Malafaosse A, Genton P, Hirsch E, Marescaux C, Broglin D, Bernasconi R (eds) Idiopathic generalised epilepsies. John Libbey, London, pp 73–83

Panayiotopoulos CP, Ferrie CD, Giannakodimos S, Robinson RO 1994 Perioral myoclonia with absences: a new syndrome. In: Wolf P (ed) Epileptic seizures and syndromes. John Libbey, London, pp 143–153

DISCUSSION

Robinson: Do these patients' seizures resemble seizures in the rat model?

Marescaux: Just a comment on the rat. I do not know if it is easy to see but in fact we have perioral myoclonus in the rat; we have twitches of the vibrissae. Indeed in the same strain, which is very homogeneous from a genetic point of view, we find 30–50% of the rats with this perioral myoclonus. Usually it is the one that we choose for the video; we can see something during the absence. Otherwise there is nothing to see in the rat, they are not counting or over-breathing.

Our impression when we have looked at the rat is that the myoclonic component of the facial muscles is not a very specific characteristic of absences. We have always considered our rats as typical absence with some complex components, but we do not believe that – in the same strain – the fact of having or not having perioral myoclonus is something very important in classifying the rats, and I wonder if it is different in humans. Moreover, it is difficult if we have to look to the video to try to produce a classification on such mild components. How is it possible in practical terms to be sure that this small myoclonia does or does not exist?

Panayiotopoulos: No one would propose that one symptom makes a syndrome. It just so happens that all eight of our patients with perioral myoclonia also had other symptoms which clustered together in a non-fortuitous manner. They all had generalised tonic-clonic seizures, which is something that does not go with childhood absence epilepsy. All of them – or at least those that we know – continued to have absences in adult life, which again does not go with classical childhood absence epilepsy. What is more interesting is that four – and we suspect six – had absence status which lasts for up to two days and terminates in generalised convulsions. So it is not the symptom, it is all this cluster of symptoms which makes these patients different.

Marescaux: The patients you present have something specific because they have absence status and generalised tonic-clonic seizures. But when we read your paper we studied our data and found a lot of children with perioral myoclonia who do very well with a small dose of valproic acid. I am not sure that eyelid myoclonia or perioral myoclonia is a relevant way of classifying these patients.

Panayiotopoulos: I did not say that these patients do not respond to treatment. On the contrary, one of our patients went on having this, being slightly aware of them and not being on any treatment until the age of 36, when he had absence status and generalised tonic clonic seizures. I did not say that they are not responsive to treatment. I said that they do not remit. It would be interesting to see whether your patients with perioral myoclonia will follow the pattern of the patients we presented when they grow up.

Aicardi: I tend to hold similar opinions to Dr Marescaux. I have no precise data but it is my feeling that I have seen a number of children with quite regular childhood absences who have that sort of movement of the jaw, or perioral. It is not new to me in any way.

Panayiotopoulos: If I want to give a video figure, and this is something we see and can confirm, we had only one with perioral myoclonia. It is rare in children with absences. In adults it is proportionately more common because they persist.

Tassinari: I have the same feeling. Aicardi said he had the impression of twitching. I would agree for some this is perioral. Eyelids, yes. This is very rare indeed, I would agree. It does not mean it is a syndrome. It means it is very rare.

Hirsch: It is not so rare and we had six patients with perioral myoclonias in a few years.

Panayiotopoulos: The prevalence of perioral myoclonia with absences in our population of adults with epilepsy is 2%. It is 5.9% in all idiopathic generalised epilepsies and 9.3% in absences.

27. Epilepsy with 3 Hz spike-and-waves without clinically evident absences

Pierre Genton

According to the International Classification Epilepsies and Epileptic Syndromes (Commission, 1989), the definition of idiopathic generalised epilepsies (IGE) rests on the following criteria:

- there is no aetiology other than a genetic predisposition,
- all seizures are initially generalised,
- the inter-ictal EEG shows normal background activity and generalised discharges.

Only three seizure types can be found in IGEs:

- typical absences
- generalised tonic-clonic seizures (GTCS)
- generalised myoclonias.

The various combinations of these types of seizures, and the age of onset of epilepsy, apparently suffice to define the different syndromes recognised in this classification. The latter states that 'the various syndromes of idiopathic generalised epilepsies differ mainly in age of onset.' However, recent genetic research has shown that there is a great degree of heterogeneity within the category of IGE. It is still not clear whether the various syndromes of IGE that include absences as one of the seizure types belong to a continuum of IGE, or to discrete syndromes.

GTCS may occur in practically any type of epilepsy. Generalised myoclonias may occur in symptomatic generalised epilepsies. So-called typical absence seizures appear thus as the most specific type of seizures encountered in IGEs. This paper will try to delineate the place of absence seizures among the various syndromes of IGE and ask whether there are IGEs without absence seizures. It will also briefly review the situations in which generalised spike-wave (SW) discharges are found without associated absences.

ABSENCE SEIZURES IN THE VARIOUS SYNDROMES OF IDIOPATHIC GENERALISED EPILEPSY: OUR RECENT EXPERIENCE

Between 1986 and 1992, 253 cases of IGE were diagnosed and evaluated among 1456 consecutive newly referred patients at the Centre St Paul in

Marseille. The distribution of these cases among the various syndromes of IGE is seen in Table 27.1.

Table 27.1 Classification of 253 consecutive cases of idiopathic generalised epilepsies diagnosed at the Centre St Paul (1986–1992)

	N	%	Sex ratio (M/F)	Age at onset (years) mean	range
Neonatal benign convulsions (NNBC)	0				
Familial NNBC	1	0.4%	0 / 1	0	
Benign myoclonic epilepsy of infancy	4	1.6%	2 / 2	1.2	0.8 – 1.4
Childhood absence epilepsy	73	28.9%	34 / 39	6.0	0.8 – 13
Juvenile absence epilepsy	28	11.1%	14 / 14	13.5	10 – 23
Juvenile myoclonic epilepsy	59	23.3%	27 / 32	14.5	3 – 33
Awakening tonic-clonic	30	11.9%	12 / 18	15.3	9.5 – 23
Isolated GTCS	39	15.4%	15 / 14	19.6	1 – 46
Photogenic epilepsy	8	3.2%	2 / 6	10.0	4 – 20
Not further classified	11	4.3%	5 / 6	11.6	4 – 21

GTCS: generalised tonic-clonic seizures

The diagnosis of IGE and of the individual syndrome was made prospectively, within a year of the patient's first contact with the centre, and entered into a database that includes all the seizure types found in a given patient. Seizure types were determined by interview and/or long-term EEG recording, or inspection of data from prior EEG recordings or medical reports. The diagnosis relied on 1989 International Classification criteria and was changed in a few cases over the years. All cases were reviewed in 1993 in order to verify strict adherence to the diagnostic criteria. From a total of 268 cases, 15 were reclassified into another category of the International Classification or recorded as 'unclassifiable' due to the absence of one of the diagnostic criteria. All had manifested at some point a pattern of generalised spike-wave discharges and had never exhibited any evidence of focal epilepsy.

In addition to the clinical syndromes recognised by the International Classification, we added three categories:

1. Although a significant proportion of patients with other syndromes of IGE, especially juvenile absence or myoclonic epilepsy, had a clinical and EEG history of photo-sensitivity, a special category gathers those uncommon cases (n=8, 3.2% of the total) in which photo-sensitivity was the dominant or exclusive triggering factor of seizures, and which did not fit into one of the other categories.
2. A comparatively large grouping of patients (n= 39, 15.4% of the total) had a history of rare GTCS, with onset ranging from childhood into adulthood, and without any marked circadian feature that might have allowed us to classify them as 'awakening tonic-clonic'.
3. Lastly, a group of patients had all the clinical and EEG criteria of IGE but could not be classified properly into one of the recognised syndromes or into either supplementary category above due to lack of data.

Absence seizures were found in a varying proportion of cases (Table 27.2). Globally, 121 patients (47.8%) had a history of absences. According to the individual syndromes, absences seizures were not noted in the four cases of benign myoclonic epilepsy of infancy (BMEI), which were all still under six years of age when evaluated at our centre. They were present (by definition) in all cases of childhood or juvenile absence epilepsy. They were found in only a minority of case with juvenile myoclonic epilepsy (JME), epilepsy with GTCS on awakening or 'unclassified cases' (18.6, 13.3 and 45.5% respectively), while they were never reported in cases with isolated GTCS or in photogenic epilepsy. The distribution of the other seizure types encountered in IGEs is in accordance with the clinical definition of the respective syndrome.

Table 27.2 Seizure types found in 253 consecutive cases of IGE

	N	Absences		GTCS		Myoclonic		Other		Undet.	
Benign myoclonic epilepsy	4	0	-	0	-	4	100%	0	-	0	-
Childhood absence epilepsy	73	73	100%	32	43.8%	2	2.7%	5	6.8%	2	2.7%
Juvenile absence epilepsy	28	28	100%	21	75.0%	2	7.1%	3	10.7%	0	-
Juvenile myoclonic epilepsy	59	13	22%	51	86.4%	56	94.9%	2	3.4%	0	-
Awakening tonic-clonic	30	2	6.7%	30	100%	4	13.3%	0	-	1	3.3%
Isolated GTCS	39	0	-	39	100%	4	10.3%	0	-	1	2.6%
Photogenic epilepsy	8	0	-	5	62.5%	3	37.5%	1	12.5%	0	-
Not further classified/overlap	11	5	45.5%	11	100%	3	27.3%	1	9.1%	0	-

GTCS: generalised tonic-clonic seizures
Undet.: underdetermined seizure type

A single seizure type was found in a variable proportion of IGE cases. BMEI is characterised by the occurrence of myoclonic jerks in the absence of any other seizure type. Among childhood absence epilepsies, a majority of the cases (52%) had no history of seizure types other than absences, while this proportion falls to 18% among patients with juvenile absence epilepsy. In the latter, 75% of patients experience GTCS and 7% myoclonic jerks. In some of our cases, GTCS were the presenting symptom, while absences had been neglected by patient, family or physician, and the syndromic classification was made only after extensive EEG monitoring showing the existence of numerous absences (Fig. 27.1). Among patients with JME, only 12% have myoclonic jerks as their single seizure type, while GTCS were the only seizure type in 82% of patients reporting only rare major seizures.

In our recent experience, absence seizures are thus predominantly found in childhood-onset epilepsies, excluding the very early onset type of BMEI. It is, however, difficult to be sure that patients seen as older adolescents or as adults and reporting GTCS or myoclonias have not had previous absence seizures (Fig. 27.1).

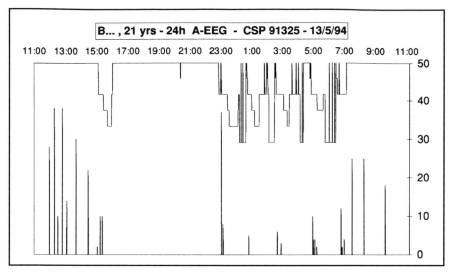

Fig. 27.1 A 21-year old male patient who probably had some isolated, rare absence seizures around age 12, and a single GTCS at age 14, for which he had been evaluated. He was reported seizure-free but treatment with phenobarbital and later valproate was maintained because of persisting inter-ictal changes. Video-EEG monitoring showed absences during hyperventilation (associated with incomplete loss of consciousness and slight jerking of the lower limbs). A 24 h ambulatory EEG recording showed very few isolated, inter-ictal SW, without activation during sleep, but several absences, in the form of prolonged SW discharges lasting up to 38 seconds. The patient, who had slight mental retardation, was classified as having juvenile absence epilepsy.

GENERALISED SW AND ABSENCES IN OTHER TYPES OF EPILEPSIES AND IN OTHER SITUATIONS

Absence seizures can be seen in epilepsies that do not belong to the IGE group. However, such absences, considered to be atypical, are always associated with other seizure types and with other neurological symptoms. They do not represent the major presenting type of seizures in these types of epilepsies. In the Lennox–Gastaut syndrome (LGS) and other symptomatic generalised epilepsies, atypical absences may represent the major seizure type, at least during part of the evolution. However, these absences are 'atypical' in their clinical and neurophysiological presentation. and the seizures that are characteristic for these syndromes are different: for the LGS, the tonic seizures that occur during sleep (Beaumanoir & Dravet, 1992);

In the syndrome of continuous spike-wave during slow-wave sleep, an age-related syndrome in which seizures always remit before puberty, the active phase of the disease is characterised by numerous, often sub-clinical, diffuse, often slow (< 3 Hz) SW discharges that are or are not associated with clinical symptoms and that are or are not considered to represent absences. Here again, the characteristic feature of the syndrome is represented by the abnormal, dramatic EEG finding during sleep and the associated neuropsy-

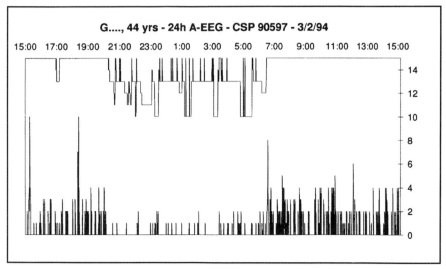

Fig. 27.2 A 44-year old female patient with onset around age 20 of episodes of slight mental confusion that lasted for hours; some shorter absences may have occurred around age 13–14. No ictal episode was ever recorded. Inter-ictal changes are represented by short, sub-clinical generalised fast SW discharges. Quantification of duration (in seconds) of SW discharges over 24 h, including night sleep (from top to bottom: awake, slow-wave sleep stages 1–4, REM sleep). Note the diffuse distribution of SW discharges over the 24 h, without major activation during sleep, and the slight increase after morning awakening. Also note the short duration of SW discharges that were sub-clinical.

chological deficit (Tassinari et al, 1992). In benign rolandic epilepsy, generalised SW discharges may be found in a proportion of patients that ranges from 40–100% according to various authors (Lerman, 1992). However, such EEG abnormalities have been ascribed to secondary bilateral synchrony and are not thought to be associated with typical absences.

Finally, there are cases characterised by a major presenting symptom: absence status. In the elderly such situations may be considered to constitute an acute, situation-related epileptic condition (Thomas et al, 1990). In younger patients such cases are not clearly understood. When inter-ictal EEG changes are generalised, they may be considered as a particular form of IGE (Fig. 27.2).

Thus 'absences' may be seen, or may occur without being noticed, in several types of epilepsies and epileptic syndromes that do not belong to the category of IGEs. The same applies to subjects not considered to be epileptic, either normals (control population in genetic studies, for instance) or siblings or offspring of patients with IGE.

In the normal population and in IGE family members the prevalence of generalised SW discharges has been evaluated at different levels, according to the methodology, to the criteria used for the identification of SW and, last but not least, to the age of subjects (Doose & Baier, 1989; Tsuboi, 1989). It has been seen to range from a low of 1.8% in children aged 1–16 to as high as 14%. Among siblings of patients with absence epilepsy, 13–40% have generalised SW discharges without evident seizures. This prevalence is close to 100% in symptomatic or asymptomatic monozygotic twins of patients with childhood absence epilepsy. In offspring of IGE patients the prevalence of sub-clinical SW range between 7–17.5%. However, 'SW carriers' have a high risk of subsequent seizures, around 18%.

IDIOPATHIC GENERALISED EPILEPSIES WITHOUT ABSENCES: THE SYNDROMIC APPROACH

The occurrence of absence seizures, typical or not, in IGEs is a major clinical feature that is a condition for the syndromic classification. The list of age-dependent types of IGEs recognised by the international classification will be used here to discuss the presence, absence and significance of absence seizures within the IGEs.

The syndromes of benign neonatal convulsions, both sporadic and familial, are distinct from the rest of IGEs: they constitute transient situations and occur at an age when absence seizures are never witnessed clinically or under EEG. The familial form is also characterised by a genetic marker on chromosome 8 or 20. Seizures that may occur later in life in some of these cases do not seem to be absences, although little is known about them. In these types of IGEs, absence seizures clearly do not represent a major clinical problem.

BMEI is probably the earliest true type of IGE. Neither the original nor the follow-up descriptions have mentioned absences as a possible seizure type, even in untreated patients followed over periods as long as 5 and 8.5 years (Dravet et al, 1992). Massive, isolated (myoclonic) jerks are the only seizure form seen in the infant, while some rare GTCS may occur occasionally in adolescence. Myoclonic epilepsies may occur in young children after the age of BMEI and long before the age of juvenile myoclonic epilepsy. In such cases, absences are not a major clinical problem either.

Among cases today classified as 'absence epilepsies', either of childood or of adolescence, there are forms in which the only seizure type is absences; there are others in which other seizure types are associated (Table 27.2). Absences, which may or may not be typical, can also be found in a percentage of cases with JME (10–31%, Wolf, 1992a) or awakening tonic-clonic seizures (13–63%, Wolf, 1992). The prognostic significance of the presence of absence seizures in these patients is not known.

A comparatively large group of patients experience only isolated, infrequent generalised tonic-clonic seizures that are not particularly associated with awakening. If their inter-ictal EEG also shows generalised SW discharges, they clearly belong to the group of IGEs, but not necessarily to the category described as awakening tonic-clonic. Such patients were considered to have 'benign Grand Mal epilepsy in adults' by Oller-Daurella & Sorel

Table 27.3 Distributions of seizure types in patients with IGEs: cases with only one seizure type GTCS: generalised tonic-clonic seizure

	N	Absences		GTCS		Myoclonic		Clonic	
Benign myoclonic epilepsy	4					4	100%		
Childhood absence epilepsy	73	38	52%						
Juvenile absence epilepsy	28	5	18%						
Juvenile myoclonic epilepsy	59			2	3%	7	12%		
Awakening tonic-clonic	30			24	80%				
Isolated GTCS	39			32	82.1%				
Photogenic epilepsy	8			4	50%	2	25%	1	25.0%
Not further classified/overlap	11			2	18%	1	9%		

(1989), who found inter-ictal generalised SW discharges in only a minority of their cases (only three typical findings among 59 patients), while most authors include them in the category of awakening tonic-clonic (Wolf, 1992). In our experience, this type of 'non-syndromic' tonic-clonic epilepsy should be diagnosed only in the presence of inter-ictal generalised EEG changes. Clinical absences are never reported by such patients or by their families, even if the age of onset of seizures is in the age group associated with the absence syndromes,i.e., between the ages of 3 and 15. This type may thus represent the most frequently encountered type of IGE without absences.

CONCLUSIONS

Typical absences are one of the seizure types considered characteristic of idiopathic generalised epilepsy (IGE). There are two IGE syndromes where absences are the main seizure type: childhood and juvenile absence epilepsies. Among these, there are (comparatively uncommon) cases in which absences are the only seizure type. Probably a better assessment of the semiology, triggering factors, course and pharmacological sensitivity of these types of absence epilepsies will result in a more accurate subclassification. Absences are also part of other epileptic syndromes, but their diagnostic or prognostic significance in such syndromes is not known.

It is difficult to be certain that absences are really absent, i.e., retrospectively to ascertain that a patient has not had, at some early stage of his condition, infrequent absences that may have escaped attention. This may be due to the fact that absences are not always 'typical', in the sense that they are not all accompanied by total loss of consciousness. Only systematic, long-term EEGs, including those conducted during sleep and, possibly, sleep deprivation, will permit a closer approximation of the actual prevalence of absence seizures in patients with IGE or with apparently asymptomatic SW.

However, there are idiopathic generalised epilepsies that never include absences. This is particularly true for most of the cases in which GTCS are both the only seizure type and infrequent. A common situation is also represented by the presence of generalised SW discharges in subjects who never experience seizures, but who may or may not be related to patients with epilepsy.

REFERENCES

Commission on Classification and Terminology of the International League Against Epilepsy 1989 Proposal for revised classification of epilepsies and epileptic syndromes. Epilepsia 30: 389–399

Beaumanoir A, Dravet C 1992 The Lennox–Gastaut syndrome. In: Roger J, Bureau M, Dravet C, Dreifuss FE, Wolf P, Perret A (eds) Epileptic syndromes in infancy, childhood and adolescence, 2nd edn. John Libbey Eurotext, London, pp115–133

Dravet C, Bureau M, Roger J 1992 Benign myoclonic epilepsy in infants. In: Roger J, Bureau M, Dravet C, Dreifuss FE, Wolf P, Perret A (eds) Epileptic syndromes in infancy, childhood and adolescence, 2nd edn. John Libbey Eurotext, London, 67–74

Doose H, Baier WK 1989 Generalized spikes and waves. In: Beck-Managetta G, Anderson VE, Doose H, Janz D (eds) Genetics of the epilepsies. Springer Berlin, pp95–103

Grünewald RA, Panayiotopoulos CP (1993) Juvenile myoclonic epilepsy: a review. Arch Neurol 50: 594–598

Oller -Daurella L, Sorel L 1989 L'épilepsie grand mal bénigne de l'adulte. Acta Neurol Belg 89: 38–45

Tassinari CA, Bureau M, Dravet C, Dalla Bernardina B, Roger J 1992 Epilepsy with continuous spikes and waves during slow sleep – otherwise described as ESES (epilepsy with electrical status epilepticus during slow sleep). In: Roger J, Bureau M, Dravet C, Dreifuss FE, Wolf P, Perret A (eds) Epileptic syndromes in infancy, childhood and adolescence, 2nd edn. John Libbey Eurotext, London, pp245–256

Thomas P, Beaumanoir A, Genton P, Dolisi C, Chatel M 1992 'De novo' absence status of late onset: report of 11 cases. Neurology 42: 104–110

Tsuboi T 1989 Genetic risk in offspring of epileptic patients. In: Beck-Managetta G, Anderson VE, Doose H, Janz D (eds) Genetics of the epilepsies. Springer, Berlin, pp111–118

Wolf P 1992 Epilepsy with grand mal on awakening. In: Roger J, Bureau M, Dravet C, Dreifuss FE, Wolf P, Perret A (eds) Epileptic syndromes in infancy, childhood and adolescence, 2nd edn. John Libbey Eurotext, London, pp329–341

Wolf P 1992 Juvenile myoclonic epilepsy. In: Roger J, Bureau M, Dravet C, Dreifuss FE, Wolf P, Perret A (eds) Epileptic syndromes in infancy, childhood and adolescence, 2nd edn. John Libbey Eurotext, London, pp67–74

28. Clinical aspects of typical absences and related syndromes – consensus statement

R. O. Robinson

Myoclonus may not only be an associated feature of typical absence syndromes. It may be so prominent that it becomes the defining feature. As with juvenile myoclonic epilepsy, its characteristics help the clinician towards a prognosis both in terms of its likely responsiveness (or unresponsiveness) to medication as well as the likelihood of remission. Unlike juvenile myoclonic epilepsy, the outcomes of the syndromes discussed in this session are less good. Since the pathogenesis of myoclonus may be generated at any point from the cortex to the spinal cord, speculation as to why this might be so is at best tentative. However, it is worth noting that in juvenile myoclonic epilepsy the myoclonus is often erratic and fragmentary, and not associated with the absence ictus, while what is described in these syndromes is an ictal manifestation of the absences and may be massive (as in myoclonic absence epilepsy) or stereotyped and bilateral as in eyelid and perioral myoclonia with absences.

As a general point, it is likely that careful observation of patients, with video-EEG combined with other features such as psycho-social development and family history (which may include EEG in asymptomatic first degree relatives), will allow further delineation of 'new' syndromes with clinical and biological relevance.

The status of perioral myoclonus remains to be established. Here I have to confess to bias as I was involved in the initial description. I think I should not have been had the rhythmic pouting movements not struck me as so unusual and distinctive.

Eyelid myoclonia with absences can apparently resemble self-induced seizures in photo-sensitive patients, but it is undoubtedly distinguishable on careful observation. The area of photo-sensitivity remains a rich field for further research. We are not clear whether the photo-sensitivity associated with typical absence syndromes is the same as that seen in 'pure' photo-sensitive epilepsy. The type of stimuli need to be much more strictly defined. Both transient movement as well as transient luminosity may play a part. The observations of Wilkins on the effect of tinted light and its possible role in the generation of seizures must provoke further work.

Another area which remains to be clarified is the variable loss of consciousness in the myoclonic absence syndromes. As a rule this is not as profound as in childhood absence epilepsy and juvenile absence epilepsy. However, our tools for measuring this are as yet crude. Generally, patients are shown objects during the absence and then asked what was shown following the absence. This, however, tests declarative memory only. If one object is shown during the absence and then a choice of objects is offered afterwards (the 'forced choice' paradigm), the correct choice is made more often than by chance, demonstrating that some consciousness was preserved and some form of memory retained. We need better tools for assessing what degree of consciousness is lost, for this may help further in our understanding and delineation of these syndromes.

29. Symptomatic typical absence seizures

C. D. Ferrie   S. Giannakodimos   R. O. Robinson
C. P. Panayiotopoulos

Typical absence seizures (TAS) are considered the paradigm seizure type of the idiopathic generalised epilepsies (IGE) but may occasionally be symptomatic, arising as a consequence of a known disorder of the CNS. Patients with cerebral disease may develop TAS coincidentally and additional evidence of an aetiological link should be sought before classifying them as symptomatic typical absences (STAS). This might be: an increased prevalence of TAS in the condition over that in the general population, clinical features distinguishing the patient's symptoms from any of the recognised absence epilepsy syndromes, electrophysiological evidence of focal onset; or disappearance of absences following treatment of the other condition. Absences are sometimes reported in patients with evidence of brain dysfunction, such as minor neurological or radiological signs or mental retardation, in which the underlying disorder is obscure. Such TAS should not be classified as symptomatic but may be considered cryptogenic. TAS are classified as generalised seizures. However, STAS arising by secondary bilateral synchrony (SBS) are actually partial seizures with rapid generalisation. STAS are often considered phenocopies of genetically determined TAS.

EPIDEMIOLOGY

Older studies of 'petit mal' often used imprecise definitions and included patients without diagnostic EEG abnormalities, causing difficulty when attempting to quantify the prevalence of STAS.

Dalby (1969) found wide discrepancies (0–38%) in the prevalence of 'brain damage' in series reported up to the 1960s of patients with petit mal. In his study, which used today's EEG criteria, 49 (14%) out of 346 patients had an 'aetiological diagnosis with reference to the central nervous system'. Holowach et al (1962) found nine out of 88 children (10%) had brain damage of recognised aetiology. However, fewer than 50% had spike and wave EEG paroxysms documented. Six of 117 patients (5.1%) with 'true petit mal' reported by Livingston et al (1965) had evidence of brain damage prior to the onset of petit mal and in a prospective study of 300 patients with generalised epilepsies, Niedermeyer (1972) found seven with petit mal due to secondary bilateral synchrony (SBS), one due to a 'deep seated lesion' and two due to metabolic causes. Lugaresi (1973) reported that 20% of his patients with petit mal had a history of 'nonphysiological childbirth or neonatal disturbance', 4.7% of cranial trauma and 2.8% of encephalitis and post-natal encephalopathies. In a recent population-based study of absence epilepsies, 12 out of 119 (10.1%) Swedish children selected on EEG criteria had evidence of encephalopathy (Olsson & Hedstrom, 1991).

Epidemiological studies suggest that 5–14% of patients with TAS may have additional CNS pathology. Often, however, these studies fail to distinguish patients in whom the two conditions are genuinely related from those in whom they are coincidental. We found two patients with absences which we considered symptomatic and another two as cryptogenic out of 101 patients with TAS seen in one of our epilepsy clinics.

SYNDROMES WITH STAS AND CEREBRAL PATHOLOGIES LINKED TO TAS

The range of pathologies reported with TAS is shown in the box. The ILAE recognises one syndrome of cryptogenic/symptomatic absences: epilepsy with myoclonic absences. Intermediate petit mal and petit mal with focal component are other proposed symptomatic/cryptogenic epilepsy syndromes. The majority of reported cases had no proven cerebral lesion, making them cryptogenic. Epilepsy with myoclonic absences is discussed elsewhere and all were recently reviewed (Aicardi, 1994).

ABSENCES ASSOCIATED WITH DIFFUSE CEREBRAL PATHOLOGIES

The best-documented reports of TAS in patients with diffuse cerebral pathology are case studies in patients with juvenile Batten's disease (Andermann, 1967) and SSPE (Broughton et al, 1973), in which apparent classical pyknolepsy preceded onset of typical symptoms of the underlying disease. TAS have also been reported following specific viral infections and generalised encephalitides, including measles, chicken pox, vaccinia, mumps and influenza (Dalby, 1969; Gastaut, 1969). Mild cerebral trauma without evidence of focal pathology has been linked to absences by a number of authors (see also Fig. 29.1) and Gastaut (1969) reported induction of EEG photo-sensitivity. Most series also include patients with perinatal problems, minor neuro-radiological abnormalities or neurological signs or varying degrees of mental retardation.

Biochemical and endocrine disturbances (Gastaut, 1969) have rarely been associated with TAS, despite hypoglycaemia being a precipitating factor for 3 Hz spike and wave discharges (Niedermeyer, 1993). A reported link with precocious puberty (Scherman & Abrahams, 1963) is probably related to lesions in the hypothalamic region rather than a direct endocrine effect. TAS and absence status have occasionally been associated with drugs and drug withdrawal (Yohai & Barnett, 1989; Thomas et al, 1992; Jackson & Berkovic, 1992).

Range of cerebral pathologies linked to TAS. Not included are the numerous reports of associations with non-specific perinatal problems, mental retardation and minor neurological signs

- Diffuse cerebral pathologies

autism	Gillberg & Schaumann 1983
biochemical/endocrine disturbances	Gastaut 1969, Niedermeyer 1972
congenital microcephaly	Holowach et al 1962
craniosynostosis	Holowach et al 1962
Down's syndrome	Ollson & Hestrom 1991
drugs/drug withdrawal	Yohai & Barnett 1989, Jackson & Berkovic 1992
encephalitis/encephalomeyelitis	O'Brien et al 1959, Holowach et al 1962, Dalby 1969, Gastaut 1969
head injury	O'Brien et al 1959, Gordon 1959, Varcelletto 1966, Dalby 1969, Gastaut 1969
juvenile Batten's disease	Andermann 1967
MERRF	Ollson & Hedstrom 1991
progressive myoclonus epilepsy	Ollson & Hedstrom 1991
shunted-post haemorrhagic hydrocephalus	Aicardi 1994
Sturge–Weber syndrome	Holowach et al 1962
subacute sclerosing panencephalitis (SSPE)	Broughton et al 1973
tuberous sclerosis	Holowach et al 1962

- Focal cerebral pathology

A-V malformation	Niedermeyer et al 1969
cerebral abscess (old)	Gabor & Ajmone Marsan 1969
cerebral tumour	Ajmone Marsan & Lewis 1960, Scherman & Abraham 1963, Madsen & Bray 1966, Stewart & Dreifuss 1967, Millichap et al 1962, Page et al 1969, Gabor & Ajmone Marsan 1969, Dalby 1969, Stevens 1970, Loiseau et al 1971, Niedermeyer 1972, Farwell & Stuntz 1984, Panayiotopoulos et al 1992
hemiplegia	Dalby 1969, Gastaut 1969, Niedermeyer 1972, Sato et al 1983, Gastaut et al 1987
subcortical (hypothalamic/pineal/brain stem lesions, associated with tumours, Sotos syndrome and precocious puberty)	Scherman & Abraham 1963, Dalby 1969, Niedermeyer 1972
neonatal intracranial haemorrhage	Holowach et al 1962
tuberculous meningitis	Niedermeyer 1972

There are reports of TAS occurring in patients with many diffuse cereb-ral conditions. However, as TAS are not considered characteristic of any of them, caution is required in ascribing cause and effect. The mere occurrence of TAS in patients with diffuse CNS disorders does not prove an aetiological association. With the exception of Batten's disease and SSPE, all these conditions are common. In the majority TAS are probably coincidental. However, cerebral pathology may modify the expression of a predominantly genetic epilepsy, e.g. causing absences to begin earlier, to be associated with other seizure types, or to show a poor response to treatment.

Patients with a variety of severe symptomatic generalised epilepsies characterised by diffusely slow EEG and slow spike and wave patterns may have

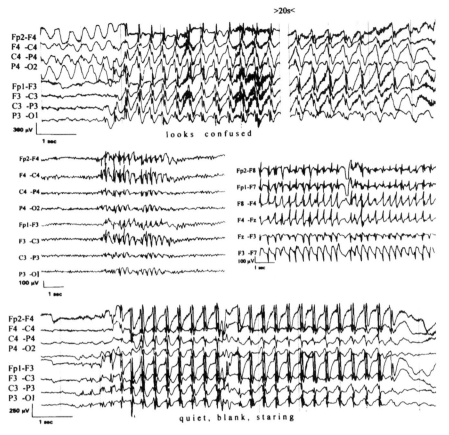

Fig. 29.1 Typical absences and 3 Hz spike and wave patterns recorded in patients with definite/possible diffuse cerebral pathology. **Top**: TAS recorded from Case 1. The patient presented one week after being concussed in a road traffic accident. Absences were of pyknolepsy frequency, lasted up to 35 s and were associated with profound impairment of consciousness, tonic upward eye deviation, fast eyelid flutter and at times walking in circles. They were partially controlled by valproate and ethosuximide. MRI was normal. Note that the spike wave discharge was consistently preceded by long runs of 3 Hz rhythmic slow maximal in the right posterior temporal electrode. **Centre left**: TAS recorded from Case 2. TAS had their onset at 10 years and were successfully treated, medication being withdrawn at 25 years. At 34 years they recurred two weeks after being hit on the head by a machine cover. Impairment of consciousness was mild, causing 'sudden discontinuation of thoughts and speech'. CT was normal and the patient showed a partial response to valproate. **Centre right**: Electrical absence status. This was recorded from a comatose middle-aged woman (Case 4). The day before she had had a cardiac arrest with four minutes elapsing before resuscitation began. Brainstem reflexes were preserved and infrequent myoclonic jerks were observed. She died one day later. **Bottom**: TAS recorded from Case 3. This Bangladeshi girl with a family history of schizophrenia and retardation developed GTCS and severe global retardation at three years of age. Occasional absences began at 12 years. They lasted into the 20s, consisting of psychomotor arrest, upward eye deviation, swallowing movements and sometimes apnoea and cyanosis. All ended abruptly, usually with immediate recovery but sometimes with brief post-ictal tiredness. EEG showed discharges consistently started in the left parasagittal region. MRI was normal. In Cases 1 and 2 there was little or no evidence of an aetiological link between the head injury and TAS. These are probably cases of IGE, the expression of which has been modified by cerebral trauma. In Case 3, an aetiological link is more likely, with the possibility of SBS. This patient's epilepsy may be classified as cryptogenic.

episodes of 3 Hz spike and wave associated with TAS (Fig. 29.1, Case 3) (Aicardi, 1994; Niedermeyer, 1992; Olsson & Hedstrom, 1991). The clinical picture in these patients, however, is dominated by other features and they are not classified among the typical absence epilepsies. It is not clear if TAS alters their prognosis. Figure 29.1 (Case 4) illustrates electrical 'absence' status in a comatose patient following anoxic brain damage. These cases show the potential for diffusely damaged cortex to generate spike wave discharges at 3 Hz as well as at slower frequencies.

ABSENCES ASSOCIATED WITH FOCAL CEREBRAL PATHOLOGY

The association of TAS with focal cerebral pathologies is better documented. Most reports are of cerebral tumours, with infantile hemiplegia being the only other pathology frequently implicated. As the latter is common, many cases may be chance associations, although in some there is additional evidence of an aetiological link (Fig 29.2, Case 5).

Ajmone Marsan & Lewis (1960) calculated that cerebral tumours were associated with 3 Hz spike and wave patterns more often than by chance. A review by us of the literature (Marsden & Bray, 1966; Stewart & Dreifuss, 1967; Dalby, 1969; Gabor & Ajmone Marsan, 1969; Page et al, 1969; Stevens, 1970; Loiseau et al, 1971; Farwell & Stuntz, 1984) found 22 patients with brain tumours and EEG evidence of TAS. Only 12 had clinical absences, suggesting tumours may produce bilaterally synchronous 3 Hz spike and wave discharges without clinical accompaniments. A large majority of cases reported in detail had features (either clinical or on EEG) suggesting the patients did not have IGE, although some (eg, Stevens, 1970; Case 1) were compatible with IGE. Figure 29.2 (Case 6) illustrates TAS in a patient with a slow-growing frontal glioma.

Most early authors considered that only lesions involving sub-cortical midline structures generated TAS (Ajmone Marsan & Lewis, 1960; Scherman & Abraham, 1963; Gastaut, 1969). This was not supported by later evidence and frontal lobe lesions, particularly those involving the medial surfaces of the intermediate frontal region, are implicated most often as giving rise to STAS (Bancaud & Talairach, 1992). Mazar (1970) emphasised the role of the cingulate gyrii. There are, however, well-documented reports of TAS associated with cortical lesions elsewhere, particularly in the temporal lobes (Stevens, 1970). Four out of five cases we have seen with absences which appeared to have a focal origin arose in the frontal lobes with a temporal lobe origin possible in one (Case 7, Fig. 29.2).

MECHANISMS OF SYMPTOMATIC ABSENCES

The 3 Hz spike and wave discharge is generated by cortical neurons but debate continues as to whether its origin is sub-cortical (centrocephalic), in

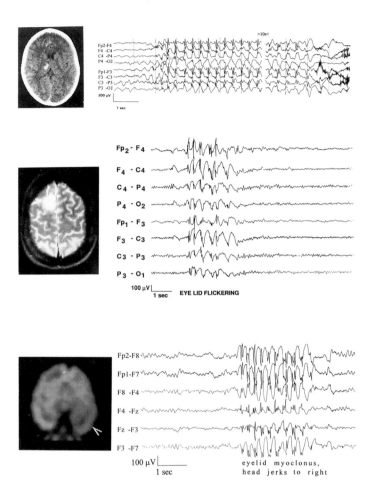

Fig. 29.2 Absences in patients with focal cerebral pathology. **Top** (Case 5): This boy developed a right hemiplegia and behavioural and learning difficulties following a road traffic accident at 4 years of age, in which he sustained an extensive frontal intra-cerebral contusion extending into the right thalamus (CT). Pyknolepsy-type absences, lasting up to 10 s, began at 9 years. Impairment of consciousness was moderate, with a 'glazed expression' accompanied by small rhythmic upward eye movements. EEG showed that discharges were preceded by left-sided slow activity. **Centre** (Case 6): This woman developed absences at 28 years. Initially infrequent but later occurring daily, they lasted up to 1 minute and consisted of 'losing control of thoughts', repeating simple phrases and sometimes mild jerking of the head to the right. Rare GTCS and an episode of probable absence status with expressive dysphasia occurred. MRI showed an extensive, slow-growing right frontal lobe glioma (Panayiotopoulos et al, 1992). **Bottom** (Case 7): This patient, with a family history of 'epilepsy', had some respiratory problems in the neonatal period. Absences began at 3 years of age, and GTCS, including episodes of convulsive status, began shortly afterwards. She was moderately retarded and of short stature; she developed hypothyroidism. Absences, which occurred daily, consisted of moderate impairment of consciousness and were of variable duration; during the absences, adversive movement of the head, usually to the right, occurred. MRI was normal but inter-ictal PET showed hypoperfusion of the right temporal lobe (arrow).

the cortex (cortico-reticular) or at multiple points on an oscillating circuit between cortex and sub-cortical structures. The evidence from STAS favours the latter.

SBS denotes the generation of a bilateral synchronous discharge from a unilateral cortical focus and may be associated with various seizure types, including TAS. Generalisation occurs through interconnecting neural networks within the cortex and between it and sub-cortical structures. Scalp EEG may not detect the focal discharge, either because it arises in cortex 'hidden' to it or because generalisation is so rapid. Lesions in the mesial or orbital surfaces of a hemisphere were initially proposed as giving rise to SBS (Tukel & Jasper, 1951). Gabor & Ajmone Marsan (1969) and Blume & Pilley (1985) found the frontal lobe to be involved in the majority of cases, with the latter authors reporting the origin to be in superior frontal, frontal polar, inferior frontal and sagittal regions in that order. Others found almost equal involvement of frontal and temporal lobes (Niedermeyer, 1972) or a predominance in the temporal lobes (Gastaut et al, 1987).

In most cases of supposed SBS there is no neuro-radiological or pathological confirmation of a lesion and focal EEG abnormalities are common in patients with IGE. Nevertheless, cases with clear and consistent surface or depth EEG focal abnormalities and associated generalised EEG discharges (Fig. 29.3) support the concept, as do reports of electrical stimulation of cortical areas identified on EEG (in all cases located in the frontal lobes) giving rise to generalised 3 Hz spike and wave discharges (Bancaud et al, 1974) and patients in whom surgical removal of such areas was curative (Gloor, 1969; Niedermeyer, 1969).

SBS may not explain all cases. Interruption of ascending midbrain inhibitory systems may be involved in patients with brainstem lesions (Stevens, 1970).

CLINICAL AND EEG CHARACTERISTICS OF STAS

It is crucial to distinguish TAS occurring as part of an IGE from those with a lesional basis (Roger & Bureau, 1992). TAS are often syndrome-related and it has been suggested that STAS may constitute a separate epilepsy syndrome (Aicardi, 1994). The wide range of causative pathologies may make this unlikely but there are no detailed analyses of the clinical, EEG or video-EEG features of STAS.

We reviewed 28 cases in the English literature with EEG evidence supportive of TAS and with definite or probable causative cerebral pathology. In 10 no seizures resembling TAS were described. The median age of onset of TAS was eight years (range 2–30), similar to that seen in IGE. Almost two-thirds of patients had seizures other than TAS. Absence status has been reported (Stevens, 1970). TAS often occurred for only a short period during a longer seizure disorder. In few cases is the description of ictal events

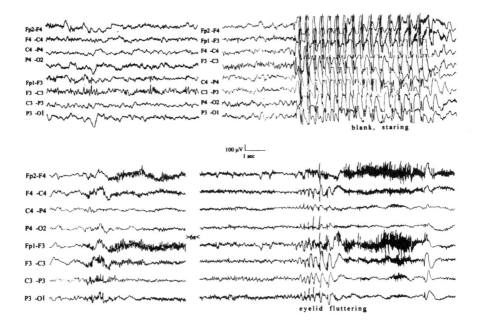

Fig. 29.3 Absences in association with consistent focal EEG abnormalities (SBS). **Top** (Case 7): This patient, with language delay, presented at two years of age with occasional episodes when he would drop to the floor 'dazed'. Three EEGs (including video-EEG) showed continuous high-amplitude fast and sharp activity highly localised around the left frontal electrode. On two occasions this was interrupted by generalised discharges lasting 7 and 9 s. In one of these (not shown) a myoclonic jerk occurred, followed by a rhythmic head nodding. At the end of the generalised discharges the left frontal fast and sharp activity ceased for around 30 s. CT showed atrophic changes only. Response to valproate was good. **Bottom** (Case 9): This patient presented at nine years of age with frontal lobe complex partial seizures. At 19 years of age, following addition of vigabatrin, her habitual seizures changed and resembled TAS. Shown is a seizure recorded by video-EEG during sleep. The seizure begins with a recruiting response followed by a generalised discharge of 4 Hz spike and wave.

accompanying EEG discharges detailed, but in some the description only superficially resembles TAS. Discharges were usually irregular, with only five patients having regular 3 Hz bilaterally symmetrical discharges. A positive response to hyperventilation was seen in eight out of 16 patients. Only one patient was photo-sensitive.

Among our own patients we consider Cases 3 and 5–9 to be definite or possible cases of STAS. The median age of onset of absences was 10.5 years (range 1–28). Four patients also had other seizure types; two had partial seizures and one absence status. In no cases were regular 3 Hz symmetrical spike and wave discharges seen and all cases had multiple spikes. Consistent focal abnormalities occurred in five cases. A positive response to hyperventilation was common but only one patient (Case 7) was photo-sensitive. Only Case 5 was compatible with a recognised syndrome of IGE.

The prognosis of patients with STAS depends on the underlying pathology. The prospect for control of absences and the likelihood of development of other seizure types is poorer in the presence of a low IQ or neurological signs (Sato et al, 1983) and if associated with partial seizures (Loiseau et al, 1983). Appropriate drug strategies will vary and may include drugs effective in both generalised and partial seizures. Talairach et al (1992) reported their experience in surgical treatment of 100 patients with frontal lobe epilepsies. Patients with apparently generalised seizures, especially if spike-wave discharges were symmetrical, did less well than those with clearly localised seizures. The success rate was least favourable for seizures originating in the intermediate medial frontal region, the area particularly associated with frontal absences. Wider excisions, with interruption of radiating fibres, increased the success rate.

CONCLUSIONS

TAS have been reported in patients with many different cerebral conditions. In most cases an aetiological link is not proved and it is likely that many are coincidental. Population-based epidemiological studies are required to determine whether TAS are more common following head injury, viral encephalitis, congenital hemiplegias, etc. If they are, investigating why may help elucidate the pathogenesis of TAS in IGE.

Evidence that TAS may arise as a consequence of focal brain pathology is stronger, but still not proved. Given the predominance of reports with brain tumours a large multi-centre study should give a conclusive answer to this question. The evidence for SBS is strong but an explanation is still needed as to why it occurs in some patients and not others. Attention has focused on the site of lesions, with evidence suggesting lesions in the mesial surfaces of the frontal lobes as most likely to give rise to SBS. Another possibility is that a genetic predisposition is also necessary. Advances in genetics should allow this question to be answered.

Techniques already applied in IGE should be extended to STAS. Video-EEG studies will determine if STAS show quantitative and qualitative differences from other TAS and whether a seperate syndrome(s) can be defined. Functional scanning may also prove fruitful.

ACKNOWLEDGEMENTS

We thank Marion Merrell Dow, British Telecom Charitable Organisation and the Research (Endowments) Committee of the Special Trustees of St Thomas' Hospital for their support.

REFERENCES

Aicardi J 1994 Epilepsies with typical absence seizures. In: Aicardi J (ed) Epilepsy in children, Raven Press, New York, pp94–117

Ajmone Marsan C, Lewis WR 1960 Pathologic findings in patients with 'centrencephalic' electroencephalographic patterns. Neurology 10: 922–930

Andermann F 1967 Absence attacks and diffuse neuronal disease. Neurology 17: 205–212

Bancaud J, Talairach J, Morel P et al 1974 'Generalised' epileptic seizures elicited by electrical stimulation of the frontal lobe in man. Electroencephalography and Clinical Neurophysiology 37: 275–282

Blume WT, Pillay N 1985 Electrographic and clinical correlates of secondary bilateral synchrony. Epilepsia 26: 636–641

Broughton R, Nelson R, Gloor P, Andermann F 1973 Petit mal epilepsy evolving to subacute panencephalitis. In: Lugaresi E, Pazzaglia P, Tassinari CA (eds) Evolution and prognosis of epilepsies (XIXeme Reunion Europeenne D' Enseignement Electroencephalographique). Aulo Gaggi Editore, Bologna, pp63–72

Dalby MA 1969 Epilepsy and 3 per second spike and wave rhythms: a clinical, electroencephalographic and prognostic analysis of 346 patients. Acta Neurologica Scandinavia 45 (Suppl. 40)

Farwell JR, Stuntz JT 1984 Frontoparietal astrocytoma causing absence seizures and bilaterally synchronous epileptiform discharges. Epilepsia 25: 695–698

Gabor AJ, Ajmone Marsan C 1969 Co-existence of focal and bilateral diffuse paroxysmal discharges in epileptics. Epilepsia 10: 453–472

Gastaut H 1969 Introduction to the study of organic generalised epilepsies. In: Gastaut H, Jasper H, Bancaud J, Waltregny A (eds) The physiopathogenesis of the epilepsies. Charles C Thomas, Springfield, Ill., pp147–157

Gastaut H, Zifkin B, Maggauda A, Mariani E 1987 Symptomatic partial epilepsies with secondary bilateral synchrony: differentiation from symptomatic generalised epilepsies of the Lennox-Gastaut type. In: Wieser HG, Elgar CE (eds) Presurgical evaluation of epileptics, Springer-Verlag, Berlin, pp308–316

Gillberg C, Schaumann H 1983 Epilepsy presenting as infantile autism? Two case studies. Neuropediatrics 14: 206–212

Gloor P 1969 Neurophysiological bases of generalised seizures termed centrencephalic. In: Gastaut H, Jasper H, Bancaud J, Waltregny A (eds) The physiopathogenesis of the epilepsies. Charles C Thomas, Springfield, Ill., pp209–236

Gordon N 1959 Petit mal epilepsy and cortical epileptogenic foci. Electroencephalography and Clinical Neurophysiology 11: 151–153

Holowach J, Thurston DL, O'Leary JL 1962 Petit mal epilepsy. Pediatrics 30: 893–901

Jackson GD, Berkovic SF 1992 Ceftazidime encephalopathy: absence status and toxic hallucinations. Journal of Neurology, Neurosurgery and Psychiatry 55: 333–334

Livingston S, Torres I, Pauli LL, Rider RV 1965 Petit mal epilepsy: results of a prolonged follow-up study of 117 patients. Journal of the American Medical Association 194: 113–119

Loiseau P, Cohadon F, Cohadon S 1971 Recording of absences of petit mal type in a man of 40, with epileptic attacks since the age of 3, who had a frontal glioma. Electroencephalography and Clinical Neurophysiology 30: 248

Loiseau P, Pestre M, Partigues JF, Commenges D, Barberger-Gateau C, Cohadon S 1983 Long term prognosis in two forms of childhood epilepsy: typical absence seizures and epilepsy with rolandic (centrotemporal) EEG foci. Annals of Neurology 13: 642–648

Lugaresi E, Pazzaglia P, Frank L et al 1973 Evolution and prognosis of primary generalised epilepsies of the petit mal absence type. In: Lugaresi E, Pazzaglia P, Tassinari CA (eds) Evolution and prognosis of epilepsies (XIXeme Réunion Européenne D'Enseignement Electroencephalographique). Aulo Gaggi Editore, Bologna, pp3–22

Madsen JA, Bray PF 1966 The coincidence of diffuse electroencephalographic spike-wave paroxysms and brain tumours. Neurology 16: 546–555

Mazars G 1970 Criteria for identifying cingulate epilepsies. Epilepsia 11: 41–47

Millichap JG, Bickford RG, Miller RH, Backus RE 1962 The electroencephalogram in children with intracranial tumors and seizures. Neurology 12: 329–336

Niedermeyer E, Laws ER, Walker AE 1969 Depth EEG findings in epileptics with generalised spike-wave complexes. Archives of Neurology 21: 51–58

Niedermeyer E 1972 The generalised epilepsies: a clinical electroencephalographic study. Charles C. Thomas, Springfield, Ill.

Niedermeyer E, Fineyre F, Rilley T, Uematsu S 1979 Absence status (petit mal status) with focal characteristics. Archives of Neurology 36: 417–421

Niedermeyer E, Da Silva FL 1993 Electroencephalography: basic principles, clinical applications and related fields, 3rd edn. Williams & Wilkins, Baltimore

O'Brien JL, Goldensohn ES, Hoefer FA 1959 Electroencephalographic abnormalities in addition to bilaterally synchronous 3 per second spike and wave activity in petit mal. Electroencephalography and Clinical Neurophysiology 11: 747–761

Olsson I, Hedstrom A 1991 Epidemiology of absence epilepsy II. Typical absences in children with encephalopathies. Acta Paediatrica Scandinavica 80: 235–242

Page LK, Lombroso CT, Matson DD 1969 Childhood epilepsy with late detection of cerebral glioma. Journal of Neurosurgery 31: 253–261

Panayiotopoulos CP, Chroni E, Daskalopoulos C, Baker A, Rowlinson S, Walsh P 1992 Typical absence seizures in adults: clinical, EEG, video-EEG findings and diagnostic/syndromic considerations. Journal of Neurology, Neurosurgery and Psychiatry 55: 1002–1008

Roger J, Bureau M 1992 Distinctive characteristics of frontal lobe epilepsy versus idiopathic generalised epilepsy. In: Chauvel P, Delgado-Escueta AV, Halgren E, Bancaud J (eds) Frontal lobe seizures and epilepsies. Raven Press, New York, pp399–410

Sato S, Dreifuss FE, Penry JK, Kirby DD, Palesch Y 1983 Long-term follow-up of absence seizures. Neurology 33: 1590–1595

Scherman RG, Abraham K 1963 'Centrencephalic' electroencephalographic patterns in precocious puberty. Electroencephalography and Clinical Neurophysiology 15: 559–567

Stevens JR 1970 Focal abnormality in petit mal epilepsy: intracranial recordings and pathological findings. Neurology 20: 1069–1076

Stewart LF, Dreifuss FE 1967 'Centrencephalic' seizure discharges in focal hemispheral lesions. Archives of Neurology 17: 60–68

Talairach J, Bancaud J, Bonis A et al 1992 Surgical therapy for frontal epilepsies. In: Chauvel P, Delgado-Escueta AV, Halgren E, Bancaud J (eds) Frontal lobe seizures and epilepsies. Raven Press, New York, pp 707–732

Thomas P, Beaumonoir A, Genton P, Dolisi C, Chatel M 1992 'De novo' absence status of late onset: report of 11 cases. Neurology 42: 104–110

Tukel K, Jasper H 1952 The electroencephalogram in parasagittal lesions. Electroencephalography and Clinical Neurophysiology 4: 481–494

Varcelletto MP 1966 A propos d'une observation de petit mal 'post-traumatique' chez un adulte. Le Journal de Medecine de Lyon 5 November: 1567–1569

Yohai D, Barnett SH 1989 Absence and atonic seizures induced by piperazine. Pediatric Neurology 5: 393–394

DISCUSSION

Prendergast: Does carbamazepine make these patients worse?

Ferrie: There is very little evidence in the literature on what the best treatment should be. There is no doubt from the cases in the literature and from our own cases that the majority were more resistant to treatment than typical absences as part of idiopathic generalised epilepsies, although some of the cases seemed to respond very well to treatment. Good arguments can be made for treatment with carbamazepine or with valproate and the answer is that we do not know if carbamazepine will make things worse or not.

Gloor: I am familiar with the two cases, the Batten's disease and the SSPE. It was suggested en passant that these patients may have had a genetic predisposition. In both these cases we can exclude this because we see the progressive change of a typical classical spike and wave, especially clearly in the SSPE case, where the spike and wave gradually becomes slower, becomes more disorganised, and finally becomes very disorganised and then begins to be periodic. It is a continuum of the change. I think the underlying pathophysiology is such that at the early stages there was some diffuse grey matter disease cortically and sub-cortically and we know that this sets up a change of having bilateral asynchronous discharge, not necessarily the spike and wave type but in these cases it was of that type, and it is just the natural history of the disease which gradually transforms this into other forms of bilateral synchronous discharges.

Ferrie: I was trying to make the point that these cases have been known for many years now. From the literature search I did I could not find any other cases reported, and from asking paediatric neurologists with many years of experience nobody had seen 3 Hz spike and wave with absences in these cases.

Gloor: It is there. No question.

Ferrie: Therefore it is difficult to say that these are aetiologically linked. It is true to say that these patients may have had an underlying genetic predisposition that was modified by the other condition and modified the seizure, but whether we can say that they are genuinely caused by the underlying condition: that is, if these children had not developed SSPE and Batten's disease would they have had absences? I suspect they may have done.

30. Blank spells that are not typical absences

D. R. Fish

For the most part typical absences are readily differentiated from other causes of blank spells on the basis of the history, ictal semiology, and EEG findings. There is a small area of potential diagnostic difficulty relating to absences that are: atypical; due to non-epileptic events; or symptomatic or due to partial seizures (Fig. 30.1).

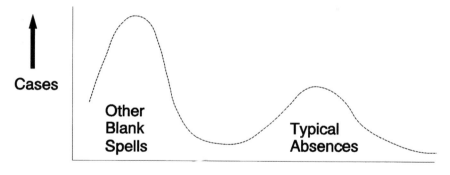

Fig. 30.1 Schematic representation to demonstrate the clinical differentiation between typical absences and other blank spells. There is a small area of clinical difficulty when the separation of typical absences from other causes of blank spells is uncertain or impossible.

Atypical absences are characterised by a predominance of clinical attacks with prolonged ictal semiology and slow spike and wave. Although individual attacks may last only a few s, they often occur in clusters, sometimes going on for hours or days (see Ch. 1). The attacks themselves may be clinically very subtle. They are not usually affected by over-breathing or photic stimulation. Often there is mental retardation. Neuro-imaging may reveal an underlying structural basis (Fig. 30.2).

Non-epileptic causes of brief blank spells include: psychological attacks; cardiac disorders; transient cerebral ischaemia; and syncope. Psychologically mediated attacks are usually much more prolonged than typical absences with additional features, either motor or behavioural. This temporal differ-

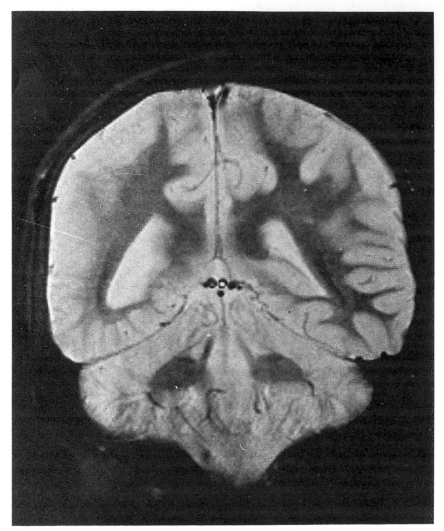

Fig. 30.2 MRI scan of a child with mental retardation and prolonged episodes of staring, sometimes eye deviation, lack of responsiveness, facial automatisms and showing extensive gyral abnormalities. EEG shows slow (approximately 2.5 Hz) generalised spike and wave activity.

ence also applies to transient ischaemic attacks. The latter often last for hours, or at least several minutes, and rarely have the frequency of typical absences. Occasionally critical vascular occlusion may present with flurries of attacks but there are usually focal neurological features, and an older age group is normally affected.

Cardiac arrhythmias can cause diagnostic confusion. They may be brief, recurrent, and present in a young age group. The nature of the events may be such that the cardiac output is not reduced to the degree required to cause complete loss of consciousness and collapse. However, usually there is a history of palpitations, change in colour, or complaints such as light-headedness, dizziness or tiredness that may last for several minutes (or longer) and may be partially relieved by lying down. Simple faints that do not progress to complete loss of consciousness often have characteristic features such as a postural relationship, ringing in the ears, blurring or darkening of vision, light-headedness, sweating, and colour changes. In abortive cases, however, there may be confusion with brief absences.

Partial seizures may mimic some aspects of typical absences, but it is very unusual for them simultaneously to mimic the full constellation of clinical and EEG features (Fig. 30.3).

BLANK SPELLS : NOT TYPICAL ABSENCES

● Altered Consciousness

● Arrest of Activity

● Eyelid Twitching

● Myoclonic Jerks

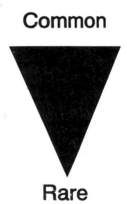

Common

Rare

Fig. 30.3 Constellation of clinical features in typical absences that may be seen in isolation, or rarely combined in partial epilepsies.

In terms of the ictal semiology, seizures arising in many different cerebral locations may be associated with: arrest of activity and/or impaired awareness and sometimes simple automatisms. These are most often apparent in brief temporal or frontal lobe seizures. Usually, however, other ictal semiology is also present such as experiential phenomena or motor activity, at least in some of the patient's attacks. Tonic axial seizures may cause apparent arrest of activity through contraction of the axial musculature, mimicking typical absences if too mild to cause falls.

Eyelid flicker or blinking can be seen in partial seizures, but these are not usual features of temporal or frontal lobe seizures. When present they are more often found in patients with posterior seizures (Fig. 30.4). For

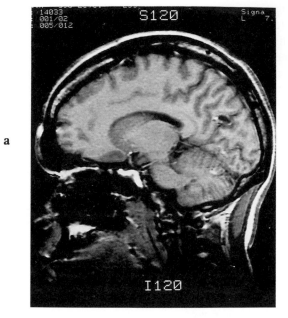

a

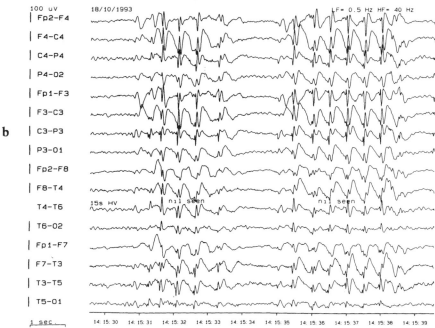

b

Fig. 30.4 A 19-year-old male with onset of seizures at age nine. Attacks consist of arrest of activity and eyelid blinking lasting for up to 1 min. During some of the earlier episodes he also had head turning to the right. Parasagittal T_1-weighted MRI (a) showing small circumscribed left mesial parietal lesion (subsequently shown to be an oligodendroglioma). Inter-ictal EEG (b) shows generalised spike and slow wave activity at 2–2.5Hz.

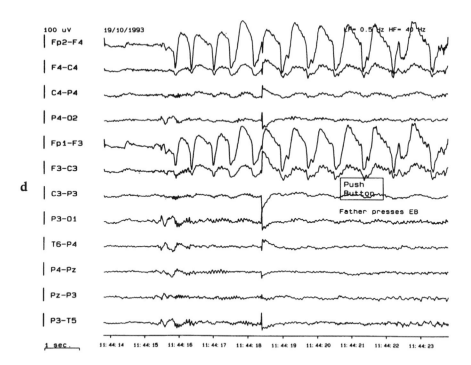

Fig 30.4 Ictal EEG (c) shows onset of low-amplitude fast activity in the left centro-parietal region. Note the slow eye blink artefacts (d) towards the end of another seizure.

example, Williamson et al (1992) reported eye blinking in 14/25 patients with occipital seizures. Seizures arising in the posterior cerebral regions, however, are usually associated with other additional clinical features such as visual or somatosensory phenomena that clearly differentiate the attacks from typical absences. In consequence, partial seizures may mimic isolated aspects of typical absences, but rarely mimic the full constellation of clinical features.

In terms of the EEG findings it is well known that some patients with partial epilepsy may show 3 Hz spike and wave activity on the EEG. This is usually associated with other more focal features. In a review of pre-surgical patients we identified 3/81 patients with MRI-defined hippocampal atrophy, and 3/28 patients with non-dysplastic frontal lobe lesions who displayed approximately 3 Hz generalised spike and slow wave activity (in addition to any focal features) (Fig. 30.5). The occurrence of this EEG finding may represent a co-existent susceptibility to primary generalised seizures, or secondary bilateral synchrony, especially with parasagittal lesions (Tukel & Jasper, 1952).

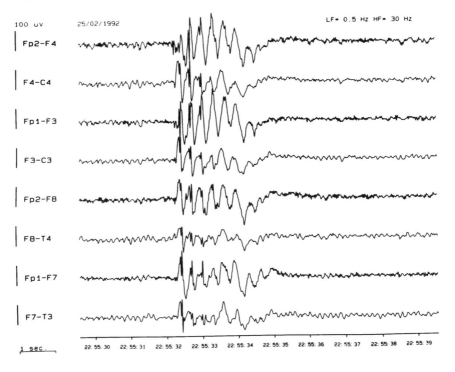

Fig. 30.5 A 30-year-old female with a positive family history of epilepsy and prolonged childhood febrile seizures. The patient subsequently had frequent seizures with a rising epigastric sensation, sometimes proceeding to loss of awareness and manual automatisms. MRI showed right hippocampal sclerosis, confirmed at subsequent histology of excised surgical specimen. Resting EEG showed frequent episodes of generalised spike and wave activity without obvious clinical change (example shown) and only rare right temporal discharges.

There has been much recent interest in the pathological finding of cortical dysgenesis (microdysgenesis) in patients with childhood absence epilepsy (see Ch. 15). As part of a larger study we reviewed the EEGs of 100 adult patients with cortical dysgenesis of various types and epilepsy (Raymond et al, 1994). These were classified as: abnormalities of gyration (39 cases), heterotopias (28 cases), tuberous sclerosis (5 cases), focal cortical dysplasia/microdysgenesis (7 cases), duplication of the fascia dentata (1 case) and dysembryoplastic neuro-epithelial tumours (21 cases).

Fourteen patients had episodes of approximately 3 per s generalised spike and slow wave activity in one or more of the EEG records. The abnormalities in these cases were sub-ependymal heterotopia (5 cases), band heterotopia (3 cases), macrogyria (4 cases), tuberous sclerosis (1 case) and microdysgenesis (1 case). We have recently reported the diagnostic difficulties that may arise in patients with sub-ependymal heterotopia (Raymond et al, 1994a) and these form the largest sub-group. Sub-ependymal heterotopia may be familial, is much commoner in females than males and the seizures usually commence in the second decade of life. Clearly some of these features may overlap with idiopathic generalised epilepsy and typical absences. Although not all of these 14 cases had video-EEG monitoring of clinical attacks, several did report brief blank spells without other ictal semiology to suggest a partial onset (Fig. 30.6). The pathogenetic relationship between neuronal migration defects and idiopathic generalised epilepsy is not yet clear and needs further study.

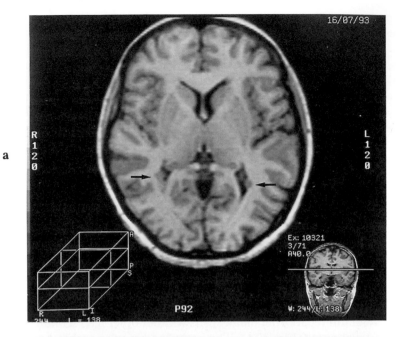

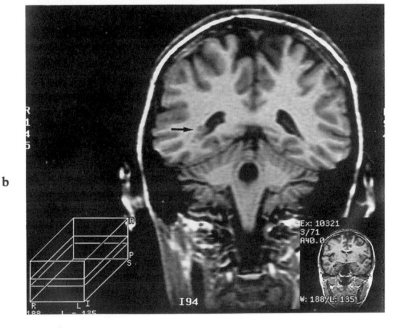

Fig. 30.6 A 33-year-old female with onset of attacks in early adolescence. Predominant seizure type was absences. Occasional generalised tonic-clonic seizures. In addition she had some episodes of fear and anxiety lasting for up to an hour. Axial MRI (a) with arrows shows bilateral sub-ependymal heterotopia; coronal MRI (b) demonstrates the more extensive right-sided sub-ependymal heterotopia.

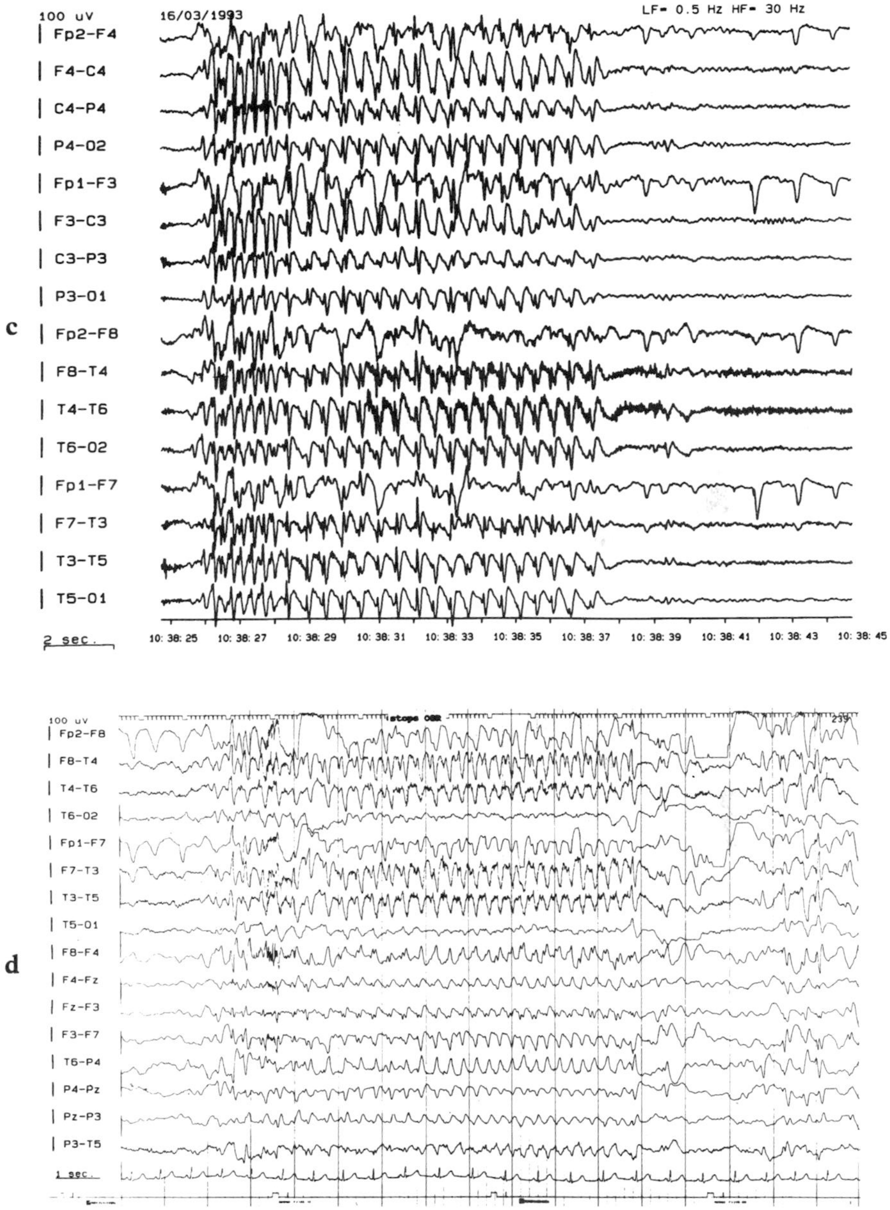

Fig. 30.6 Resting EEG (c) shows bursts of generalised 3 Hz spike and slow-wave activity; EEG during an attack (d) shows generalised 3 Hz spike and slow-wave activity. Clinically this seizure involved arrest of activity, blank stare and small, shuffling lower limb movements.

REFERENCES

Tukel K, Jasper HH 1952 The electroencephalogram in parasagittal lesions. Electroencephalography and Clinical Neurophysiology 4: 481–494

Raymond AA, Sisodiya S, Fish DR, Shorvon SD, Stevens J 1994 Subependymal heterotopia: a distinct neuronal migration disorder associated with epilepsy. Journal of Neurology, Neurosurgery and Psychiatry 57: 1195–1202

Raymond AA, Fish DR, Sisodiya S, Sanjari NA, Shorvon SD, Stevens J 1994a The clinical and investigative features of 100 adults with epilepsy and cortical dysgenesis. Brain (in press)

Williamson PD, Thadani VM, Danney TH, Spencer DD, Spencer SS, Mattson R 1992 Occipital lobe epilepsy: clinical characteristics, seizure spread patterns, and results of surgery. Annals of Neurology 31: 3–13

DISCUSSION

Andermann: The co-existence of generalised spike and wave and temporal lobe discharges is very interesting. Many of these people have spike and wave and yet it does not seem to be clinically significant as far as the introduction of seizures is concerned. We had one patient where there seemed to be a clinically correlated spike and wave. She would push the button when she had a temporal lobe attack and when she had a burst of spike and wave she would also push the button. The lady you presented comes about as close to classical absences or typical absences as we can get. Did she have multiple contiguous periventricular nodules or only isolated ones? The implication is that, if the nodules are contiguous along with the whole ventricular wall, then the cortex diffusely must be abnormal because obviously some of the cells that should be going there are not going there.

Fish: No. Hers are relatively low class but bilateral. It is important to say the way we identify these patients. The starting point for nearly everyone in the meeting is video-telemetry to identify the patient. These patients are identified from the MRI scan first and working backwards. So the finding of 5/20 with spike and wave is quite a high figure.

31. Absence status epilepticus

Simon Shorvon

Episodes of non-convulsive status were well-recognised curiosities in the 19th and early 20th centuries. Controversy abounded about the nature of these epileptic conditions and their relationship to epilepsy, a debate which was clarified only with the introduction of the EEG into clinical practice in the 1930s. The identification of the 3 Hz spike-wave EEG pattern underlying the generalised absence seizure was a landmark in 20th-century neurology. The first description of petit mal status came in 1938, in a cousin of Lennox who had continuous spike-wave recorded on an EEG following insulin-induced hypoglycaemia (Lennox, 1945). The term petit mal status was first used by Lennox (1945).

For a time, all cases of non-convulsive status were grouped together under the single rubric of petit mal, a unified approach which became evidently untenable when epileptic confusional states without concurrent EEG spike-wave discharges were described, and when prolonged spike-wave was observed in some patients without overt seizures. Classification has since been revised in the light of a better physiological understanding of the range of prolonged absence states, and a suggested classification scheme is shown in the box below (Shorvon, 1994). Here non-convulsive status is divided into three categories: absence status, partial status and boundary syndromes. In this paper only generalised absence status will be considered.

Classification of non-convulsive status epilepticus

- Generalised absence SE
  - Typical absence SE
  - Atypical absence SE
  - De novo absence SE of late onset
  - Absence SE in other epileptic syndromes

- Partial SE
  - Non-convulsive complex partial SE
  - Non-convulsive simple partial SE

- Boundary syndromes
  - Electrographic SE
  - Prolonged post-ictal confusional states
  - Epileptic behavioural disturbances and psychosis

The sub-categorisation of 'absence status' is contentious. A particular problem concerns the differentiation of typical and atypical absence status epilepticus. Some authorities, in recognition of the overlap between the clinical and EEG features of absence status in a variety of clinical contexts, view absence status as a spectrum (a 'biological continuum'). Among those taking this view are: Gastaut (1983), who used the term absence status to encompass all cases on the basis that the clinical and EEG semiology can be indistinguishable and that aetiology is only 'a relative phenomenon'; Porter & Penry (1983), who nevertheless confusingly prefer the appellation 'petit mal status' (this term would perhaps better be confined to absence status in idiopathic generalised epilepsy); and Berkovic et al (1987). Others (Gibberd, 1972; Doose, 1983; Ohtahara et al, 1979; Shorvon, 1994) feel it appropriate to split the condition into typical and atypical forms. Doose (1983) complicates the matter further by admitting a category of atypical idiopathic generalised cases into the typical absence category ('primary myoclonic-astatic epilepsy').

In this chapter the view is taken that, in spite of the overlap between clinical and EEG forms, typical and atypical absence status should be differentiated because of the dissimilarity of their general clinical features, natural history, pathological basis, response to treatment and prognosis. For the same reasons, cases of absence status occurring in other clinical contexts (eg, in other epileptic encephalopathies and myoclonic-astatic epilepsy) should also be categorised separately.

The differentiation between generalised and partial absence status has been another source of confusion. Cases of what were undoubtedly complex partial status were recounted sporadically as 'interesting freaks' in the 19th century. Authentication by EEG of the first case had to wait until 1956 (Gastaut et al, 1956). More recently most cases have been lumped together under the rubric absence status and barely differentiated from status in idiopathic and secondarily generalised epilepsies. This confusion is not helped by the fact that there is considerable overlap in clinical features between partial and generalised status. Furthermore, although detailed EEG recording (including depth EEG) has elucidated essential physiological differences between partial and generalised absence status, focal lesions (particularly frontal lesions) can result in clinical and EEG seizures which are indistinguishable from absence seizures. How many cases of apparently generalised absence status (particularly atypical absence status) are in fact partial and not generalised is unclear.

In this chapter the author has adhered to the traditional division between generalised and partial epilepsy (and status), with the suspicion that this is an often simplistic and false division. The differentiation between absence status and the epileptic boundary syndromes is also difficult (Shorvon, 1994).

In this chapter generalised absence status is sub-divided into four separate categories:

1. Typical absence status epilepticus: non-convulsive status, occurring in the syndrome of idiopathic generalised epilepsy.
2. Atypical absence status epilepticus: non-convulsive status that occurs largely in secondarily generalised epilepsy of the Lennox–Gastaut type and also in similar patients with compromised cerebral function and transitional cases.
3. De novo absence status epilepticus of late onset: non-convulsive status arising de novo in adults without a history of epilepsy.
4. Absence status epilepticus occurring in other epileptic syndromes: non-convulsive generalised status in other symptomatic epilepsies and other epileptic syndromes.

TYPICAL ABSENCE STATUS EPILEPTICUS

Assessment of the published literature of absence status is complicated by three factors. First is the fact that many authorities have failed to separate typical and atypical absences (Roger et al, 1974; Bendix, 1964; Dalby, 1969; Hajnsek & Durrigl, 1970; Gastaut, 1983; Lob et al, 1967). Secondly there is the confusion with complex partial status, due in part to the erroneous yet once prevalent view that all generalised spike-wave discharges imply a generalised rather than focal epilepsy (Niedermeyer & Khalifeh, 1965). Finally, there is the difficulty that exists with regard to patients with electrographic spike-wave status in whom there are also focal EEG changes greater than would normally be accepted for a truly generalised epilepsy, but who have no other focal clinical features. Such cases are not uncommon, particularly in adult practice, conforming neither to the classical picture of idiopathic generalised nor of secondary generalised epilepsy, and these patients are difficult to classify (Hess et al, 1971; Niedermeyer et al, 1979; Shorvon, 1994). The largest series was reported by Roger et al (1974).

Lennox (1960) reported a history of petit mal status in 2.6% of his 1039 petit mal patients, and Livingston et al (1965) in 9.9% and Loiseau & Cohadon (1970) in 5.8% in their own clinic series. Dalby (1969) reported petit mal status (on historical grounds) in 6.2% of patients with EEGs showing spike-wave (not all of whom have idiopathic generalised epilepsy) and in 9.3% of those with a history of petit mal absences.

Clinical features

Males and females seem equally affected. Absence status usually occurs in patients with a history of idiopathic generalised epilepsy, although it may be the first and occasionally the only epileptic manifestation. Repeated attacks can occur. The status lasts 12 h or less in over 50% of episodes, but it can persist for days, weeks or possibly months. An episode of absence status is often terminated, and less commonly initiated, by a grand mal seizure.

Identifiable precipitants, commoner in typical absence status than in complex partial status, include: menstruation, withdrawal of medication, hypoglycaemia, hyperventilation, flashing or bright lights, sleep deprivation, fatigue, stress or grief. Often, though, status seems to occur spontaneously.

Clouding of consciousness

This can vary from slight clouding to profound stupor. About 20% of patients show slowing of ideation and expression only, with psychological effects noted, particularly on activities requiring sustained attention, sequential organisation or spatial structuring. Amnesia may be slight or even absent (Andermann & Robb, 1972). Occasionally psychometric testing may be required to document specific isolated psychometric impairments during spike-wave status (Geier, 1978). A notable feature in generalised absence status is the relative preservation of verbal functioning, in marked contrast to complex partial status. In over 50% of cases there is much more marked clouding of consciousness. These patients are immobile, able to perform simple voluntary actions only after repeated requests, and often mute or almost mute with long delays in verbal responses or with monosyllabic and hesitant speech. Mental state examination shows confusion, disorientation and widespread impairment of intellectual functioning. The expression may be blank or puzzled, the eyes may be partially closed, and the patient appears groggy or trance-like. The pseudo-ataxic gait may be hesitant and stumbling. Automatisms can occur and even ambulatory epileptic fugues (absence status may be the commonest cause of ictal fugue; Vizioli & Magliocco, 1953). Amnesia is usual but variable and may be punctuated by short patches of recall. About 20% of patients show more severe psychomotor retardation, with incontinence of urine, pseudo-dementia, bradyphrenia or stupor.

Other motor features

About 50% of patients show other motor features such as myoclonus, atonia, hippus, rhythmical blinking of the eyelids and quivering of the lips, facial grimacing and smiling. Facial, especially eyelid, myoclonus is a common feature of absence status, but rare in complex partial status (an important consideration in differential diagnosis).

Other psychological features

Psychotic and behavioural changes are less frequent and severe than those encountered in complex partial status. Hebephrenia, catatonia, paranoia, hallucinations and episodic quarrelsome, irascible, impulsive and regressive behaviour can occur (Dongier, 1959).

Only Rohr-le Floch et al (1988) have directly compared the symptomatology of typical absence and complex partial status. The most characteristic presentation of petit mal status was a fluctuating confusional state with altered consciousness, psychomotor retardation, myoclonus, indifference and mutism (Table 31.1).

Table 31.1 Comparison of the clinical features of petit mal, psychomotor and frontal polar status epilepticus (from the series of Rohr-Le Floch et al, 1988)

	Petit Mal status (n=32)	Psychomotor status (n=9)	Frontal Polar status (n=19)
Intellectual features:			
Altered consciousness	100%	66%	58%
Fluctuating consciousness	29(90%)	3(33%)	6(32%)
Poverty of speech	8(34%)	0	4(22%)
Slowness of speech	3(21%)	0	3(16%)
Feeble voice	3	0	1
Slowness of gesture	4	1	3
Confabulation	0	0	4(22%)
Ideas of persecution	0	3(33%)	0
Myoclonus (facial/global)	18(59%)	0	0
Psychiatric misdiagnosis	3	2	4
Attitude:			
Indifferent, peevish	7(22%)	0	4(22%)
Perplexed/mute	7(22%)	1	7(37%)
Sly, ironic	0	0	6(32%)
Smiling/hilarious	0	0	8(42%)
Sad	1	0	1
Anxious, frightened	3	4(44%)	1
Negativistic	1	2(22%)	2
Irritable, aggressive	1	5(56%)	2
Agitated	4	1	1
Automatism:			
Simple gestural	7(22%)	1	3
Complex gestural	2	4(44%)	2
Stereotyped gestural	0	1	3
Ambulatory	1	2(22%)	0
Verbal	1	2(22%)	0
Echolalia	0	0	3
Jargon aphasia	0	1	0
Defect in programming	0	0	2

(percentages are of the number of cases in which it was possible to test the patient)

The numbers investigated were small and the cases selected; this is, however, the only direct published comparison of the clinical appearances of status in the three patient groups (table from Shorvon, 1994).

Electroencephalographic features

The diagnostic electrographic pattern is continuous or almost continuous bilaterally synchronous and symmetrical 3 Hz spike-wave activity, with little or no reactivity to sensory stimuli. This classical EEG appearance is usually seen in the setting of a prior history of clear-cut idiopathic generalised epilepsy. The closer the EEG is to this classic pattern the more typical are the clinical features. Other forms have been described, including irregular and slow spike-wave (1.5–4 Hz), prolonged bursts of spike activity, generalised periodic triphasic sharp waves, and polyspike and wave at frequencies from 2–6 Hz, but whether or not to include such cases within the rubric of absence status and quite where to draw the nosological line is uncertain. The cycling of EEG changes common in complex partial status is not usual in spike-wave status, but does occur; in some patients the spike-wave is not continuous, but rather broken into frequent bursts (Schwab, 1953).

A detailed EEG description of 148 patients for the Marseilles symposium was reported by Gastaut & Tassinari (1975). In about 40% the spike-wave rhythm was continuous and in about 30% broken up into frequent bursts. In about 15% of patients, arrhythmic spike/wave bursts were repeated and in 10% the EEG showed underlying slow activity with bursts of spikes or spike-wave. The type or degree of clouding of consciousness does not in general strongly correlate with the form of the EEG.

Cause

Strictly speaking, episodes of typical absence status occur only in idiopathic generalised epilepsy. Probably they can develop in any of the sub-categories of this condition.

Treatment and outcome

Typical absence status is rapidly terminated by intravenous benzodiazepine. It is usual to give: diazepam at a dose of 0.2–0.3 mg/kg, clonazepam 1 mg (0.5 mg or 0.02 mg/kg in children) or lorazepam 0.07 mg/kg (children 0.1 mg/kg), repeated as required. In the rare cases in which this is ineffectual, valproate or chlormethiazole can be given. So effective is benzodiazepine treatment that if the patient does not respond, the diagnosis is likely in fact to be atypical absence or complex partial status. The outcome of absence status is good, with most patients making a full recovery without sequelae. The occurrence of absence status does not imply a poorer longer-term prognosis for the epilepsy.

ATYPICAL ABSENCE STATUS EPILEPTICUS

This is a term best reserved to decribe the absence status which occurs in patients with secondarily generalised epilepsy of the Lennox–Gastaut type and in other cryptogenic or symptomatic generalised syndromes, especially those associated with mental handicap and diffuse cerebral damage. It seems sensible to categorise these cases separately in view of the greatly different clinical context, prognosis and aetiology.

Clinical features

The clinical phenomenology of typical and atypical absence status overlaps considerably, but, because many studies mix the two conditions, the extent of this overlap is not known. Certain features are more characteristic of atypical absence status, however (Shorvon, 1994):

1. Episodes of atypical absence status are generally longer and more frequent than those of typical absence status.
2. Atypical absence status often has a gradual onset and offset. An episode of atypical absence status is usually preceded by a deterioration in the general physical and psychical state of the patient before overt seizures develop.
3. Atypical absence status tends to fluctuate, and may evolve into minor motor, myoclonic or tonic seizures. In some patients, the mental state fluctuates gradually in and out of this ill-defined epileptic state over long periods of time (some attacks last weeks or even months), with little distinction possible between ictal and inter-ictal phases. Initiation or termination of the status with a tonic-clonic seizure is unusual in atypical absence.
4. Atypical absence status is precipitated by drowsiness or under-stimulation and is commoner in over-medicated patients.
5. Some cases have a striking and unexplained periodicity.
6. The EEG during absence status may show continuous irregular slow (2 Hz) spike-wave, or hypsarrhythmia, or other ictal patterns not seen in idiopathic generalised epilepsy (Beaumanoir et al, 1988).

Cause

Any condition which can result in the Lennox–Gastaut syndrome or in other forms of diffuse or multifocal epileptic encephalopathy can result in atypical absence status.

Treatment and outcome

In acute atypical absence status, intravenous benzodiazepine therapy can be given, although the response is less satisfactory than in typical absence status. Paraldehyde, chlormethiazole, phenobarbitone or steroid therapy can also be helpful. In patients whose level of consciousness is not severely impaired, oral rather than intravenous treatment is more appropriate, and any of the conventional anti-epileptic drugs can be tried, the drugs of first choice being valproate, lamotrigine, clonazepam and clobazam. In some cases, the drugs seem ineffective and the condition fluctuates and runs its course irrespective of treatment. Carbamazepine has been said to worsen seizures in some cases. Although the atypical absence status can persist for long periods of time, there are usually no permanent sequelae. The overall outcome depends on the underlying epileptic condition.

DE NOVO ABSENCE STATUS EPILEPTICUS OF LATE ONSET

Absence status can occur in adult (especially late adult) life. In some cases this is typical absence status occurring in patients with pre-existing idiopathic generalised epilepsy. In a series of 18 adults admitted to a general hospital over a 28-month period with absence status (20% of all cases of status in adults), 10 had a history of idiopathic generalised epilepsy (Dunne et al, 1987). The status developed between the ages of 18–81 and five patients were >50. The epilepsy has often been in long remission prior to onset of status (Neidermeyer & Khalifeh, 1965; Lob et al, 1967; Andermann & Robb, 1972; Gall et al, 1978; Nightingale & Welch, 1982); between 2–40 years in four of the 10 patients reported by Dunne et al (1987). Why status suddenly recurs after long seizure-free intervals is not known, and in only a minority of patients are precipitating factors obvious. The onset is acute, often ushered in by a tonic-clonic seizure, and the duration of status varies from hours to days.

In most published cases, however, there is no prior history of epilepsy (Shorvon, 1994). The EEG changes, although showing spike-wave, are atypical, and the clinical precipitation, course, response to treatment, and prognosis differ from typical absence status. In a review of 64 such cases from the literature (Thomas et al, 1992), 66% were female, with a mean age of 62 years (range 42–88). Late-onset absence status presents, like ordinary absence status, as acute confusion with variable alteration of consciousness, ranging from profound stupor with catatonia and loss of sphincteric control at one extreme through mental dullness and abulia to mild motor retardation and isolated intellectual disturbances at the other. Amnesia may be total, patchy or occasionally not apparent. Changes in affect are common and, almost invariably, a primary psychiatric misdiagnosis is initially made. Motor retardation or perseveration are common, the gait is often pseudo-ataxic and slow; and other motor features include myoclonic jerking, posturing, automatisms, catatonia or myoclonus. There is usually no cycling of signs as in complex partial status. Generalised tonic-clonic seizures are reported in about 50% of cases, but not initiating nor terminating the status, as in typical absence status. The EEG is usually diagnostic, showing continuous or frequent generalised spike-wave activity at frequencies between 1–4 Hz, or less often other, less well-defined epileptic abnormalities.

Precipitating factors

In a high proportion of published cases, precipitating factors were identified. Benzodiazepine (or other drug or alcohol) withdrawal is the commonest cause – for instance, in 16 of 29 cases in three series (Dunne et al, 1987; Van Sweden & Mellerio, 1988; Thomas et al, 1992). As there is a high incidence of pre-existing psychiatric disorder in adult onset non-convulsive status, psychotropic drug withdrawal may have passed unrecognised in other reported cases. Other precipitants include ECT (Weiner et al, 1980; Varma & Lee, 1992), metrizamide myelography (Pritchard & O'Neal, 1984; Vollmer et al, 1985), cerebral angiography, lithium therapy, acute metabolic disturbances, toxic or other pharmacological agents (Schwartz & Scott, 1971; Vignaendra et al, 1976; Ellis & Lee, 1977; Beaumanoir, Jenny & Jekiel, 1980; Richard & Brenner, 1980; Rumpl & Hinterhuber, 1981; Van Sweden, 1985; Lee, 1985; Bourrat et al, 1986; Dunne et al, 1987; Hersch & Billings, 1988; Thomas et al, 1992).

Treatment and outcome

The status invariably responds to intravenous benzodiazepine, with rapid and complete resolution of the epilepsy. The prognosis is excellent when the precipitating factors are removed. The overall outcome is dependent upon the underlying psychiatric condition. Long-term anti-epileptic drug therapy is not usually required.

The nosological position of such cases is controversial, but as a relatively homogeneous and distinctive core syndrome exists, it seems reasonable to distinguish these cases from other forms of absence status. In view of the fact that the condition is often precipitated by drug withdrawal, metabolic or toxic factors, Thomas et al (1992) suggest the designation 'situational-related non-convulsive generalised status epilepticus', and include these cases among the category of 'Special syndromes – situation-related seizures' in the 1985 ILAE classification of the epilepsies and epileptic syndromes.

ABSENCE STATUS EPILEPTICUS IN OTHER SYNDROMES

Absence status can occur in a variety of other contexts, with a clinical form very similar to other categories of absence status. Because the associated clinical aspects are so different, it is sensible to sub-categorise these cases separately. Included here are non-convulsive status: in other forms of mental handicap (many perhaps best considered as cases of atypical absence status), in the severe myoclonic epilepsies of infancy and early childhood, in the syndrome of myoclonic-astatic epilepsy, in the progressive myoclonic epilepsies, in ESES, in the Landau–Kleffner syndrome, in the symptomatic epilepsies with focal and multifocal pathologies (eg, metabolic and degenerative disorders), and in electrographic status with subtle clinical signs. The clinical and EEG features overlap with other forms of absence and complex partial status. The principles of treatment are similar to those in atypical absence status, and the overall prognosis depends on the underlying epileptic condition.

REFERENCES

Andermann F, Robb JP 1972 Absence status: a reappraisal following a review of thirty-eight cases. Epilepsia 13: 177–187

Beaumanoir A, Foletti G, Magistris M, Volanschi D 1988 Status epilepticus in the Lennox-Gastaut syndrome. In: Niedermeyer E, Degen E, Degen R (eds) The Lennox-Gastaut syndrome. Neurology and neurobiology, Vol 45. Alan Liss, New York, pp283–300

Beaumanoir A, Jenny P, Jekiel M 1980 Etude de quatre "petit mal status" post-partum. Revue d'Electroencéphalographie et de Neurophysiologie Clinique 10: 381–385

Bendix T 1964 Petit mal status. Electroencephalography and Clinical Neurophysiology 17: 210–211

Berkovic SF, Bladin PF 1982 Absence status in adults. Clinical and Experimental Neurology 19: 198–207

Bourrat Ch, Garde P, Boucher M, Fournet A. 1986 Etats d'absence prolongée chez des patients agés sans passé épileptique. Revue Neurologique 142: 696–702

Dalby MA 1969 Epilepsy and 3 per second spike and wave rhythms; a clinical, electrographic, and prognostic analysis of 346 patients. Acta Neurologica Scandinavica 45 (Suppl. 40): 1–183

Dongier S 1959 Statistical study of clinical and electroencephalographic manifestations of 536 psychotic episodes occurring in 516 epileptics between clinical seizures. Epilepsia 1: 117–142

Doose H 1983 Non-convulsive status epilepticus in childhood: clinical aspects and classification. In: Delgado-Escueta AV, Wasterlain CG, Tremain DM, Porter RJ (eds) Status epilepticus: mechanisms of brain damage and treatment. Advances in neurology, Vol. 34. Raven Press, New York, pp83–92

Dunne JW, Summers QA, Stewart-Wynne EG 1987 Non-convulsive status epilepticus: a prospective study in an adult general hospital. Quarterly Journal of Medicine 62: 117–126

Ellis JM, Lee SI 1978 Acute prolonged confusion in later life as an ictal state. Epilepsia 19: 119–128

Gall M, Scollo-Lavizzari G, Becker H 1978 Absence status in the adult. European Neurology 17: 121–128

Gastaut H 1983 Classification of status epilepticus. In: Delgado-Escueta AV, Wasterlain CG, Treiman DM, Porter RJ (eds) Status epilepticus: mechanisms of brain damage and treatment. Advances in neurology, Vol 34. Raven Press, New York, pp15–35

Gastaut H, Roger J, Roger A 1956 Sur la signification de certaines fugues épileptiques: état de mal temporal. Revue Neurologique 94: 298–301

Gastaut H, Tassinari C 1975 Status epilepticus. In: Redmond A (ed) Handbook of electroencephalography and clinical neurophysiology, Vol 13A. Elsevier, Amsterdam, pp39–45

Geier S 1978 Prolonged psychic epileptic seizures: a study of the absence status. Epilepsia 19: 431–445

Gibberd FB 1972 Petit mal status presenting in middle age. Lancet i: 269

Hajnsek F, Durrigl V 1970 Some aspects of so-called 'petit mal status'. Electroencephalography and Clinical Neurophysiology 28: 322

Hess R, Scollo-Lavizzari G, Wyss FE 1971 Borderline cases of petit mal status. European Neurology 5: 137–154

Hersch EL, Billings RF 1988 Acute confusional state with status petit mal as a withdrawal syndrome – and five year follow-up. Canadian Journal of Psychiatry 33: 157–159

Lee SI 1985 Nonconvulsive status epilepticus: ictal confusion in later life. Archives of Neurology 42: 787–781

Lennox W 1945 The petit mal epilepsies: their treatment with tridione. Journal of the American Medical Association 129: 1069–1073

Lennox W 1960 Epilepsy and related disorders. Little, Brown, Boston

Livingston S, Torres I, Pauli L, Rider RV 1965 Petit mal epilepsy: results of a prolonged follow up study of 117 patients. Journal of the American Medical Association 194: 227–232

Lob H, Roger J, Soulayrol R, Regis H, Gastaut H 1967 Les états de mal généralisés à expression confusionelle. In: Gastaut H, Roger J, Lob H (eds) Les états de mal epileptiques. Masson, Paris, pp91–128

Loiseau P, Cohadon F 1970 Le petit mal et les frontières. Masson, Paris

Niedermeyer E, Khalifeh R 1965 Petit mal status ('spike-wave stupor'): an electro-clinical appraisal. Epilepsia 6: 250–262

Niedermeyer E, Fineyre F, Riley T, Uematsu S 1979 Absence status (petit mal status) with focal characteristics. Archives of Neurology 36: 417–421

Nightingale S, Welch J 1982 Psychometric assessment in absence status. Archives of Neurology 39: 516–519

Ohtahara S, Oka E, Yamatogi Y et al 1979 Non-convulsive status epilepticus in childhood. Folia Psychiatrica et Neurologica Japonica 3: 345–351

Porter RJ, Penry JK 1983 Petit mal status. In: Delgado-Escueta AV, Wasterlain CG, Treiman FDM, Porter RJ (eds) Status epilepticus: mechanisms of brain damage and treatment. Advances in neurology, Vol 34. Raven Press, New York, pp61–67

Pritchard PB, O'Neal DB 1984 Nonconvulsive status epilepticus following metrizamide myelography. Annals of Neurology 16: 252–254

Richard P, Brenner RP 1980 Absence status: case reports and a review of the literature. L'Encephale 6: 385–392

Rohr-Le Floch J, Gauthier G, Beaumanoir A 1988 Etats confusionnels d'origine épileptique intérêt de l'EEG fait en urgence. Revue Neurologique 144: 6–7; 425–436

Roger J, Lob H, Tassinari CA 1974 Status epilepticus. In: Magnus O, Lorentz de Haas AM (eds) Handbook of clinical neurology, Vol 15. The epilepsies. North Holland Publishing, Amsterdam, pp145–188

Rumpl E, Hinterhuber H 1981 Unusual 'spike-wave stupor' in a patient with manic-depressive psychosis treated with amitriptylline. Journal of Neurology 226: 131–135

Schwab RS 1953 A case of status epilepticus in petit mal. Electroencephalography and Clinical Neurophysiology 5: 441–442

Schwartz MS, Scott DF 1971 Isolated petit mal status presenting de novo in middle age. Lancet 2: 1399–1401

Shorvon SD 1994 Status epilepticus: its clinical features and treatment in children and adults. Cambridge University Press, Cambridge

Thomas P, Beaumanoir A, Genton P, Dolisi C, Chatel M 1992 'De novo' absence status of late onset: report of 11 cases. Neurology 42: 104–110

Van Sweden B 1985 Toxic 'ictal' confusion in middle age: treatment with benzodiazepines. Journal of Neurology, Neurosurgery and Psychiatry 48: 472–476

Varma NK, Lee SI 1992 Nonconvulsive status epilepticus following electroconvulsive therapy. Neurology 42: 263–264

Vignaendra V, Loh TG, Lim CL 1976 Petit mal status in a patient with chronic renal failure. Medical Journal of Australia 2: 258–259

Vizioli R, Magliocco EB 1953 Clinical and laboratory notes: a case of prolonged petit mal seizures. Electroencephalography and Clinical Neurophysiology 5: 439–440

Vollmer ME, Weiss H, Beanland C, Krumholz A 1985 Prolonged confusion due to absence status following metrizamide myelography. Archives of Neurology 42: 1005–1008

Weiner RD, Volow MR, Gianturco DT, Cavenar JO 1980 Seizures terminable and interminable with ECT. Neuroscience Letters 87: 23–28

DISCUSSION

Stephenson: One of the symptomatic ones is perhaps an Angelman's syndrome which is not much seen but is important; they may be at a low level but they go even lower in their absence status.

Nothing has been said about de novo absence status in young children. One has seen a number who have no history of typical absences.

Shorvon: I know what the literature reports, that childhood absences sometimes present as status, it is the first epileptic manifestation. But do they get the same thing?

Stephenson: They may remain only with having status episodes.

Shorvon: And is it caused by drug withdrawal?

Stephenson: No. It may be genetic of some sort.

Stores: The impression gained is that non-convulsive status is often overlooked, not recognised for what it really is. Or, even when it is correctly recognised, it is often treated rather casually, certainly when compared with convulsive status. Is that other people's impression?

Shorvon: Probably it is overlooked, although I see in myself, and colleagues perhaps, a strong danger that we attribute all epileptic disturbances to subclinical epilepsy. I see myself doing this when we see a patient with a history of epilepsy who goes off in some way. It does cross one's mind it might be non-convulsive status. Undoubtedly some the these cases are, but I am not sure to what extent they all are. But Dr Stores is quite right. The frequency of non-convulsive status is completely unknown. It is probably more common than is recognised. Complex partial status is certainly commoner than is recognised.

One of the striking features of people who have long episodes of complex partial status is how they do not seem to have brain damage, in contrast to, say, tonic-clonic status. Having said that, we see patients with atypical absences, particularly the Lennox–Gastaut patients, having frequent attacks of absence status. How many of those are slowly deteriorating because of the status is difficult to say.

32. Biorhythms in the occurrence of absence seizures

Gregory Stores

Patterns in the occurrence of epileptic attacks have been described from the earliest times. Temkin (1971) cites several examples such as the periodicity attributed by Galen to the influence of the moon. In more recent times many factors have been identified, apparently acting as precipitating or inhibitory influences on seizures. However, history-taking often still neglects the circumstances in which seizures seem more or less likely to occur. Detailed enquiry may reveal many possible examples (Verduyn et al, 1988), although, of course, objective confirmation is needed.

Patterns of occurrence can be important both clinically and theoretically:

1. EEG and other special investigations are best undertaken at times at which the seizures are most likely to occur.
2. Influences on seizure occurrence (eg, emotional factors) might be suggested which can be modified to prevent or reduce the likelihood of further attacks.
3. Satisfactory seizure control may only be achieved by attention to such factors in combination with the use of anti-epileptic medication.
4. The timing or dosage of anti-epileptic drugs might need to be related to patterns of occurrence.
5. Different patterns can raise the possibility of sub-groups within an otherwise apparently homogeneous type of seizure disorder such as childhood absence epilepsy (Stores & Lwin, 1981).
6. The distribution of intervals between seizures can suggest the nature of underlying mechanisms (Stevens et al, 1971).

There are many factors that can facilitate or inhibit seizures, some physical or physiological, others psychological. Patterns of occurrence may be regular (or periodic) or irregular. Within the regular group are circadian and other biorhythms which are the subject of the present account.

Studies employing long-term EEG recordings to investigate patterns of occurrence in patients with absence seizures have the advantages that the frequency of such attacks is usually high, the generalised spike wave discharge is easy to identify, and the correlation between clinical and electrographic features is close. However, the number of such studies is small and the types of absence epilepsy are not always described precisely. It is only comparatively recently that it has been appreciated that absences can feature in different epilepsy syndromes. Systematic studies of patterns of occurrence in any form of absence epilepsy have not been carried out, still less comparisons of the various absence epilepsies. Some clinical accounts give an indication of the time of day in which attacks are most likely to occur but this aspect is often not given much prominence, even in the comprehensive and up-to-date reviews of childhood absence epilepsy, epilepsy with myoclonic absences, juvenile absence epilepsy and juvenile myoclonic epilepsy in Roger et al (1992). Most merely note that absences syndromes tend to occur mainly on awakening.

BIORHYTHMS

This term refers to periodically recurring events whose periodicity is the result of an endogenous pacemaker. Three basic types of biorhythm have been described: circadian, with periodicity of about 24 h; ultradian, especially those based on a cycle of about 100 min; and the less often discussed infradian rhythms with a periodicity longer than a day and possibly extending over weeks, as in so-called catamenial epilepsy.

The key issues in the epilepsies are: a) how convincingly such biorhythms can be demonstrated; and b) whether the rhythmicity is the result of an endogenous pacemaker for the epilepsy itself or whether it is secondary to the sleep–wake cycle, which has its own endogenous controls (Webb, 1994). Important discussions, mainly of circadian and ultradian rhythms in relation to the epilepsies, are contained in Martins da Silva et al (1985). The present account is confined, as far as possible, to the patterns of occurrence of typical absence seizures.

Circadian rhythms

Shouse (1989) has pointed out the consistency with which writers have classified seizures according to their occurrence in the sleep–wake cycle. There has been general agreement that in about two-thirds of patients seizures occur predominantly in the awake state ('diurnal or awakening epilepsy') or predominantly during sleep ('sleep epilepsy').

In this grouping, absences are seen as a form of awakening epilepsy, sharing the general characteristics of awakening epilepsies as being idiopathic generalised, age-dependent, idiopathic or hereditary in origin, and with a benign course. Janz (1962) reported that the seizures of patients with absences alone occurred particularly on waking in two-thirds of cases; this figure rose to over 90% if absences were combined with tonic-clonic seizures. This strong clinical impression of an association between absences and awakening appears to apply to the absences of childhood absence epilepsy and also to those in juvenile myoclonic epilepsy.

There have been relatively few attempts to confirm these clinical impressions of a circadian rhythm by long-term EEG monitoring. Studies have been concerned mainly with the distribution over 24 h of spike or spike-wave discharges of variable duration, including many which are very brief and unlikely to be accompanied by obvious clinical seizures (Stevens et al, 1972; Kellaway & Frost, 1983; Martins da Silva et al, 1984). The various findings generally provide some evidence of a circadian pattern, perhaps especially in generalised regular spike wave discharge. In some studies, monitoring has taken place overnight in order to assess the relationship between sleep stages and the nature of the seizure discharge, rather than patterns of occurrence. A few investigations have been concerned specifically with absence seizures but some have been confined to daytime recordings of between 3–12 h duration (Guey et al, 1969; Sato et al, 1976). In these and studies extending over approximately 24 h (Stores & Lwin, 1981; Horita et al, 1991) no obvious circadian patterns were seen consistently and variations in the distribution of seizure activity were prominent.

Assuming that more appropriate and sophisticated studies would demonstrate a circadian biorhythmicity in the absence epilepsies, the question would still arise: what is the origin of this rhythmicity? Webb (1985a) points out that circadian rhythms which might appear to be truly biorhythmic (in the sense of reflecting an intrinsic pacemaker of the epileptic process itself) may, in fact, be the result of some other independent periodic process. In the case of epilepsy, alternative explanations for a circadian pattern would be: a) an intrinsic pacemaker for the seizure activity itself (a 'state-related periodicity' in Webb's terms); or b) an influence external to the epileptic process itself but with its own pattern in time ('time-related periodicity') eg, the sleep–wake cycle. The frequent occurrence of absences on awakening in the morning is likely to be state-related, or secondary to the provocative effect on seizures of awakening, as the available evidence suggests that this association between the seizures and awakening is seen whatever the time of that awakening. Webb recommends the use of the various experimental methodologies developed in chronobiological sleep research in further attempts to determine the biological basis of circadian rhythms in epilepsy.

Ultradian rhythms

The difficulty of separating state-dependent from time-dependent effects applies no less to ultradian patterns. An endogenous 'basic rest–activity cycle' (BRAC), continuous through each 24 h, was postulated by Kleitman (1969). In sleep this is expressed as the NREM/REM cycle, and during wakefulness and fluctuations in level of arousal. Each cycle in this ultradian rhythm is considered to last about 100 min. Many biological, psychological and medical variables are thought to show this type of periodicity during wakefulness. The possibility that such a rhythm applies to epilepsy is more contentious.

Stevens et al (1972) used telemetry to record mainly inter-ictal discharges in various forms of epilepsy and described an approximately 90-min periodicity of these discharges during sleep, related to the NREM/REM cycle. There was some evidence that this pattern extended into the awake state. Binnie et al (1984) also reported ultradian periodicity, mainly during sleep, in the inter-ictal discharges of some patients with various forms of epilepsy, although the cycles were usually shorter or longer than 100 min.

Kellaway and his colleagues (Kellaway & Frost, 1983) have maintained that both focal and generalised epileptic activity display patterns of occurrence that can be explained in terms of the interaction of two independent pacemakers, one with a period of about 24 h and the other with a period of about 100 min, each influencing the production of spike wave activity. Different patterns of occurrence of seizure discharge are considered to arise from different phase relationships of these two cyclic processes, the phase relationships being determined by the time of sleep onset.

Investigation of ultradian rhythms in actual absence seizures seems limited to the single case report by Broughton et al (1985). The patient was an 8-year-old girl of normal intelligence with frequent absences. Ambulatory EEG monitoring, performed continuously over 84.5 h, revealed that night-time discharges were increased in NREM sleep and decreased in REM sleep (in keeping with earlier reports). The daytime fluctuations of the patient's spike-wave discharges (almost always >5 s in duration and, therefore, likely to have been accompanied by clinical changes) were generally at the NREM/REM cycle rate appropriate for the child's age. This correspondence between the patterns of discharges during the day and the NREM/REM sleep cycle tend to support the idea that both are modulated by the basic rest-activity cycle.

Broughton (1975) has also drawn attention to a 12 h biorhythm involving Stage 3–4 NREM sleep ('slow-wave sleep') mechanisms. This 'circasemidian' rhythm is thought to produce the afternoon drop in vigilance associated in some patients with seizures without the actual onset of sleep.

Arousal levels and mechanisms in epilepsy

Other findings in the Broughton study highlight the importance of arousal (ie, changes in alertness, rather than the sustained awake state) in the occurrence of seizures and the way in which patterns of occurrence can be dictated, at least partly, by changes in arousal level. The authors reported that when their patient's spike wave discharges were frequent the EEG showed evidence of drowsiness, with an increase in discharges immediately preceding daytime naps. In contrast, suppression of the discharges was associated with increased alertness.

The relationship between seizures, including absences, and level of alertness is well documented. Lennox and his colleagues (1936) described how seizure activity was reduced during tasks requiring concentration, although when the demands of the task became stressful seizure activity increased. Ounsted & Hutt (1964) also showed that some children with epilepsy had more seizures when bored or when tasks made excessive demands on them. Additional evidence that boredom and inattention are associated with an increased rate of absences was provided by Mirsky & van Buren (1965) and Guey et al (1969).

Further examples of an association between an increase in seizure frequency and extremes of arousal level were reported by Sato et al (1976) and Stores & Lwin (1981) in their studies of children with absence seizures using long-term EEG monitoring. In neither of the latter studies was any periodicity of seizure occurrence reported but both serve to illustrate how any endogenous rhythm might well be obscured by other influences on seizure occurrence, such as type of activity or emotional state. Also relevant is the fact that some patients have more seizures not only soon after awakening but also in the evening, when presumably their alertness is decreased, and that seizure frequency seems to increase as a result of sedation induced by anti-epileptic drugs or other medication.

A number of authors have sought to identify the precise aspect of arousal that is provocative of seizures. Niedermeyer (1982) placed special emphasis on the K complex (usually considered to be an arousal phenomenon) in light NREM sleep as the trigger to increased seizure discharge. He considered there is a counterpart in the seizure discharge during wakefulness to the frontal voltage maximum seen in the 'epileptic' K complexes of people with idiopathic generalised epilepsy. Seizure discharge is seen as an abnormal response to arousal ('dyshormia').

Halasz (1982) was concerned with changes in arousal or vigilance levels in periods of 'intermediate sleep' between the awake state, NREM and REM sleep. Fluctuations of arousal in intermediate sleep are said to be more pronounced in patients with generalised epilepsy compared with the general population. These fluctuations can be external or internal in origin and they result in spike wave discharge which itself exaggerates further fluctuations in levels of arousal. In Halasz's view, K complexes during light NREM sleep (or the corresponding V potential during transitional periods) are not so much an arousal reaction as a sign of either increased or decreased arousal level. This is in keeping with clinical observations that seizures can have a predilection for certain periods, namely awakening during the morning, during light NREM sleep at the time of transient awakenings during the night, and also when falling asleep in the evening. The activating effect on seizure discharge of sleep deprivation might also be explicable in these terms in that it induces a transitional sleep state. Halasz also reports an increase in ictal events in transitional periods, with fluctuating arousal levels, between periods of REM and NREM sleep.

Infradian rhythm

Catamenial epilepsy is the example usually given of an infradian pattern of occurrence of seizures in general, including absence seizures in some cases. In spite of the belief by many women with epilepsy that most of their seizures occur near or at the time of menstruation, objective recording of seizures seem to confirm that belief in only a few cases (Duncan et al, 1993). Even in such cases, the present evidence does not distinguish between possible endocrine or emotional factors.

It is possible that further long-term documentation of seizures would demonstrate ultradian rhythms reflecting patterns of change in sleep–wake states, themselves affecting seizure occurrence.

CONCLUSIONS

Clinically, there is a need for separate studies of the epilepsy syndromes of which absences are a part or, at least, clear definition of the type of absence epilepsy under investigation. The results of studies across a range of absence epilepsies could be relevant to the issue discussed elsewhere in this symposium of whether or not they are discrete syndromes or a continuum. Possible effects of anti-epileptic medication on patterns of seizure occurrence also deserve more attention. The pharmacology of such drugs may have its own biorhythmicity (Aronson, 1990).

One basic conceptual issue concerns the practice in some studies of combining ictal and inter-ictal events. Horita et al (1991) argue that when exploring circadian rhythms in childhood absence epilepsy only seizure discharge typically associated with daytime absences should be considered. They feel that the degraded form of discharge typically seen during NREM sleep represents the effect of other influences, the results of which might confound analysis of the typical seizure discharge alone.

A similar point has been made by Wolf (1985) concerning the relevance of inter-ictal discharges in general for the study of biorhythms and epilepsy. He contends that clinical seizures and epileptiform discharges are two different classes of events. The former have not been sufficiently inhibited; the latter reflect periods of particularly strong inhibition. Against these views is the argument that the distinction between ictal and inter-ictal events is false because, with sufficiently sensitive assessment, even very brief discharges can often be shown to have transient psychological accompaniments (Binnie, 1993).

It seems appropriate to consider separately different categories of spike wave discharge, defined in terms of duration, in biorhythmic research rather than risk confounding the issue by combining events with possibly different underlying mechanisms.

There are also suggestions that a more sophisticated view of sleep physiology needs to be taken. Replying to concerns that some ultradian periodicities detected in the epilepsies have been shorter than the classically described basic rest-activity cycle, Webb (1985b) remarked that 'the so-called 90 to 100 minute REM cycle is something of a myth' and pointed out that within an individual there is considerable variation in the duration of the NREM/REM cycle on a given night. Differences in NREM/REM cycle length between adults and children are especially relevant to the absence epilepsies. On a different point, Halasz (1982) has argued the need to consider intermediate categories of sleep (to which he attributes much significance as the time of important fluctuations in arousal) rather than being preoccupied with phases of sleep which fully meet the conventional criteria for NREM or REM sleep.

Of fundamental importance is Webb's (1985a) distinction between state-related and time-related periodicities. In a recent article (Webb, 1994) he has demonstrated the value of applying chronobiological research methods to demonstrate that sleep is a biological rhythm. Although there are clinical and logistical constraints to applying such methods in studying the occurrence of epileptic attacks, it seems appropriate to approximate to these experimental designs as closely as is feasible.

Other aspects of research methodology and procedure concern the extent of EEG recording required adequately to detect patterns of occurrence, the circumstances in which such recordings need to be taken, and the mathematical methods for analysing the findings.

Long-term EEG monitoring by means of telemetry or ambulatory recording may need to extend over at least several days in order reliably to detect patterns of occurrence. Significant day to day variations in generalised seizure discharge, including that accompanying clinical absences, has been demonstrated by such investigators as Milligan & Richens (1981). Although the concern of these authors was the implications for evaluation of anti-epileptic drug treatment effectiveness by means of EEG recordings, the implications are no less important in the present context.

From the mathematical point of view, Smith (1985) has suggested that, because of the multiplicity of factors that might influence seizure occurrence in addition to biorhythms, 20–30 days of recording might be required convincingly to detect periodicity. This is a daunting prospect as ideally an attempt should be made to standardise the activities, experiences and sleep habits (insofar as they affect the pattern of daytime arousal levels) of subjects from one day to another over the period of investigation. This is desirable in order to minimise the largely sporadic fluctuations in seizure occurrence caused by extraneous factors.

Smith's point relates to another main issue of the mathematical operations required reliably to identify rhythmic patterns of occurrence which may be concealed within the 'noise' of seizure occurrence caused by irregular influences such as emotional or attentional factors. A wide variety of techniques for time series analysis have been suggested for detecting biorhythms. As it remains unclear which are the most appropriate, there seems some merit in using several techniques in parallel to see if they yield consistent evidence of periodicity. This area of enquiry requires very close collaboration between clinical and non-clinical disciplines.

REFERENCES

Aronson JK 1990 Chronopharmacology: reflections on time and a new text. Lancet 335: 1515–1516

Binnie CD 1993 Significance and management of transitory cognitive impairment due to subclinical discharge in children. Brain and Development 15: 23–30

Binnie CD, Aarts JHP, Houtkooper MA et al 1984 Temporal characteristics of seizures and epileptiform discharges. Electroencephalography and Clinical Neurophysiology 58: 498–505

Broughton R 1975 Biorhythmic variations in consciousness and psychological functions. Canadian Psychological Review 16: 217–239

Broughton R, Stampi C, Romano S, Cirignotta F, Baruzzi A, Lugaresi E 1985 Do waking ultradian rhythms exist for petit mal absences? A case report. In: Martins da Silva A, Binnie CD, Meinardi H (eds) Biorhythms and epilepsy. Raven Press, New York, pp95–107

Daly DD 1973 Circadian cycles and seizures. In: Brazier MA (ed) Epilepsy its phenomena in man. Academic Press, New York, pp215–233

Duncan S, Read CL, Brodie MJ 1993 How common is catamenial epilepsy? Epilepsia 34: 827–831

Guey J, Bureau M, Dravet C, Roger J 1969 A study of the rhythm of petit mal absences in children in relation to prevailing situations. The use of EEG telemetry during psychological examination, school exercises and periods of inactivity. Epilepsia 10: 441–451

Halasz P 1982 Generalised epilepsy with spike wave pattern (GESW) and intermediate states of sleep. In: Sterman MB, Shouse MN, Passouant P (eds) Sleep and epilepsy. Academic Press, New York, pp219–237

Horita H, Uchida E, Maekawa K 1991 Circadian rhythm of regular spike wave discharges in childhood absence epilepsy. Brain and Development 13: 200–202

Janz D 1962 The grand mal epilepsies and the sleep–waking cycle. Epilepsia 3: 69–109

Kellaway P, Frost JD 1983 Biorhythmic modulation of epileptic events. In: Pedley TA, Meldrum BS (eds) Recent advances in epilepsy, 1. Churchill Livingstone, Edinburgh, pp139–154

Kleitman N 1969 Basic rest–activity cycle in relation to sleep and wakefulness. In: Kales A (ed) Sleep: physiology and pathology. Lippincott, Philadelphia, pp33–38

Lennox WG, Gibbs FA, Gibbs EL 1936 The effect on the electroencephalogram of drugs and conditions which influence seizures. Archives of Neurology and Psychiatry 35: 1236–1250

Martins da Silva A, Aarts JHP, Binnie CD et al 1984 The circadian distribution of interictal epileptiform EEG activity. Electroencephalography and Clinical Neurophysiology 58: 1–13

Martins da Silva A, Binnie CD, Meinardi H 1985 Biorhythms and Epilepsy. Raven Press, New York

Milligan N, Richens A 1981 Methods of assessment of antiepileptic drugs. British Journal of Clinical Pharmacology 11: 443–456

Mirsky AF, van Buren JM 1965 On the nature of the "absence" in centrencephalic epilepsy: a study of some behavioural, electroencephalographic and autonomic factors. Electroencephalography and Clinical Neurophysiology 18: 334–348

Niedermeyer E 1982 Petit mal, primary generalised epilepsy and sleep. In: Sterman MB, Shouse MN, Passouant P (eds) Sleep and epilepsy. Academic Press, New York, pp191–207

Ounsted C, Hutt SJ 1964 The effect of attentive factors on bio-electrical paroxysms in epileptic children. Proceedings of the Royal Society of Medicine 57: 1178

Roger J, Bureau M, Dravet Ch, Dreifuss FE, Peret A, Wolf P 1992 Epileptic syndromes in infancy, childhood and adolescence, 2nd edn. John Libbey, London

Sato S, Penry JK, Dreifuss FE 1976 Electroencephalographic monitoring of generalised spike–wave paroxysms in the hospital and at home. In: Kellaway P, Petersen I (eds) Quantitative analytic studies in epilepsy. Raven Press, New York, pp237–251

Shouse MN 1989 Epilepsy and seizures during sleep. In: Kryger MH, Roth T, Dement WE (eds) Principles and practice of sleep medicine. Saunders, Philadelphia, pp364–376

Smith JR 1985 Discussion following Martins da Silva A, Binnie CD Ultradian variation of epileptiform EEG activity. In: Martins da Silva A, Binnie CD (eds) Biorhythms and epilepsy. New York, Raven Press, p78

Stevens JR, Kodama H, Lonsbury B, Mills L 1971 Ultradian characteristics of spontaneous seizure discharges recorded by radio telemetry in man. Electroencephalography and Clinical Neurophysiology 31: 313–325

Stevens JR, Lonsbury BL, Goel SL 1972 Seizure occurrence and interspike interval telemetered electroencephalogram studies. Archives of Neurology 26: 409–419

Stores G, Lwin R 1981 A study of factors associated with the occurrence of generalised seizure discharge in children with epilepsy using the Oxford Medilog system for ambulatory monitoring. In: Dam M, Gram L, Penry JK (eds) Advances in epileptology: XIIth epilepsy international symposium. Raven Press, New York, pp421–422

Tempkin O 1971 The falling sickness, 2nd edn. John Hopkins Press, Baltimore

Verduyn CM, Stores G, Missen A 1988 A survey of mothers' impressions of seizure precipitants in children with epilepsy. Epilepsia 29: 251–255

Webb WB 1985a Circadian biological rhythm aspects of sleep and epilepsy. In: Martins da Silva A, Binnie CD, Meinardi H (eds) Biorhythms and epilepsy. Raven Press, New York, pp13–27

Webb WB 1985b Discussion following Martins da Silva A, Binnie CD Ultradian variation of epileptiform EEG activity. In: Martins da Silva A, Binnie CD, Meinardi H (eds) Biorhythms and epilepsy. Raven Press, New York, p78

Webb WB 1994 Sleep as a biological rhythm: a historical review. Sleep 17: 188–194

Wolf P 1985 Plenary discussion. In: Martins da Silva A, Binnie CD, Meinardi H (eds) Biorhythms and epilepsy. Raven Press, New York, p208

33. Typical absences in the first two years of life

Jean Aicardi

The onset of typical absence epilepsy is usually between 3–12 years of age, with a peak frequency at 6–7 years and a mean age of onset of seven years (Loiseau, 1992). Published series of typical absences include only rare or occasional cases with onset before two years. This chapter briefly reviews cases of early onset previously reported as typical absences or typical 'petit mal' and presents five additional cases observed by the author.

PREVIOUSLY REPORTED CASES

Large series of typical absence epilepsy mention occasional cases of early onset. Lugaresi & Volterra (1963) had only two patients of less than two years of age in a series of 85 cases (2.4%); Livingston et al (1965) had only three patients in a series of 117 (2.6%). Several of the early onset cases had unusual features. In two of the 194 patients described by Dieterich et al (1985), the absences had been preceded by generalised tonic-clonic seizures. One patient of Manoumani & Wallace (1994) and one of Tassinari et al (1992) had myoclonic absences, and one of the 119 patients reported by Olsson and Hedström (1991) had a progressive encephalopathy. More precise data are available for a few isolated cases of typical absences with onset under the age of two years (Beaumanoir, 1976; Cavazzuti et al, 1989; De Marco, 1980), but only one publication has dealt with a series of patients under three years (12 of whom were under two years) with typical absences (Cavazzuti & Cappella, 1970). These 12 patients, along with the single case later reported by the same group (Cavazzuti et al, 1989), are presented together, as individual details cannot be ascribed to individual patients.

The onset of absences occurred at six months in one infant, between 12–18 months in seven and between 19–24 months in five. In 11 children the onset was between 2–3 years.

The absences were described as clinically typical in 13 cases, with apparent loss of awareness, staring and sometimes twitching of eyelids and slight elevation of the eyeballs. Eleven patients had more marked myoclonic jerking; this was limited to the face and upper limbs in nine cases. The EEG showed paroxysmal discharges on a normal background tracing. In three patients the discharges were described as typical spike-waves at 3 Hz. Two of these patients were 35 months of age at recording. One patient, first recorded at nine months of age, had in addition to runs of typical spike-waves, theta rhythms sometimes preceding or following some of the spike-wave discharges. On video-EEG the theta rhythms were shown to be associated with loss of awareness preceding the spike-wave discharges by approximately 1 s or following it for 3–4 s. Twelve patients had brief runs of rhythmical slow waves at 2.5–3.0 Hz with only 'abortive' spikes. Two others had brief runs of atypical, irregular 2.5 Hz spike-waves. Four had atypical spike-wave complexes and polyspike-wave paroxysms and one had long rhythmical discharges at 2.5 Hz. Three infants had had febrile seizures preceding or accompanying these absences and three more had febrile convulsions. Only two patients had 'modest' mental retardation and the outcome was favourable also with respect to the seizures in several cases.

PERSONALLY OBSERVED PATIENTS

Five infants with apparently typical absences were seen at the Hôpital des Enfants Malades, Paris, between 1980 and 1991. Patient 1 was a 22-month-old girl at onset of typical absences with 3 Hz rhythmical EEG discharges. Her absences were easily controlled with sodium valproate and she had a normal development when last seen at five years of age.

Patient 2 had brief (2–3 s) absences with a marked myoclonic component. The jerks involved the face, head, upper and lower limbs and responded only partially to a combination of sodium valproate and ethosuximide. This girl was moderately mentally retarded. At 12 years her absences remained poorly controlled and she had repeatedly shown brief (1–3 s), rhythmical discharges at 3 Hz.

Patients 3 and 4 both had absences consistently associated with eyes and head deviation to the right side. Patient 3, a girl, who had onset of absences at 20 months, had marked myoclonic activity during absences. The jerks sometimes involved the lower limbs and could then result in falls. She was retarded mentally and her absences remained uncontrolled when last seen at the age of five years despite multiple therapeutic attempts. Her EEGs were quite typical, with discharges lasting 3–8 s but the amplitude of the spike-wave complexes was higher on the left side. Patient 4, a boy began to have absences without myoclonic components at 19 months of age. These were easily controlled by ethosuximide treatment and his development was only mildly delayed. EEG discharges were clearly asymmetrical in amplitude but synchronous; they lasted up to 20 s.

Patient 5, a boy, had his first attacks at the age of nine months. Clinically, they were typical absences, with loss of awareness lasting 5–6 s, without any associated motor component. He also had isolated atonic attacks with falls. His EEG repeatedly showed runs of slow waves at 2.5–3.0 Hz, with only occasional and often abortive spikes interspersed among the slow waves, between 9–23 months of age. Later on, the EEG discharges became typical spike-wave runs with fronto-central predominance, indistinguishable from typical absences but sometimes of very long duration, up to 90 s. From the age of four years he also had generalised tonic or tonic-clonic seizures. His development was slow and autistic features became increasingly striking as he grew older. At age 16 years he was markedly autistic and still had infrequent seizures.

DISCUSSION

Our personal cases and review of the literature indicate that typical absence seizures can have their onset in children under two years of age, although this is an infrequent occurrence. It appears that there are two different categories of patients in this age group. A first category includes a small number of patients whose absences have classical clinical and EEG features and respond readily to treatment. Such cases are unassociated with neurological or mental difficulties. They apparently run uncomplicated courses and probably have a favourable outcome. Our Case 1 and the case of Cavazzuti et al (1989) are typical examples.

The second category includes a larger number of patients with features that are not usually present in typical absence epilepsy of later childhood. One feature mentioned in several patients (our Cases 2 and 3 and several patients of Cavazzuti & Cappella, 1970) is the occurrence of prominent myoclonic jerking during attacks. Myoclonias can be limited to the face and head or they may involve also the upper and lower limbs; they are more prominent than the simple eyelid blinking frequently seen in classical absences. Such cases are reminiscent of the myoclonic absences described by Tassinari et al (1992). Whether they belong to the syndrome of myoclonic absences cannot be decided as not enough details are available in the reports that antedate the definition of myoclonic absences in the International Classification of Seizures (1981) and of Epileptic Syndromes (1989). Two recent cases (Tassinari et al, 1992; Manoumani & Wallace, 1994) have been reported in series of myoclonic absences.

Another frequent feature of early onset absences is their association with developmental delay or mental retardation. This was the case in our Patients 2, 3, 4 and 5, in two patients of Cavazzuti & Cappella (1970) and in the patients of Olsson & Hedström (1991). The neurodevelopmental difficulties are probably dependent on lesional brain damage that was demonstrated in our Patient 3 by the presence of diffuse brain atrophy on CT scanning.

It thus appears that a high proportion of the cases reported as typical absences with onset in the first two years of life have special characteristics and probably do not belong to the syndrome of childhood absences epilepsy (CAE) as defined in the International Classification (1989). In this syndrome, absences are not associated with neurological or mental abnormalities and genetic factors play a major aetiological role. Most cases of early onset absences exhibit some unusual features, such as prominent myoclonic activity, brief duration of attacks or evidence of lateralisation. The EEG discharges usually last less than 3–5 s. They are less regularly rhythmical and the spike component may be poorly developed, although spikes may appear secondarily, as illustrated in our Patient 5. Developmental abnormalities are common. One may hypothesise that such cases are mainly related to more or less diffuse organic brain damage and can be regarded as 'phenocopies' of the syndrome of CAE.

The remaining and probably rarer cases with typical features may represent the extreme end of the age distribution curve of CAE and share the same natural history and prognosis.

REFERENCES

Beaumanoir A 1976 Les épilepsies infantiles. Problèmes de diagnostic et de traitement. Editions Roche, Basle
Cavazzuti GB, Cappella L 1970 Quadri di piccolo male precoce. Rivista Neurologica (Napoli) 40: 242–249
Cavazzuti GB, Ferrari P, Galli V, Benatti A 1989 Epilepsy with typical absence seizures with onset during the first year of life. Epilepsia 30: 802–806
Commission on Classification and Terminology of the International League Against Epilepsy 1981 Proposal for revised clinical and electroencephalographic classification of epileptic seizures. Epilepsia 22: 489–501
Commission on Classification and Terminology of the International League Against Epilepsy 1989 Proposal for revised classification of epilepsies and epileptic syndromes. Epilepsia 30: 389–399
De Marco P 1980 Petit mal epilepsy during early infancy. Clinical Electroencephalography 11: 38–40
Dieterich E, Baier WK, Doose H, Tuxhorn I, Fichsel H 1985 Long term follow up of childhood epilepsy with absences. I Epilepsy with absences at onset. Neuropediatrics 16: 149–154
Dieterich E, Doose H, Baier WK, Fichsel H 1985 Long term follow up of childhood epilepsy with absences. II Absence epilepsy with initial grand mal. Neuropediatrics 16: 155–158
Livingston S, Torres I, Pauli LL, Rider RV 1965 Petit mal epilepsy. Results of a prolonged follow up study of 117 patients. Journal of the American Medical Association 194: 227–232
Loiseau P 1992 Childhood absence epilepsy. In: Roger J, Bureau M, Dravet C, Dreifuss FE, Perret A, Wolf P (eds) Epileptic syndromes in Infancy, childhood and adolescence, 2nd edn. John Libbey, London, pp135–150
Lugaresi E, Volterra V 1963 Considerazione cliniche ed EEG sull'assenza piccolo male. Clinica Pediatrica 45: 3–18
Manoumani V, Wallace SJ 1994 Epilepsy with myoclonic absences. Archives of Disease in Childhood 70: 288–290
Olsson I, Hedström A 1991 Epidemiology of absence epilepsy. II Typical absences in children with encephalopathies. Acta Paediatrica Scandinavica 80: 235–242
Tassinari CA, Bureau M, Thomas P 1992 Epilepsy with myoclonic absences. In: Roger J, Bureau M, Dravet C, Dreifuss FE, Perret A, Wolf P (eds) Epileptic syndromes in Infancy, childhood and adolescence, 2nd edn. John Libbey, London, pp151–160

DISCUSSION

Stephenson: I had three children between the ages of 1–2 years. With one of them we did not believe it until, in due course, when she was aged approximately two-and-a-half, prolonged cassette recording revealed typical absences, although with some polyspikes. She is seizure free and of normal intelligence.

The one who started at one year of age was precipitated by startle: if she got a fright she had an absence with slight myoclonus. I do not suppose myoclonic absence – typical absence with a little bit of myoclonus. That patient remitted spontaneously at 18 months of age.

The third is slightly intellectually delayed (IQ of about 90 but normal) who had remitted by about the age of five without treatment.

Marescaux: A comment on the idea that it is perhaps more frequent to see absences in very young children. We have only one case. The mother was a nurse and she told us her seven-month-old son was having absences once a week. We did an EEG and we saw nothing, but she insisted that every week she saw it at least once. We had to wait until he was three years old before we confirmed absence for the first time. If she had not been a nurse she would have been unable to see these small absences. This is perhaps a reason for which there is an over-representation of absences with myoclonic component at a very young age, because these are striking for the family.

Aicardi: I certainly think that some of the absences at this age are difficult to detect because of the subtlety of the symptoms.

Mirsky: Supposing we assume that the majority of cases develop at around the age of six and that earlier development is somewhat unusual. What might this mean in terms of the pathogenesis of the disorder? In terms of that cortico-reticular model? Does the cortex have to reach a certain level of myelinisation in order to support absence epilepsy?

Aicardi: I am unable to answer that sort of question. I certainly think that even a young cortex, at the age of six months, is capable apparently, occasionally, of producing 3 Hz relatively typical spike wave activity, even if it is not entirely typical. The fact is that in one of my patients the appearance of the discharges changed over time and they became more typical as the patient grew older, but this is an isolated experience.

Tassinari: Absences with myoclonic jerks are probably frequent at this age. It is quite interesting. Probably the myoclonic jerking is some other group. It is not a situation that can be missed, rhythmic jerking in children. Probably it is more frequent.

34. Typical absences in adults

C. P. Panayiotopoulos   S. Giannakodimos   E. Chroni

There is a widely held misconception that typical absences (TA) are rare in adults. This is despite well-documented reports that 7–81% of children with TA continue having absences in adult life, with other types of generalised seizures often occurring in the course of the disease (Lennox & Lennox, 1960; Lees & Liversedge, 1962; Currier et al, 1963; Livingston et al, 1965; Charlton & Yahr, 1967; Dalby, 1969; Gibbert, 1972; Lugaresi et al, 1973; Sato et al, 1983; Loiseau et al, 1983; Dieterich et al, 1985; Gastaut et al, 1986). From studies on the prognosis of TA the following general conclusions can be drawn:

1. The prognosis of TA in children with an early onset (mean 6 years) is better than those with onset later in childhood or adolescence, particularly if they are of normal intelligence. Approximately half will continue to experience TA in adult life.
2. Absences with ictal myoclonic or atonic components, photo-sensitivity and poor response to treatment are more likely to continue, combined with other generalised seizures. Motor or versive seizures caused by frontal epilepsies may develop in a few cases.
3. Generalised tonic-clonic seizures (GTCS) preceding or coinciding with the onset of TA indicate a worse prognosis.
4. GTCS are nearly inevitable in patients (90%) who continue having absences in adult life. GTCS are usually infrequent, onset is in mid-teens and they respond well to treatment.
5. Absences become less frequent and less severe with age.

All the above studies involve long-term follow-up of patients with onset of absences in childhood or adolescence. Most were based on clinico-EEG documented 'absences', mainly with severe impairment of consciousness, without reference to syndromic classification and without the help of video-EEG recordings. Myoclonic jerks occurring independently of absences, severity of impairment of consciousness during the absence ictus, syndromic criteria of epilepsies and video-EEG documentation have not been considered in the evaluation process of patients with absences.

Furthermore, these studies are mainly dealing with TA where impairment of consciousness is very severe, although others (Aarts et al, 1984; Giannakodimos et al, 1994) have shown that the EEG manifestations of 3–4 Hz spike and slow-wave discharges are frequently associated with mild cognitive impairment which may not be clinically discernible. The reported low prevalence of TA in adults (1–2%) may be influenced by the above selection criteria. Prevalence of absences among 15 102 adults and children with epilepsies was 2.34% (Charlton & Yahr, 1967; see also Ch. 17), while in a more recent study with video-EEG documentation the prevalence was 10% (Panayiotopoulos et al, 1992).

DIAGNOSING ABSENCES IN ADULTS: CLINICAL ASPECTS

Diagnosing absences in adults is an art. In our studies, absence seizures had frequently been unrecognised for years or misdiagnosed as complex partial seizures (Panayiotopoulos et al, 1992). Absences are perceived by patients as transient sensations of 'momentary lack of concentration', 'flashes of black-outs', 'going to a distance' or 'lack of awareness' – descriptions which may be misinterpreted as normal sensations, or drug-induced phenomena in patients who are often overmedicated or as complex partial seizures. De-realisation and fear may occasionally be experienced (Panayiotopoulos et al, 1992; Ferner & Panayiotopoulos, 1993).

Trained to identify absences in their classic form, the child with transient episodes of severe impairment/loss of consciousness, we are not familiar with absences in an adult whose level of awareness is not conspicuously impaired during the ictus. Similarly, episodes of impairment of consciousness preced-ing GTCS or independently occurring in an adult with GTCS are more likely to be interpreted as complex partial seizures than as absences. Even absence status may remain unrecognised or misdiagnosed in adults.

In our clinic, patients with GTCS and/or myoclonic jerks are specifically questioned for brief episodes of altered cognition. Patients with IGE often reveal such episodes, which may precede onset of GTCS by years. Also, it is not uncommon for patients to describe clusters of absences or prolonged episodes of altered consciousness or slowing in mental activity (absence sta-tus) preceding GTCS. However, these episodes should not automatically be interpreted as absences without EEG or video-EEG documentation.

'Phantom absences' is the term we have coined to denote TA which are so mild that they are inconspicuous to the patient and imperceptible to the observer (Ferner & Panayiotopoulos, 1993). They are disclosed by video-EEG recording and breath counting during hyperventilation. They mani-fest as brief (usually 3–4 s) 3–4 Hz spike/multiple spike and slow wave discharges. The absences are simple, occasionally with eyelid blinking. They are common in patients with idiopathic generalised epilepsies but are often unrecognised.

DIAGNOSING ABSENCES IN ADULTS: EEG ASPECTS

Absences may escape clinical detection even if conventional EEG shows 3 Hz spike/multiple spike and slow wave discharges. This is because current practice is to test the patient's ability to recall a phrase or number given by the technician during spike-wave discharges. For those patients with mild absences who pass this test successfully, the EEG discharges are interpreted as 'sub-clinical abnormalities indicating low threshold to seizures' or, in the presence of co-existing focal abnormalities, as secondary generalisation.

For practical purposes we propose that patients with spike-wave paroxysms should be asked to count their breaths during hyperventilation (Panayiotopoulos et al, 1993). This may reveal signs of impairment of consciousness and speech which otherwise would escape recognition. This method is sensitive, easy to perform and evaluate and clinically relevant, in that it may reflect impaired performance in daily life (Giannakodimos et al, 1994).

In our studies, all patients with generalised epilepsies and TA have their absences studied and classified with video-EEG as previously reported (Panayiotopoulos et al, 1989a; Panayiotopoulos et al, 1989b; Panayiotopoulos et al, 1992; Ferner & Panayiotopoulos, 1993; Panayiotopoulos et al, 1993; Giannakodimos et al, 1994). Partial sleep deprivation with video-EEG during sleep and at least half an hour of awakening is obtained if routine long video-EEG fails to record suspected absences. This is important in detecting absences in patients with infrequent generalised seizures on awakening after sleep deprivation and fatigue. Absences in patients with a history of specific precipitation (somatosensory, pattern, video-games, calculations) are tested with the appropriate mode of excitation.

THE SYNDROMIC CLASSIFICATION OF ABSENCE EPILEPSIES IN ADULTS

In a previous clinical, electroencephalographic (EEG) and video-EEG study of absences in adults (age range 21–67 years, mean 35.9 years), (Panayiotopoulos et al, 1992) we showed that:

1. There was a 10% prevalence of absences among adult patients with epilepsies. Females were 3.6 times more frequently affected than males.
2. Clinically, the absences showed considerable quantitative and qualitative variations. Automatisms, occurring only when impairment of consciouness was profound, were rare.
3. Onset of absences ranged from 7–46 years (mean ± SD = 18.3 ± 10.5); six patients reported onset of absences after the age of 20 years.
4. Generalised tonic-clonic seizures occurred in 20 patients; frequency varied from a few per lifetime to as many as one per month. Myoclonic jerking of the limbs occurred in 11 patients but was not associated with the absence ictus. In contrast, eyelid myoclonia (four patients) and perioral myoclonia (two patients) were consistent clinical manifestations of the absence ictus. Absence status occurred in five patients with EEG documentation in four.

5. Absence seizures were frequently unrecognised or misdiagnosed as complex partial seizures. The most commonly used drug was carbamazepine, with 10 patients on polypharmacy. Satisfactory control was achieved with sodium valproate.
6. The EEG, particularly video-EEG, was invaluable in the diagnosis, but focal abnormalities (seven patients) might have been misinterpreted as indicative of partial seizures.
7. A syndromic classification showed that absences were syndrome-related. Seven patients had juvenile myoclonic epilepsy, four juvenile absence epilepsy, three eyelid myoclonia with absences, one symptomatic absence epilepsy, and one photo-pattern reflex absence epilepsy. Two of the six unclassified patients had what we now classify as perioral myoclonia with absences (see Ch. 26) and two had features probably of atypical JME. Two of the remaining unclassified patients and an additional one with 'de novo absence status' can now be diagnosed as suffering from the syndrome of phantom absences with GTCS (see below).

RECENT STUDIES

We have identified 75 patients with TA from 391 adults with epileptic disorders who were older than 20 years of age; 119 suffered from idiopathic generalised epilepsies. All patients were referred and studied in our epilepsy clinic at St Thomas' Hospital between April 1989 and April 1994 (Panayiotopoulos et al, 1992). All patients had normal neurological and mental state except for two with cryptogenic absences who had learning difficulties.

RESULTS

Patients were syndromically classified as follows:

Juvenile myoclonic epilepsy (JME)

Twenty-three patients (30.7%) had JME; all had absences and myoclonic jerks on awakening. All but one had GTCS. The clinical and EEG manifestations of TA in JME have been extensively reported (Panayiotopoulos et al, 1989a; Panayiotopoulos et al, 1989b; Panayiotopoulos et al, 1994).

Briefly, the absences in JME are simple typical absences with brief impairment of consciousness and 3–4 Hz spike/multiple spike and slow wave discharges. The characteristic JME patient does not jerk, nor have automatisms or other motor manifestations such as eyelid or perioral myoclonia during the absence ictus. Furthermore, and unlike in childhood absence epilepsy (CAE) or JAE, impairment of consciousness is mild. The EEG discharge is characteristically different from that of childhood or juvenile absence epilepsy. In JME it is usually short and fragmented; the spike and slow wave complexes show intra-discharge frequency variations with multiple spike components (Ws). Longer discharges with fragmentations and Ws may occur without clinical manifestations but are much less common.

Typical absences pre-dated myoclonic jerks and GTCS in all patients; nine had onset of absences before the age of 10 years. The clinical severity of absences appeared to be age-related. Early onset absences (before the age of 10 years) are often superficially similar to those of childhood or juvenile absence epilepsy. They may be pyknoleptic in frequency with severe impairment of consciousness and occasionally with automatisms. Absences decrease in frequency and severity with age. Late onset absences are usually mild. It is exceptional for patients to show overt interruption of mental and physical activity and there are no automatisms. Patients usually complain of brief impairment of concentration only. Frequency is difficult to assess; they are usually reported by patients as being rare but occasionally there may be up to 10 per day.

Juvenile absence epilepsy (JAE)

Ten patients (13.3%) were diagnosed as suffering from JAE. Their mean age was 36 years (range 22–48). All had absences (mean±SD age at onset was 11.8±4.5 years) which interfered with daily life, with severe impairment of consciousness often associated with rhythmic or random eyelid blinking and occasionally with automatisms. Infrequent GTCS occurred in all but one patient (mean±SD age at onset was 17.1±7.8 years). Two patients had additional infrequent and mild myoclonic jerks randomly distributed during the day. Only one patient was sensitive to flickering lights, at the onset of the disease.

The main differentiation between JAE and JME is that in JAE the absences are severe and constitute the predominant seizure type; GTCS are usually infrequent and myoclonic jerks, when present, are mild or rare and random. In JME myoclonic jerks are the hallmark of the disease; absences, if present, are mild and often inconspicuous.

Eyelid myoclonia with absences (EMA)

Nine patients had eyelid myoclonia with absences. Absences were usually brief (3–4 s), impairment of consciousness was mild and often the myoclonic jerking of the eyelids was the dominant clinical manifestation. All patients were female, all were photo-sensitive and all had eye closure-related EEG abnormalities. None employed self-induction. Infrequent GTCS developed in all patients; these were usually evoked by lights or were associated with sleep deprivation, fatigue or alcohol or were catamenial. Three patients had infrequent and mild myoclonic jerks. Photo-sensitivity usually declined with age but eye closure EEG abnormalities persisted (Giannakodimos & Panayiotopoulos, 1994). One patient had benign childhood epilepsy with centro-temporal spikes before the development of EMA (Aliberti et al, 1992).

Perioral myoclonia with absences (PMA)

Seven patients had PMA and are described separately in this volume (see Ch. 26).

Photo/pattern induced absences

Four patients had TA with onset in childhood which were consistently induced by flickering lights and/or patterns; they could also occur spontaneously. They all had usually infrequent GTCS at some stage of their disease.

Absences with single myoclonic jerks during the absence ictus

There was one female patient, aged 25 years, with early childhood onset (three years of age) of frequent TA during which single myoclonic jerks were consistently observed and confirmed with video-EEG. GTCS started at the same age as absences. Absences and GTCS are resistant to treatment and continue in adulthood. Our experience is that children having TA and single myoclonic jerks are usually resistant to treatment and remission is probably not expected.

Symptomatic and cryptogenic absences

One patient had TA due to a frontal low-grade glioma (Panayiotopoulos et al, 1992). One patient with a mild degree of retardation had cryptogenic eyelid myoclonia with fixation-off sensitivity (Panayiotopoulos, 1987). The third patient with eyelid myoclonia, absences and GTCS but without photosensitivity, is described in Ch. 25.

Unclassified patients with TA

There were 18 patients who could not be classified in the above syndromes. However, 12 patients showed remarkably similar clinico-EEG features which occurred in a non-fortuitous manner, indicating that they probably belong to a previously unrecognised syndrome for which we propose the name of 'phantom absences with generalised tonic-clonic seizures'. This may be a dose gene dependent syndrome of IGE.

The syndrome of phantom absences and GTCS

The clinical and EEG manifestations of 12 patients (six male) can be summarised as follows. They all had:

1. Mild simple absences of which they were unaware (phantom absences) and their age of onset could not be determined. The absences were revealed on video-EEG recordings with breath counting and consisted

of brief (3–4 s) generalised discharges of 3–4 Hz spike or multiple spike and slow-wave discharges during which mild impairment of cognition manifests as consistent errors and discontinuation of breath counting. Some patients, after the video-EEG was reviewed with them, admitted brief episodes of lack of concentration and forgetfulness.

2. GTCS which were infrequent. Six patients had had one or two GTCS. The maximum frequency of GTCS did not exceed three per year. GTCS did not show any apparent circardian distribution except in two patients in whom they occurred on awakening. The age at onset of GTCS ranged from 15–56 years (median 27.5). This was by far the highest median age at onset of GTCS found among our patients with other syndromes with TA.

3. Absence status occurred in six patients, either in isolation or terminating in GTCS. In these patients GTCS were consistently preceded by absence status (Fig. 34.1). Following recognition of this sequence, GTCS were often preventable with rectal diazepam or oral sodium valproate (2 g), self-administered while in absence status.

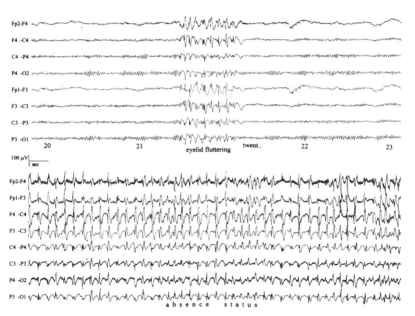

Fig. 34.1 Video-EEG (upper traces) and EEG (lower traces) of a 61-year-old female patient who had two episodes of de novo absence status at 56 years, both confirmed with EEG. She has three nephews, each from a different sister, with idiopathic generalised epilepsy (infrequent, spontaneous or provoked GTCS, mainly of late onset). The video-EEG showed brief generalised 3–4 Hz spike/multiple spike and slow-wave discharges associated with eyelid blinking and impairment of breath counting (upper traces).

4. None of the patients had myoclonic jerks and none were photo-sensitive.

Two patients had a family history of infrequent GTCS; the father of one of these patients (Fig. 34.2) had three late onset GTCS. An EEG had shown brief spike and slow-wave discharges.

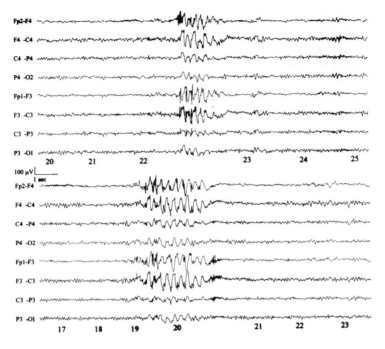

Fig. 34.2 Video-EEG of 20-year-old female patient who had a diurnal single GTCS at age 17 years. The video-EEG demonstrated 3–4 Hz brief generalised spike/multiple spike and slow wave discharges without clinically discernible manifestations. However, breath counting revealed ictal delays, indicating impairment of cognition (phantom absences). Her father, now aged 61, had three GTCS, one nocturnal and two on awakening, in his mid-50s.

CONCLUSION

Absences in adults constitute a diagnostic challenge to physicians and have important implications in the syndromic classification and management of patients.

REFERENCES

Aarts HR, Binnie CD, Smit AM, Wilkins AJ 1984 Selective cognitive impairment during focal and generalized epileptiform EEG activity. Brain 107: 293–308

Aliberti V, Grunewald R, Panayiotopoulos CP 1992 Exacerbation of typical absence seizures by progesterone. Seizure 1: 137–138

Charlton MH, Yahr MD 1967 Long term follow-up of patients with petit mal. Archives of Neurology 16: 595–598

Currier RD, Kooi KA, Saidman J 1963 Prognosis of pure petit mal: a follow-up study. Neurology 13: 959–967

Dalby MA 1969 Epilepsy and 3 per second spike and wave rhythms. A clinical, electroencephalographic and prognostic analysis of 346 patients. Acta Neurologica Scandinavia (Suppl.) 40: 45

Dieterich E, Baier WK, Doose H, Tuxhorn I, Fichsel H 1985 Long term follow-up of childhood epilepsy with absences. I. Epilepsy with absences at onset. Neuropediatrics 16: 149–154

Ferner R, Panayiotopoulos CP 1993 'Phantom' typical absences, absence status and experiential phenomena. Seizure 2: 253–256

Gastaut H, Zifkin BG, Mariani E, Puig JS 1986 The long-term course of primary generalized epilepsy with persisting absences. Neurology 36: 1021–1028

Giannakodimos S, Ferrie CD, Panayiotopoulos CP 1994 Qualitative and quantitative abnormalities of breath counting during brief generalised 3 Hz spike and slow wave 'subclinical' discharges. Electroencephalography and Clinical Neurophysiology (in press)

Giannakodimos S, Panayiotopoulos CP 1994 Eyelid myoclonia with absences: a clinical and video-EEG study in adults. Electroencephalography and Clinical Neurophysiology (in press)

Gibberd FB 1972 The prognosis of petit mal in adults. Epilepsia 3: 171–175

Lees F, Liversedge LA 1962 The prognosis of 'petit mal' and minor epilepsy. Lancet I: 797

Lennox WG, Lennox MA 1960 Epilepsy and related disorders. Little, Brown, Boston

Livingston S, Torres J, Pauli LL, Rider RV 1965 Petit mal epilepsy: Results of a prolonged follow-up study of 117 patients. Journal of the American Medical Association 194: 227–232

Loiseau P, Pestre M, Dartigues JF, Commenges D, Barberger-Gateau C, Cohadon S 1983 Long term prognosis in two forms of childhood epilepsy: typical absence seizures and epilepsy with rolandic (centrotemporal) EEG foci. Annals of Neurology 13: 642–648

Lugaresi E, Pazzaglia PP, Franck L et al 1973 Evolution and prognosis of primary generalised epilepsy of the petit mal absence type. In: Lugaresi E, Pazzaglia PP, Tassinari CA (eds) Evolution and prognosis of epilepsy. Auto Gaggi, Bologna, pp3–22

Panayiotopoulos CP 1987 Fixation-off-sensitive epilepsy in eyelid myoclonia with absence seizures. Annals of Neurology 22: 87–89

Panayiotopoulos CP, Obeid T, Waheed G 1989a Absences in juvenile myoclonic epilepsy: a clinical and video-electroencephalographic study. Annals of Neurology 25: 391–397

Panayiotopoulos CP, Obeid T, Waheed G 1989b Differentiation of typical absences in epileptic syndromes. A video EEG study of 224 seizures in 20 patients. Brain 112: 1039–1056

Panayiotopoulos CP, Chroni E, Dascalopoulos C, Baker A, Rowlinson S, Walsh P 1992 Typical absence seizures in adults: clinical, EEG, video-EEG findings and diagnostic/syndromic considerations. Journal of Neurology, Neurosurgery and Psychiatry 55: 1002–1008

Panayiotopoulos CP, Baker A, Grunewald R, Rowlinson S, Walsh P 1993 Breath counting during 3 Hz generalised spike and wave discharges. Journal of Electrophysiological Technology 19: 15–23

Panayiotopoulos CP, Obeid T, Tahan A 1994 Juvenile myoclonic epilepsy: a 5-year prospective study. Epilepsia 35(2): 285–296

Sato S, Dreifuss FE, Penry JK, Kirby DD, Palesh Y 1983 Long term follow-up of absence seizures. Neurology 33: 1590–1595

DISCUSSION

Janz: Is not childhood absence epilepsy seen in adults, or in juveniles?

Panayiotopoulous: I have tried very hard to find patients who we would classify as childhood absence epilepsy. I have not seen it. I think it is a matter of criteria. For example, if a patient had absences as a child but later develops myoclonic jerks on awakening and generalised tonic-clonic seizures, I would classify him as juvenile myoclonic epilepsy. A patient who at the age of nine has absences with severe impairment of consciousness and then develops random myoclonic jerks and continues having severe absences and infrequent generalised tonic-clonic seizures I would tend to classify as juvenile absence epilepsy.

In our data, many of the absences started before the age of ten, but we do not classify them as childhood absence epilepsy. We classify them as eyelid myoclonia with absences, juvenile myoclonic epilepsy. It is a matter of classification.

In other words, although half of these patients started having absences before ten years of age, this was not childhood absence epilepsy.

Brodie: I wonder what effect the wrong medication has on the presentation of these patients. It is very difficult to differentiate this; they have to be treated with something. If we take them off carbamazepine and put them on valproate they will improve, but it would be interesting to know what would happen if we took them off carbamazepine and left them off treatment. Is this a side-effect of the wrong treatment?

Panayiotopoulos: Certainly I do not think it is a side-effect of the treatment, although some of these patients were worse because they were on Tegretol. However, some of these patients, like those with 'phantom' absences, were first presented to us without any medication, although the majority of them improved with proper medication: sodium valproate, ethosuximide, alone or in combination. Small doses of lamotrigine added to valproate are also effective. Most of these patients are driving.

Fish: I was uncertain about the choice of the word phantom, although it is an interesting word. There were four patients out of 12 who did not have video-EEG confirmation. Does this mean you did video-EEG but did not record any attacks? How did you confirm that they had phantom absences?

Panayiotopoulos: These four patients were already on treatment when they had video-EEG. The diagnosis was based on clinical grounds and previous EEG, which showed up to 5 s 3 Hz spike and slow wave activity. For one of these patients, his secretary could tell when he was about to have a generalised tonic-clonic seizure. He slowed down in his behaviour and did not communicate very well. Occasionally he recognises himself that he is not exactly with it. His video-EEG showed brief 3 Hz spike and slow wave activity but he did not make any mistakes during this activity.

Fish: You recorded bursts of spike and wave?

Panayiotopoulos: All of them have 3 Hz spike and slow wave activity, but we could not prove that they also had cognitive disturbances.

Duncan: Would Genton make a comparison between what he presented (see Ch. 27), with the spike and wave without absences, with the phantom absences that Panayiotopoulos has described?

Genton: The main clinical phenomenon we see in these patients is absence status. They have very rare generalised tonic-clonic seizures, with onset usually in adolescence and early adulthood, but the characteristic trait is absence status. Children with absence epilepsy do not have absence status very often. Practically the only evident clinical manifestation is absence status.

What I showed was a 24-hour continuous Oxford Medilog EEG record that shows that they have continuous small spike and wave discharges that are completely sub-clinical in daily life; they do not feel anything and the people around them do not see anything. It is quite possible that a subtle neuropsychological examination would show something.

Panayiotopoulos: We showed this.

Genton: That was not so subtle but it did show something. We did not do it. They did not have typical absences in the sense that absences last at least 6, 8 or 10 s. They have very short discharges and widespread through the day.

Panayiotopoulos: But they are still called typical absences, even if they are for 4 s.

Genton: One or two seconds. I do not know whether that is typical absence. And the clinical picture is characterised, I repeat, by absence status for hours or days.

Panayiotopoulos: In our cases it was absence status in half of them. I like the term 'phantom' absences. We used to call them phantom absences; every time someone came in with absences that were not recognised we would say another 'phantom'. Then we tried very hard to find why we called them phantom. This is newly defined.

I agree with Genton. We try very hard to find these absences. It is not unusual for them to have absences only if the video-EEG is on upon awakening, after partial sleep deprivation. I do not think we need Dr Mirsky's psychological testing to prove this because then it would be very expensive and everyone would resist. We do routine EEG. The only addition is that we ask the patient to count his or her breaths.

Marescaux: When you presented perioral myoclonia this morning you said that all the patients displayed absence status. The patients this afternoon also have absence status with this milder absence and also tonic-clonic generalised seizures. If they have something huge and simple to recognise, which is absence status, then why classify the patient according to the subtle manifestations during absences and not according to the huge manifestation that is absence status?

Panayiotopoulos: Fifty percent of them will not have absence status. Where are these going to be classified?

35. Debate on classification of epileptic syndromes with typical absences

SECTION 1: INTRODUCTION

E H Reynolds

This debate goes back well into the last century. In the 1860s, two physicians at the National Hospital in London, Russell Reynolds and Henry Sievking, were both interested in the classification of epilepsy. Reynolds was a 'splitter.' He said there was only one true form of epilepsy: the idiopathic variety, which has to be separated off from the symptomatic variety. Sievking said this was an impossibility and that essential could not be separated from non-essential epilepsy, or idiopathic from symptomatic epilepsy. That debate is continuing now, at a more complicated and sophisticated level.

Today we shall hear from Dr Frederick Andermann and Dr Panayiotopoulos. Dr Andermann is Chairman of the International League's Commission on Classification and is a representative of the 'lumper' school. Dr Panayiotopoulos is also a member of the ILAE Commission on Classification, and favours a more splitting approach.

Next, Dr Hirsch and Prof. Marescaux give their views on the classification of syndromes with typical absences, and the difficulties encountered. Finally, there is a discussion of the topic by the other participants in the Symposium.

SECTION 2: TYPICAL ABSENCES ARE ALL PART OF THE SAME DISEASE

F Andermann

Until the advent of electroencephalography there was still considerable discussion as to whether absences were indeed epileptic in nature (Friedmann, 1906). The development of the EEG clarified this and demonstrated that absences are part of many idiopathic generalised epileptic syndromes and that they may be correlated with either classical, 3 Hz spike and wave discharge, or with what Lennox called atypical, slow spike and wave, or as he termed it, petit mal variant (Lennox, 1945; Lennox & Davis, 1950; Lennox & Lennox, 1960).

Are all absences part of the same disease? Clearly, closely related mechanisms are involved and similar seizure patterns are found in different generalised epilepsy syndromes but the clinical manifestations associated with the spike and wave discharge may be quite varied. The absences themselves range from the very brief to the prolonged. Discharges which last 2 or 3 s may not lead to clinical changes which can be perceived by the observer but they may be noticed by the patient and described as 'jolts in the mind', or brief interruptions in thought. As the discharges become longer they may be obvious to the witness as a simple absence or there may be additional manifestations such as automatisms, myoclonus, or loss of tone.

The presence of automatisms is closely correlated with the duration of the absence. This is best seen in children who, when hyperventilating on command, very often rub their nose, move their face, or fiddle with their hands. The parents will then comment that this is the longest absence they have ever witnessed. Should one then classify these two forms of absence as separate entities since in the same individual automatisms may be more or less apparent?

The same variability exists in the association with myoclonus. Some mild myoclonic components, usually involving the bulbar musculature and at times the hands, are often present in children with absence though they are of course much more striking in myoclonic absences (MA). For reasons of convenience and in order to clarify prognosis it has been accepted for some years that MA should be considered as a separate subgroup, but the possibility of splitting off several further categories according to the severity of the myoclonus persists. This could lead to confusion not only in the understanding of the non-epileptologist but even in the mind of absence devotees.

The degree of impairment of awareness in absence is also quite variable. We have all seen children who are completely out of touch and unable to react during a clinical absence and the accompanying spike and wave. On the other hand, many children can be aroused and their absence terminated when they are stimulated during such an attack. The same variability exists in memory mechanisms during the episode. Many children remember words which they hear during the attack. It is quite possible that they remember mostly what they hear in the latter part of the attack when the spike components have dropped out. However this has not been conclusively shown. Others have no recollection of what they hear during the entire episode. Some are aware of having had an absence because of the break in the conversation or in their experience of the environment. Others appear to be unaware of having had an absence. Apart from the obvious role of the duration of discharge the neurophysiological correlates of these different variables are not very clearly established. Thus in childhood absence the impairment of awareness, to a variable degree, is the dominant feature.

So far two major determinants of the classification of absence have been the prognostic value of the clinical pattern and the coexistence, and at times the predominance, of additional seizure types. In children with the myoclonic astatic epilepsy of Doose the myoclonic and falling attacks predominate. In juvenile absence epilepsy (JAE) myoclonus and generalised tonic-clonic seizures are fairly common. Occasionally absences may also be seen in patients with juvenile myoclonic epilepsy (JME). In all these epileptic syndromes the absence has a variable clinical significance and probably reflects more the duration of the spike and wave discharges than anything else.

The slow spike and wave described by Lennox and colleagues (Lennox, 1945; Lennox & Davis, 1950; Lennox & Lennox, 1960) may also be associated with absence at different ages in many of the secondary generalised epilepsies. The current term of 'atypical absence' indicates mainly that there is no clear onset and offset of the clinical manifestations. It is difficult to determine the beginning and end of a behavioural change in patients whose spike and wave discharges are extremely abundant and at times ongoing. It would be difficult to speak of atypical absences without taking into account the whole clinical picture of the different forms of secondary generalised epilepsy. The significance of these attacks must be taken into account in the light of the coexistence of several different epileptic seizure patterns. It is thus justified to consider the atypical absences separately from those found in the idiopathic generalised epilepsies and this is reflected in the conclusions of successive Classification Commissions of the International League Against Epilepsy over the years.

Similarly, it has been apparent for a long time that ongoing spike and wave discharge, even in patients with normal intelligence and normal EEG background, is not associated primarily with absence. When the discharge is of the order of 10–15 min automatisms are quite prominent and may lead even experienced epileptologists to a wrong diagnosis of partial seizures. The spectrum of petit mal status is characterised by extreme variability in the level of arousal and of attention. This ranges from merely self perceived lack of ability to think clearly to deep stupor. It thus appears that we are dealing with a wide spectrum of manifestations associated with spike and wave discharge and that the clinical accompaniment depends among other factors on the length of the epileptic discharge.

Absences may be triggered by hyperventilation and by intermittent photic stimulation. In some patients both mechanisms are operative. The pathophysiological basis however is probably quite different: metabolic in one and related to generalisation of focal cortical activation in the other. Though there may be some clinical differences in the two types of absence the striking feature has been the considerable similarity of these events occurring in one and the same individual. Quesney and Andermann (Quesney & Andermann, 1987) have shown that apomorphine, a dopaminergic agonist, will block photosensitivity. It does not however block non-photosensitive generalised spike and wave. Mervaala and the same group (Mervaala et al, 1990) demonstrated, in a group of patients with different forms of progressive myoclonus epilepsy who were all photosensitive, that apomorphine also blocked the epileptic discharge. Thus, photosensitive spike and wave, irrespective of the cause, shares a dopaminergic mechanism. There is even the possibility of a therapeutic approach related to these findings. Despite physiological and genetic differences between photosensitive and nonphotosensitive epilepsy there is a considerable resemblance in some of the clinical manifestations.

Absences, which are clinically practically indistinguishable from those seen in childhood absence epilepsy (CAE), may be encountered in diffuse neuronal diseases as presented by Ferrie in this volume (Ch. 29). Batten's disease (Andermann, 1967), Lafora body disease (Broughton et al, 1973), and subacute sclerosing panencephalitis (Roger et al, 1983) have been described to present in this way and only later has the diagnosis of diffuse brain disease become apparent. Even patients with partial epilepsy may present with absence attacks. This is not unusual in patients with temporal lobe epilepsy and can also be seen in patients with partial attacks of frontal origin. Just as in the case of absences as a manifestation of diffuse cerebral disease, it is the clinical context, the frequency of attacks in relation to the patient's age, and not least the electroclinical correlation, which provide clarification.

The maturational aspects of CAE are well known though not very well explained. The clinical patterns of persistence of absence into adult life with multiple or only occasional isolated absences in some individuals are as yet unexplained.

In recent years there has been some reduction in interest in the study of absence. This may well be due to the much more effective treatment which has permitted complete control with valproic acid monotherapy in a majority of patients with childhood absence or with absence, myoclonus and generalised seizures. What distinguishes these easily controlled patients from the ones in whom valproate alone is ineffective? To speak of more severe epilepsy or greater acquired brain dysfunction leads to a circular argument. It is thus clear that absences are manifestations of a wide range of generalised epilepsies and even of some partial epilepsies. They may be activated by a variety of stimuli and may be associated with a wide range of primary and secondary generalised epileptic syndromes. Their response to medication is equally variable as is their prognosis over time. The neuropsychological correlates have recently been neglected and we hope that further investigation will throw some light on the significance of brief but frequent spike and wave discharges occurring without grossly obvious clinical absence. The severity of the cognitive manifestations in patients with obvious absence attacks is equally variable.

Should we then discard all attempts at classification and return to the concept of the late Roland MacKay that 'All epilepsy is one'? This would certainly be a retrograde step and would negate all the advances that the Syndromic Classification has brought about leading to improved diagnosis and prognosis in many patients. On the other hand, one must avoid over-classification and the temptation to create additional syndromes distinguished by minor variables. This would represent a veritable invitation to confusion and to non-acceptance majority of such an excessively complex classification.

Perhaps the ideal approach lies in looking at each patient both from a syndromic point of view and by trying to understand his or her epilepsy in the light of a biological continuum in which both genetic and acquired components interact and contribute to the clinical and electrographic pattern. Such a dual approach, similar to that which has been suggested by Berkovic and his colleagues (1987) for absence attacks, is equally applicable to other forms of epilepsy and epileptic syndromes. We can postulate a spectrum of clinical manifestations associated with generalised spike and wave discharge patterns in idiopathic generalised epilepsy (IGE) with variable genetic and acquired components. Such a spectrum also appears to be present between primary and secondary generalised corticoreticular epileptic disorders and between focal discharge and secondary bilateral synchrony with a hemispheric predominance.

This view of absence does not of course suggest that further electroclinical study of IGE is now unnecessary. The application of modern video telemetry to the study of absence begun by the NIH Cooperative Absence Study (Penry, 1973; Penry et al, 1975), and now continued by Dr Panayiotopoulos and his colleagues, has done much to clarify our understanding of the epileptic absence. We hope that in the near future progress in our understanding of the pathophysiology and genetic basis of absence and other manifestations of IGE will permit an even more rational classification.

SECTION 3: TYPICAL ABSENCES ARE SYNDROME-RELATED

C P Panayiotopoulos

Fundamental rules of medicine which apply in all other physical diseases are often ignored in epilepsies. Vague and broad terms, such as 'patient with seizures', are bandied about, irrespective of aetiology, type of seizures, prognosis or appropriateness of treatment. The result is avoidable morbidity and mortality.

The description of epileptic seizures is usually limited to the events surrounding generalised tonic-clonic seizures (GTCS), while less dramatic 'minor' seizures, although more important than GTCS for diagnosis and management, are not considered.

Attempts to encourage differential diagnosis are met with comments to the effect that they are all the same, or they may be genetically linked, or the treatment is the same. Treatment of different epileptic syndromes is not the same. Simplistic rules and advice on what drug, when to start and when to stop treatment of epilepsy are often detrimental to the care of patients. Even for a phenotypically uniform and short-lived disease such as benign familial neonatal convulsions, genetic heterogeneity has been documented. The prognosis of different syndromes is often entirely different even if symptoms are similar (benign childhood partial epilepsies and symptomatic epilepsies of children).

One difficulty is that symptoms and signs cannot be accurately qualified and quantified. Epileptic seizures are short, transient, largely unpredictable and difficult to demonstrate publicly. This problem, however, has been overcome with video-EEG and use of the video camcorder, particularly suited to the study of absence seizures because of their frequency and precipitation by hyperventilation.

In epilepsies, the recognition of non-fortuitous clustering of symptoms and signs requires the study of clinical and laboratory data (Commission, 1989). Important clinical features include type of seizures, their localisation, frequency, sequence of events, circadian distribution, precipitating factors, response to treatment, age at onset, inheritance, physical or mental symptoms and signs. A routine EEG may not be sufficient to enable diagnosis. In some patients, high-resolution functional and structural brain imaging, biochemical and haematological tests or tissue biopsy may be needed.

A change in emphasis from 'epilepsy' to 'epilepsies' may stress that this is not simply one disease and that accurate prognostication, genetic analysis and improvement of management largely depend on a precise epileptic syndrome diagnosis.

Typical absences and related epileptic syndromes

Typical absences have attracted little attention because they are brief, often mild and usually self-limiting. They are erroneously considered as childhood-related diseases. However, even if not troublesome to the patient, absences are important clinical symptoms to consider in the differential diagnosis, genetics and treatment strategies of epilepsies.

The opinions expressed in this paper are based on an extensive review of the literature, the shared experience of distinguished colleagues and personal experience of more than 200 children and adults extensively studied, clinically and with video-EEG, over the last 10 years (Panayiotopoulos et al, 1989a; 1989b; 1992; 1993; 1994; Panayiotopoulos, 1994a; 1994c). Some of these arguments have strong statistical backing (e.g., the differences between absences in JME and JAE); others are impressions only and may need further documentation or revision.

By definition, impairment of consciousness is the cardinal clinical symptom and 3 Hz spike-wave EEG discharges the required bio-electrical feature of typical absences, but other clinical and EEG manifestations combine in a non-fortuitous manner to characterise diverse epileptic syndromes with specific prognosis and management (Commission, 1981; 1989; Panayiotopoulos et al, 1989b; 1992). The hypothesis that all absence syndromes constitute a 'neurobiological continuum' (i.e., all absences are the same disease) (Berkovic et al, 1987) may be theoretically attractive and convenient but it discourages the diagnostic precision required for correct management, prognosis and genetic analysis (Panayiotopoulos & Hirsch, 1994).

Many of the absence syndromes are entirely different in presentation, severity and prognosis. CAE will generally remit, whereas children with myoclonic absence epilepsy (MAE) suffer or may develop mental and behavioural problems. Patients with JME will, in their mid-teens, develop lifelong myoclonic jerks and GTCS. Other patients may have subtle clinical manifestations during 3 Hz spike-wave discharges of which they remain unaware (phantom absences, Ferner & Panayiotopoulos, 1993). Many of these patients seek medical consultation only after a GTCS, long after the onset of absences (Panayiotopoulos et al, 1992).

Video-EEG studies in which the level of impairment of consciousness is assessed are essential to evaluate absences fully and to classify them syndromically (Panayiotopoulos et al, 1993). The syndromic classification of absences requires details of clinical and EEG ictal features (Table 35.1) in addition to other data listed above.

Table 35.1 Clinical and ictal manifestations of absences and related data

I. Clinical ictal manifestations of absences and related data

Impairment of consciousness: severe, moderate, mild, sub-clinical (phantom)

Myoclonus: localised or generalised, rhythmic, arrhythmic or singular, brief at onset or sustained

Spontaneous behaviour: eye opening, cessation of activities, automatisms, vocalisation

Autonomic manifestations

Sequence, consistency and persistence of ictal manifestations

Frequency and duration of absences

Absence status

Precipitating factors

II. EEG ictal and inter-ictal manifestations

Frequency

Rhythmicity

Fragmentations

Relations of spikes/multiple spikes to slow waves

Multiple spikes (numbers, transient at onset or persisting throughout)

Intra-discharge variations

Topography

EEG background

Other EEG abnormalities (video-EEG during sleep and on awakening)

Precipitating factors

The manifestations/symptoms of typical absence seizures can be divided according to their significance in the syndromic diagnosis. More specific symptoms characterise certain syndromes, such as eyelid myoclonia (fast clonic eyelid movements with probably a tonic element of contraction as opposed to eyelid blinking-like movements occurring randomly or rhythmically in CAE) in eyelid myoclonia with absences (EMA), perioral myoclonia (not to be confused with perioral automatisms) in perioral myoclonia with absences (PMA), rhythmic limb and head myoclonic jerks in myoclonic absence epilepsy. Such features may develop in other epileptic conditions but their presence indicates the most likely epileptic syndrome diagnosis.

Less specific symptoms are commonly seen in more than one epileptic syndrome and are often age-related – for instance, severe impairment of consciousness occurring in CAE, JAE and childhood onset absences in other syndromes. Mild or moderate impairment of consciousness is mainly associated with syndromes which persist in adult life (EMA, PMA, the syndrome of phantom absences and GTCS, absences in adolescents and adults with JME).

The severity of impairment of consciousness often decreases with age. Severe impairment of consciousness may occur in children with absences in a variety of syndromes, although it is usually most severe in CAE. Absences with mild impairment of consciousness in children often herald syndromes persisting in adult life. Eyelid blinking or fluttering, rhythmical or arrhythmical, may be seen in CAE, JAE, reflex absences and treated EMA.

Clinical manifestations seen in the opening phase (first second) of the absence ictus (deviation of the eyes, eyelid flickering) are often not specific. Non-specific manifestations, secondary to other symptoms such as automatisms and vocalisation, cessation of voluntary or involuntary activities (over-breathing) and opening of the eyes, are primarily associated with severe impairment of consciousness and some are more likely to occur in longer absences. These symptoms do not occur if impairment of consciousness is mild even if absences are very long.

The clinical approach to identifying epileptic syndromes

Ideally, all patients with absences should be prospectively studied (with all clinical, EEG, video-EEG and other data listed above) from the onset to the end of the disease. This is impossible in clinical practice. We have therefore applied a pragmatic approach with the aim of identifying features characteristic of particular epileptic syndromes, mainly those persisting into adult life.

Patients, mainly children, developing epilepsy are prospectively studied from the onset of their disease while patients with the established condition are retrospectively investigated from the time of presentation to the onset of the disease (old medical records and EEGs, witnessed accounts).

This method has allowed us to define more closely certain characteristics of the existing syndromes and to identify two previously unrecognised syndromes: PMA and 'phantom' absences with GTCS (see Ch. 00). It should be re-emphasised that neither perioral myoclonia nor 'phantom' absences are sufficient to define these syndromes in isolation (i.e., without other combined clinico-EEG data).

Problems in the present definitions of the Commission of the ILAE (1989) for the classification of epileptic syndromes and diseases

Definitions of syndromes and diseases are currently too broad and are often based on one or two criteria which are not necessarily the most characteristic. For example, an arbitrary age of onset, before or after 10 years, has been drawn between CAE and JAE. All cases with onset of absences below the age of 10 years are considered as CAE, although other syndromes with distinct features, such as MAE and EMA, also begin in the same age group. We have previously proposed that exclusion criteria in the syndrome-definitions be as important as inclusion criteria. Application of exclusion criteria would allow a stringent definition of CAE, excluding cases with mild impairment of consciousness, eyelid, perioral and rhythmic limb and head myoclonus, photo-sensitivity, GTCS before or during the active phase of absences, brief (3 s) and fragmented generalised discharges.

CAE is defined by ILAE as an idiopathic generalised epileptic syndrome 'with onset of simple and complex absences at 4–8 years of age. Absences may be accompanied by upward deviation of the eyes and retropulsion of the head and trunk. GTCS develop in 30–40 per cent of the cases. The EEG discharge is 2.5–3.5 Hz. They are more frequent and longer lasting than the absences in JAE'. (Commission, 1989; see also Ch. 19).

This broad definition is inadequate to encapsulate an epileptic syndrome. Any child with frequent absences and 2.5–3.5 Hz spike and slow-wave discharges will be diagnosed as CAE irrespective of severity of impairment of consciousness, ictal single or repetitive myoclonic jerks, variations of the ictal EEG discharge, presence of other seizure types, prognosis and response to treatment. The definition of CAE should be revised in order to exclude other epileptic syndromes which may start with absences in childhood (Panayiotopoulos et al, 1989b; 1992).

Paradoxically, children with eyelid myoclonia and absences best fulfil the ILAE definition of CAE although they do not suffer from CAE. EMA, as in the above definition of CAE, is manifested by hundreds of typical absences per day, with onset in childhood (pyknolepsy), with clonic retropulsion of the eyelids and eyes and 3–4 Hz spike and slow-wave discharges. However, the resemblance between CAE and EMA is superficial. In EMA the absences are very short, impairment of consciousness is mild, eyelid myoclonia consistent, photo-sensitivity prominent and GTCS probably inevitable in all patients. The EEG ictal manifestations consist mainly of polyspike/slow-wave (faster than in CAE), which is more likely to be induced by eye closure. Furthermore, EMA is resistant to monotherapy and does not remit in late childhood or adolescence (Appleton et al, 1993; Giannakodimos & Panayiotopoulos, 1994; see also Chs 25 and 34).

Patients with JME may have onset of absences in childhood. These may be frequent, simple absences with usually minor but occasionally severe impairment of consciousness (Panayiotopoulos et al, 1989a). A child with frequent absences does not necessarily have CAE; nor does CAE evolve to JME.

Different syndromes may look superficially the same

It is well recognised that syndromes may look superficially the same. In IGE the triad of absences, myoclonic jerks and GTCS may occur in JME, JAE and EMA. Superficially they could be considered as the same diseases. However, closer analysis indicates that they are distinct syndromes.

The hallmark of JME is myoclonic jerking on awakening; GTCS is the next most common type of seizures (often heralded by clusters of myoclonic jerks); absences are simple and mild without myoclonic components. In contrast, the predominant features of JAE are absences with severe impairment of consciousness, relatively long duration and frequent automatisms; GTCS are infrequent (absences, not jerks, may herald them); myoclonic jerks, if present, are mild and random.

The hallmark of EMA is eyelid myoclonia. This is associated with brief absences of mild or moderate impairment of consciousness and may persist to occur without absences. The opposite is not true: absences do not occur without eyelid myoclonia. All patients are photo-sensitive. Eye closure-related EEG abnormalities which are eliminated by darkness are pronounced. GTCS and myoclonic jerks of the limbs are infrequent and may be provoked by flickering lights (Appleton et al, 1993; Giannakodimos & Panayiotopoulos, 1994).

Some syndromes may be genetically related, as is the case for Becker and Duchenne muscular dystrophy. Also, some 'specific' features of one syndrome may occur in another. However, it cannot be that there is only one brain disease responsible for this heterogeneity and complexity of clinical and EEG features of absences. This view is strongly supported by the great heterogeneity of genotypes in animal models (see Ch. 4). Even if absence syndromes were genotypically the same, differences in their prognosis and management would mandate their differential diagnosis.

Acknowledgements

The author wishes to thank the British Telecom Charitable Organisation and the Special Trustees of St Thomas' Hospital for grants towards studies on the classification of epilepsies.

SECTION 4: HOW SHOULD EPILEPTIC SYNDROMES WITH TYPICAL ABSENCES BE CLASSIFIED?

E Hirsch   C Marescaux

Epilepsies with typical absences do not constitute a homogeneous entity. In rodents, bilateral and synchronous EEG spike-and-wave discharges can be inherited either in a recessive or dominant way. Several mutations affecting distinct chromosomes are linked with the occurrence of spontaneous absence seizures. This genetic heterogeneity appears to be correlated mainly with the associated neurological symptoms such as ataxic gait, dystonic postures, etc. (Noebels, 1994; Vergnes & Marescaux, 1994). In humans the heterogeneity of absence epilepsies is well accepted and individualisation of multiple syndromes has been proposed: CAE, JAE, MAE, EMA and PMA. These classifications are based on ictal EEG and behavioural symptoms and evolution. However, similarities and discrepancies between these different syndromes raise several questions.

Should absence epilepsies be classified according to the age of onset?

The age of onset does not appear to be an absolute criterion because it allows much overlap between the different syndromes (Hirsch et al, 1994). This is consistent with data from the literature. In some cases absences starting after the age of 10–12 years are classified as CAE, whereas some others starting between 8 and 10 years are considered as JAE. In fact this classification does not take evolution or triggering factors into account and the clinical definition of CAE does not exclude patients who have absences with onset in childhood but who belong to other syndromes. Consequently, CAE is erroneously seen as a heterogeneous disease. In some cases absences are the only type of seizures; in others (which should be grouped together with JAE) GTCS occur. In some cases absences are provoked by hyperventilation; in others (which should be grouped together with EMA, see below) they are triggered by intermittent light stimulation (Aicardi, 1986; Covanis et al, 1992; Loiseau, 1992; Wolf, 1992; Berkovic, 1993a, b; Panayiotopoulos, 1994a). According to the literature, three conditions are generally associated with the occurrence of GTCS in patients suffering from typical absences: late onset after the age of 8 years; pronounced photo-sensitivity; and an inadequate response to treatment (Covanis et al, 1992; Loiseau, 1992; Hirsch et al, 1994). Thus the main characteristic of the so-called childhood absences is not the age of onset but the fact that other seizures and photo-sensitivity are not found.

Should absence epilepsies be classified according to ictal symptoms?

Discrete semiological differences appear to dissociate JAE from CAE: the intensity of loss of responsiveness, the duration and number of seizures and the EEG pattern of the discharges (Panayiotopoulos, 1994a). In a more demonstrative way three symptoms have been individualised and named according to motor symptoms observed during absence seizures.

Epilepsy with MA has been taken into account by the International Classification (Aicardi, 1986; Tassinari et al, 1992; Roger et al, 1993). The main characteristic of this type of absence seizure is the existence of marked rhythmic myoclonias of the limbs. These myoclonias may not be sufficient, however, to individualise a new form of absences and epilepsy with MA does not appear as a homogeneous entity. In some patients the seizures are easily suppressed by a combination of valproate and ethosuximide (Tassinari et al, 1992; Roger et al, 1993; Hirsch et al, 1994) and the pronounced myoclonia could correspond to a simple exaggeration of the moderate clonic component usually described during typical absence seizures (Aicardi, 1986; Loiseau, 1992; Berkovic, 1993a, b). On the contrary, some patients show mental retardation, are resistant to treatment and sometimes progress towards a Lennox–Gastaut syndrome. Bad prognosis appears to be correlated with personal antecedents, occurrence of GTCS, falls during the seizures and inappropriate treatment more than with the severity of the myoclonias (Aicardi, 1986; Tassinari et al, 1992; Roger et al, 1993).

Absences with pronounced perioral myoclonias have been individualised by Panayiotopoulos (1994a). They may not only represent a particular form of absences but also define a specific syndrome with more severe evolution. However, myoclonias of moderate intensity, involving the lips and the chin, are classically accepted as symptoms of seizures during typical childhood or JAE (Loiseau, 1992; Berkovic, 1993a, b; Serratosa & Delgado-Escueta, 1993; Hirsch et al, 1994). In a recent study (Hirsch et al, 1994) six patients having absence seizures associated with clear perioral myoclonias could not be distinguished from patients displaying other clinical symptoms during typical absence seizures.

Eyelid myoclonias with absences have been individualised for many years (Binnie & Jeavons, 1992; Panayiotopoulos, 1994a). For some authors, the marked rhythmic eyelid myoclonias consisting of fast jerks of the eyelids are clearly different from the eyelid blinking-like random movements of CAE (Panayiotopoulos, 1994a). For others, eyelid myoclonias are not specific by themselves. They may occur during CAE (Loiseau, 1992; Berkovic, 1993a, b; Serratosa & Delgado-Escueta, 1993) and are also observed during some seizures of JME (Binnie & Jeavons, 1992). Moreover eyelid myoclonias are in fact difficult to differentiate from self-triggering voluntary blinking (Berkovic, 1993a, b; Hirsch et al, 1994). Thus whether the main characteristics of this syndrome are eyelid myoclonia (Panayiotopoulos, 1994a) or the mode of transmission, evolution and photo-sensitivity with self-stimulation (Hirsch et al, 1994) remains debatable.

What are the prognostic factors of absence epilepsies?

In several studies neither the age of onset nor the ictal symptoms were corre-lated with prognosis (Covanis et al, 1992; Hirsch et al, 1994). The only char-acteristics which may have some influence on the evolution of the condition are: the type of seizures associated with absences; the nature of triggering factors; and the choice of treatment. All typical absences are sensitive to pharmacological treatment but the probability of relapses upon treatment withdrawal is higher when absence seizures are associated with GTCS, in particular in photo-sensitive patients (Covanis et al, 1992; Hirsch et al, 1994). Valproate alone or combined with ethosuximide (and/or lamotrigine) is the standard treatment. Its early and systematic use has very likely increased the number of remissions and considerably reduced the probability of secondary GTCS (Covanis et al, 1992; Loiseau, 1992; Berkovic, 1993a, b). On the con-trary, many anti-epileptic compounds (carbamazepine, phenytoin, phenobar-bital, vigabatrin) aggravate absence seizures and facilitate their persistence until adulthood (Vergnes & Marescaux, 1994; Hirsch et al, 1994).

Conclusion

There are two current approaches to the clinical conceptualisation of gener-alised absence epilepsies. The syndromic approach attempts to sub-divide the patient population into relatively homogeneous groups, largely on the basis of clinical and EEG criteria. According to this approach absence seizures occur in discrete syndromes (Panayiotopoulos, 1994a). The neuro-biological approach is based on evidence of the multifactorial origin of IGE, with a mixture of genetic and acquired factors. Moreover, patients with IGE have a spectrum of clinical and EEG features with no clear boundaries between idiopathic and secondary (symptomatic) types. In this context, gen-eralised epilepsies with absences are all part of a biological continuum (Berkovic et al, 1987).

Numerous genetic, pharmacological and semiological data suggest that the syndromic approach is logical and useful, providing that the limits of the classification are appreciated. For example, the relevant criteria for a better classification of epileptic syndromes with typical absences are still open to discussion. A precise syndromic approach to absence epilepsies, tak-ing into account age of onset, triggering factors and the main ictal signs, is certainly justified to select patients and families which can be included in molecular genetic studies. However, up to now in daily clinical practice the relevance of syndromic sub-categories to choosing a treatment or establish-ing a firm prognosis is not clearly established.

REFERENCES

Aicardi J 1986 Epilepsies with typical absence seizures. In: Aicardi J (ed) Epilepsy in children. Raven Press, New York, pp79–99

Andermann F 1967 Absence attacks and diffuse neuronal disease. Neurology 17: 205–212

Appleton RE, Panayiotopoulos CP, Acomb BA, Beirne M 1993 Eyelid myoclonia with typical absences: an epilepsy syndrome. Journal of Neurology, Neurosurgery and Psychiatry 56: 1312–1316

Berkovic SF 1993a Childhood absence epilepsy and juvenile absence epilepsy. In: Wyllie E (ed) The treatment of epilepsy: principles and practice. Lea and Febiger, Philadelphia, pp547–551

Berkovic SF 1993b Generalized absence seizures. In: Wyllie E (ed) The treatment of epilepsy: principles and practice. Lea and Febiger, Philadelphia, pp401–410

Berkovic SF, Andermann F, Andermann E, Gloor P 1987 Concepts of absence epilepsies: discrete syndromes or biological continuum? Neurology 37: 993–1000

Binnie C, Jeavons P1992 Photosensitive epilepsies. In: Roger J, Bureau M, Dravet C, Dreifuss FE, Perret A, Wolf P (eds) Epileptic syndromes in infancy, childhood and adolescence, 2nd edn. John Libbey, London, pp299–305

Broughton R, Nelson R, Gloor P, Andermann F 1973 Petit mal epilepsy evolving to subacute sclerosing panencephalitis. In: Lugaresi E, Pazzaglia P, Tassinari CA (eds) Evolution and prognosis of epilepsies. Aulo Gaggi, Bologna, pp 63–72

Commission on Classification and Terminology of the International League Against Epilepsy 1981 Proposed revisions of clinical and electroencephalographic classification of epileptic seizures. Epilepsia 22: 480–501

Commission on Classification and Terminology of the International League Against Epilepsy 1989 Proposal for classification of epilepsies and epileptic syndromes. Epilepsia 30: 389–399

Covanis A, Skiadas K, Loli N, Lada C, Theodorou V 1992 Absence epilepsy: early prognostic signs. Seizure 1: 281–289

Ferner R, Panayiotopoulos CP 1993 Phantom typical absences, absence status and experiential phenomena. Seizure 2: 253–256

Friedmann M 1906 Uber die nichtepileptischen Absencen oder kurzen narkoleptischen Anfalle. Dtsch. Z. Nervenheilk. 30: 462–492

Giannakodimos S, Panayiotopoulos CP 1994 Eyelid myoclonia with absences: a clinical and video-EEG study in adults. British EEG Society, London, 3rd June. Electroencephalography and Clinical Neurophysiology (abstract in press)

Hirsch E, Blanc-Platier A, Marescaux C 1994 What are the relevant criteria for a better classification of epileptic syndromes with typical absences? In: Malafosse A, Genton P, Hirsch E, Marescaux C, Broglin D, Bernasconi R (eds) Idiopathic generalized epilepsies: clinical, experimental and genetic aspects. John Libbey, London (in press)

Lennox WG 1945 The petit mal epilepsies. Journal of the American Medical Association 129: 1069–1073

Lennox WG, Davis JP 1950 Clinical correlates of the fast and slow spike-wave electroencephalogram. Pediatrics 5: 626–644

Lennox WG, Lennox MA 1960 Epilepsy and related disorders. Vol. 1. Little, Brown Co., Boston

Loiseau P 1992 Childhood absence epilepsy. In: Roger J, Bureau M, Dravet C, Dreifuss FE, Perret A, Wolf P (eds) Epileptic syndromes in infancy, childhood and adolescence, 2nd edn. John Libbey, London, pp 135–150

Mervaala E, Andermann F, Quesney LF, Krelina M 1990 Common dopaminergic mechanism for epileptic photosensitivity in progressive myoclonic epilepsies. Neurology 40(1): 53–56

Noebels JL 1994 Genetic and phenotypic heterogeneity of inherited spike-wave epilepsies. In: Malafosse A, Genton P, Hirsch E, Marescaux C, Broglin D, Bernasconi R (eds) Idiopathic generalized epilepsies: clinical, experimental and genetic aspects. John Libbey, London (in press)

Panayiotopoulos CP 1994a The clinical spectrum of typical absence seizures or absence epilepsies. In: Malafosse A, Genton P, Hirsch E, Marescaux C, Broglin D, Bernasconi R (eds) Idiopathic generalized epilepsies: clinical, experimental and genetic aspects. John Libbey, London (in press)

Panayiotopoulos CP 1994b Fixation-off sensitive epilepsies. In: Wolf P (ed) Epileptic seizures and syndromes. John Libbey, London (in press)

Panayiotopoulos CP 1994c Juvenile absence epilepsy. In: Wallace S (ed) Childhood Epilepsy. Chapman & Hall, London, pp 55–65

Panayiotopoulos CP, Chroni E, Daskalopoulos C, Baker A, Rowlinson S, Welsh P 1992 Typical absence seizures in adults: clinical, EEG, video-EEG findings and diagnostic/syndromic considerations. Journal of Neurology, Neurosurgery and Psychiatry 55: 1002–1008

Panayiotopoulos CP, Baker A, Grunewald R, Rowlinson S, Welsh P 1993 Breath counting during 3 Hz generalised spike and wave discharges. The Journal of Electrophysiological Technology 19: 15–23

Panayiotopoulos CP, Obeid T, Waheed G 1989b Differentiation of typical absences in epileptic syndromes. A video EEG study of 224 seizures in 20 patients. Brain 112: 1039–1056

Panayiotopoulos CP, Ferrie CD, Giannakodimos S, Robinson RO 1994 Perioral myoclonia with absences: a new syndrome? In: Wolf P (ed) Epileptic seizures and syndromes. John Libbey, London, pp 143–153

Panayiotopoulos CP, Obeid T, Waheed G 1989a Absences in juvenile myoclonic epilepsy: a clinical and video-electroencephalographic study. Annals of Neurology 25: 391–397

Penry JK 1973 Behavioural correlates of generalized spike-wave discharge in the electroencephalogram. In: Epilepsy, its phenomena in man. UCLA Forum in Medical Sciences, No. 17. Academic Press, New York, pp171–178

Penry JK, Porter RJ, Dreifus FE 1975 Simultaneous recording of absence seizures with video tape and electroencephalography: a study of 374 seizures in 48 patients. Brain 98: 427–440

Quesney LF, Andermann F 1987 A dopaminergic mechanism in photosensitive epilepsy and its possible relevance to migraine. In: Andermann F (ed) Migraine and epilepsy. Butterworth Publishers, Boston, pp380–391

Roger J, Pellissier JF, Bureau M, Dravet C, Revol M, Tinuper R 1983 Le diagnostic precoce de la maladie de Lafora: importance des manifestations paroxystiques visuelles et interet de la biopsie cutanee. Revue Neurologique 139: 115–124

Roger J, Genton P, Bureau M, Dravet C 1993 Less common epileptic syndromes. In: Wyllie E (ed) The treatment of epilepsy: principles and practice. Lea and Febiger, Philadelphia, pp624–635

Serratosa JM, Delgado-Escueta AV 1993 Generalized myoclonic seizures. In: Wyllie E (ed) The treatment of epilepsy: principles and practice. Lea and Febiger, Philadelphia, pp411–424

Tassinari CA, Bureau M, Thomas P 1992 Epilepsy with myoclonic absences. In: Roger J, Bureau M, Dravet C, Dreifus FE, Perret A, Wolf P (eds) Epileptic syndromes in infancy, childhood and adolescence. John Libbey, London, pp151–160

Vergnes M, Marescaux C 1994 Pathophysiological mechanisms underlying genetic absence epilepsy in rats. In: Malafosse A, Genton P, Hirsch E, Marescaux C, Broglin D, Bernasconi R (eds) Idiopathic generalized epilepsies: clinical, experimental and genetic aspects. John Libbey, London (in press)

Wolf P 1992 Juvenile absence epilepsy. In: Roger J, Bureau M, Dravet C, Dreifuss FE, Perret A, Wolf P (eds) Epileptic syndromes in infancy, childhood and adolescence. John Libbey, London, pp307–312

DISCUSSION

Marescaux: I am sure that in absence epilepsy we have a lot of different diseases which many of us would lump together as absence epilepsy. It is very clear that the mice and rat traits that are definable depend on different genetic bases. I am sure, however, that if I had the EEGs of the different strains of mice and rats I would be unable to differentiate them.

Let us consider a disease such as Parkinson's. If we were trying to classify on symptomatology, we would have patients with unilateral tremor, unilateral rigidity, bilateral akinesia, tremor of the tongue, and so on, although they all have the same disease. Also, sometimes we may have two patients with akinesia, one of whom has striato-nigral degeneration and the other Parkinson's disease.

Additional criteria, for example, in extrapyramidal disorders include sensitivity to DOPA, and age of onset. No single criterion is specific. If we only use certain criteria, such as the symptoms and the age of onset, we will be confused. I do not know any pathology in which relevant criteria are symptomatic.

Imagine multiple sclerosis classified by symptomatology. It is not possible. If we want a classification we need an evident biological marker. If we go in for symptomatic classification we will have a multitude of very rare cases. But is it relevant? Why is tremor in Parkinson's disease sometimes of the tongue, sometimes of the arm and sometimes of the leg? It is the same disease and it is not Parkinson's of the face, Parkinson's of the arm, Parkinson's of the leg.

However, we have to learn what the absences are like and study them using video-EEG. I would say that absence diseases are supposed to be genetic, and I stress that we cannot consider the symptomatology in an isolated manner. In each individual patient we have to have a detailed family history and genetic background. We will not be able to get an EEG for everybody but we have to consider this genetic background every time we try to describe a new syndrome. At the same time it is worthwhile trying to be better clinicians and trying to be precise about the symptomatology of every absence we see and record on video-EEG.

Prendergast: It depends on what is available. Dr Panayiotopoulos was describing definitions of syndromes which involve not just clinical manifestations but also EEG features and prognosis and family details that Marescaux just mentioned. Most of psychiatry is classified on exactly that basis and so I do not think it is sufficient to discard it on those grounds.

Berkovic: I should like to make two comments regarding the philosophy of the classification. Panayiotopoulos' point was that the division of the different types of neuromuscular diseases was important, and one cannot but agree with him. One has to remember, however, that earlier in the history of neurological diseases there are terms and diagnoses that have since been confined to the neurological wastebasket. For example, before the proper recognition of subacute sclerosing panencephalitis and its aetiology, there were a variety of syndromes which are not now considered to be of any clinical or pathophysiological utility.

In more recent times I and others have been involved, for example, in classifying the progressive myoclonus epilepsies and most of us now believe that certain terms should now be discarded, particularly with the mitochondrial diseases. There were all kinds of clinical variants that are no longer meaningful because we have made one step towards understanding the basic biology, for example, with the MERRF syndrome.

I would echo what was said before about our current purposes of looking at particular symptoms. I see three purposes: one is to aid clinical recognition and teaching, two is for prognosis, and three is for understanding the neurobiology. As far as recognition goes, it is very important that we realise that perioral myoclonus can be a manifestation of 3 Hz spike and wave, so that we can tell that this may well be an absence epilepsy. Whether this represents a different syndrome is an entirely different question, but it is important that we know that perioral myoclonus can be a symptom.

Secondly, the issue about prognosis. To my mind, apart from the age-related syndromes that are accepted, the issue about further splitting regarding prognosis has only been shown in Tassinari's syndrome of myoclonic absence, in which it seems that these are actually worse prognostically, and that is important to know when we see these patients. I remain unconvinced that any of the newer syndromes that we have heard about so far tell us anything more about prognosis.

Finally, I remain unconvinced that super-splitting will lead us to any better understanding of molecular genetics. That applies to the newer syndromes that we have heard about but I also believe it applies to the better established syndromes, such as CAE, JAE, JME. I agree that these appellations are important for clinical recognition, but it is not clear that this will help us to sort out the genetics. That will only come in retrospect. I think we have got to be very careful and get our aims right as to the purposes of these particular terms, the recognition, the prognosis and the final neurobiology, and to each three levels there may be a different rigour that is necessary for classification.

Tassinari: The relevance of a scheme of classification depends on the parameters used. Probably some are not relevant, but before we can be sure we have to apply them and examine the results. One must not pretend that any one set of parameters is the best. It is reasonable to make sub-classifications and stimulate the data. If we lump too much together we are left with a feeling that there is nothing to stimulate. On the other hand, if we split it up too much we shall be left with a lot of people who feel frustrated because they are not able to use these parameters. It is a combination of good common sense.

Duncan: I should like to ask the same question of the two main protagonists and to clarify their answers. Both speakers accept, I take it, the main categories of IGE, CAE, JAE, JME and so on?

Panayiotopoulos: I have accepted them.

Andermann: Certainly CAE and JME. JAE is reasonably useful. Epilepsy on awakening may not be that specific. That is something that needs to be clarified. With patients who have generalised epilepsy but no inter-ictal discharges and who have seizures at any time it is hard to know. We see them present time and again and it is hard to know how they should be classified.

We should further consider photo-sensitivity and eyelid myoclonia. I am not at all convinced by the perioral myoclonia syndrome.

Robinson: Most of us who are clinicians operate on two planes. We tend to classify patients accordingly. On the one hand we want to make sure that we distinguish children who have automatisms because of absences from children with complex partial seizures because we know if we give the one carbamazepine and not the other, there will be a big difference between them. From that point of view we can have a very simple and very empirical classification.

On the other hand, we want to understand the biology of the conditions that we are seeing. One may take various yardsticks for that as to what one considers fundamental. The implication here has been that if we can understand the genetics, we achieve something fairly fundamental.

To go back to Panayiotopoulos' analogy of muscle disease, it is clear that there is not one kind of Duchenne's dystrophy: each person with Duchenne's muscular dystrophy possibly has his own unique profile of DNA deletion. It may very well be that there are different phenotypes within that genotype and that may explain, for example, why some boys with Duchenne's have mental handicap and others do not.

And so in one way, although we are constitutionally lumpers in trying to help our patients in a very empirical way, in another way we are also relentlessly splitters in trying to understand what we are dealing with.

Janz: For the purpose of classification (i.e. for genetic research) one has to distinguish between childhood and juvenile absences. If we take frequency as the criterion, assuming 'daily' and 'not daily' as parameters, then we are faced with (however rare) cases of non-pyknoleptic absences beginning in childhood and correspondingly with pyknoleptic absences of juvenile onset. Or should just age be the limit: let us say, before and after ten years? Besides the biological basis for the fact of decreasing frequency with increasing age, the classification aspect has to be discussed.

But could we not now speak of childhood epilepsy with absences of varying kinds: CAE with eyelid myoclonia absences; CAE with perioral MA? Also, why should we not speak of sub-types of syndromes as suggested by Dr Genton? Not every variety should be a special syndrome. What has been described are sub-varieties, sub-types of the syndrome of CAE. This would be more practical.

Tassinari: I was very struck by some of the analogies used with regard to Parkinsonism and multiple sclerosis. Parkinsonism is not a simple disease and neither are any of the entities that we have talked about today. We have seen that they are not single gene disorders and probably a number of genes are involved. They are very much like multiple sclerosis and Parkinsonism in that respect and the complexity will continue to be quite great.

Noebels: We do not understand enough yet about the genetics of the human syndrome to say whether they are single or multiple. But I am sure that if we do not continue to grapple with the complexity and the uncertainty and go forward in the direction of splitting we shall never find the genes, whether for the diseases that exist today or for new ones that may emerge. I say this because there are probably so many that can involve destabilising the brain to cause epilepsy. I agree with the idea of simplifying things for practitioners but we must not rob ourselves of their observations, and if they are not aware how complicated experts think this group of diseases is they will not document what they are seeing and tell us more.

I would not like to see the field move in the direction of making things too simple. It is complicated. We are not talking about single types of muscle fibres. There are many different cell types in the brain. The brain expresses more genes than any other tissue in the body and we have to recognise that. The more complex it gets, the more we shall learn.

Andermann: This has been an interesting discussion. Probably the most valuable comments have been those on the molecular biology by Marescaux and Noebels and it is quite clear that this is where the clarification will come from.

Some of us have learned the hard way, like Delgado-Escueta, that when we look at the families of these patients the proband has one form of epilepsy, the cousin has another and another relative has yet another. Then there are all those who have EEG abnormalities who do not have any obvious clinical symptoms. Noebel's points are well taken, but it is not a question of simplifying things unduly; it is a question of having a classification which is clear and workable.

We should not split unreasonably. The points that Panayiotopoulos made are well taken. We have to take some of these various issues on board, whether we call them sub-groups or what we call them is an open question.

It has become clear to everybody what IGE means from a clinical point of view and how it should be approached. The main purpose of the International League and of this group is to be clear above all else, and if it is clear it will be acceptable.

What impressed me most of all this afternoon is that what is new now compared to several years ago is the enormous emphasis on clinical analysis of a type which was not possible prior to the advent of video-EEG monitoring.

Panayiotopoulos: First let me explain that I am not a phenomenologist. I simply try to apply the same medical rules in epilepsies as are applied for all other disorders. A patient with reading jaw myoclonus and two GTCS is given the same label as another patient who has intractable seizures due to severe brain damage. In my presentation I used the example of muscle diseases because a differential diagnosis is rightly required irrespective of therapeutic benefits. Why not also for epilepsies where this may also have considerable implications for treatment and prognosis?

Let us take the example of JME, which was not recognised in the early 1970s. Now, 20 years later, everyone appreciates the significance of JME. It should not take another 20 years to recognise that eyelid myoclonia is not CAE or that perioral myoclonia is not a prominent sign and may constitute a different syndrome if combined with other clinical and EEG manifestations. 'Phantom' absences are by definition mild but they should be recognised and not discarded or misdiagnosed as partial seizures. The correct diagnosis is often established by the recognition of mild symptoms. Epilepsies are no exception.

Marescaux mentioned the EEG and rightly said that he cannot identify on EEG grounds whether it is from that or another strain of rat or mouse. No one supports the idea of making a diagnosis based on single EEG or clinical factors. Let me emphasise again that it is the combined clinical and genetic, EEG, brain imaging, haematological and biochemical data which are needed for a precise diagnosis.

I agree with Noebels' comments regarding the need for a precise diagnosis (splitting may be misleading) for genetic purposes. We shall never find the genetic markers if symptomatic and idiopathic absences are grouped together, if eyelid myoclonia is considered the same as CAE, or if adult patients with absences are diagnosed as having complex partial seizures. However, even if these disorders with typical absences prove to be genetically the same, their differentiation is important for prognosis and management. In conclusion, typical absences do not constitute one symptom: they have many clinical and EEG manifestations which are syndrome related.

Reynolds: The debate has moved on from the last century. Progress is slow, but with Fred Andermann and Tom Panayiotopoulos on the ILAE Commission on Classification I expect it will be much quicker over the next four years.

36. Genetics of human typical absence syndromes

Mark Gardiner

'Because of the difficulties pertaining to such fundamental issues as precise definitions and classifications, and because of the frequent misuse of genetic methods, it is futile to attempt an assessment from the earlier literature of the role of heredity in the epilepsies. Detailed reviews of the earlier literature without critical appraisal only serve to perpetuate the confusion' (Metrakos & Metrakos, 1974).

'It is still impossible to formulate a generally valid concept of the genetics of absence epilepsies' (Doose & Baier, 1989).

Both statements remain as true today as when they were written. Most genetic studies of individuals with 'typical absence' syndromes or their apparent electrophysiological correlates have used definitions of the 'trait' under study which do not correspond to current ideas of how the epilepsies in which such seizures occur are best categorised into distinct phenotypes. It should, however, be remembered that until a molecular understanding of the inherited epilepsies emerges all phenotypic classifications are essentially arbitrary and may not reflect distinct genotypes despite the passionate conviction with which opposing camps argue their respective causes.

Recent advances in molecular genetics have emphasised how uncertain the correlation between phenotype and genotype is. For example, different mutations in the same gene (allelic heterogeneity), the receptor tyrosine kinase gene RET, have been shown to account for three phenotypically distinct familial cancer syndromes (familial medullary thyroid carcinoma and multiple endocrine neoplasia types 2A and 2B) and the developmental anomaly Hirschsprung's disease (van Heyningen, 1994). In contrast, families with tuberous sclerosis (TS) show locus heterogeneity with disease-determining genes on chromosomes 9 and 16 leading to apparently indistinguishable phenotypes (Kandt et al, 1992).

Absence epilepsy syndromes recognised at a clinical and electrophysiological level are therefore of enormous value in clinical practice and a vital starting point in genetic research. However, the extent to which they represent phenotypes determined by specific genotypes can only be surmised until their molecular genetic basis has been elucidated. Fortunately, the methods which allow testable hypotheses to be formulated about the molecular genetic basis of human typical absence syndromes are now to hand.

In this chapter, classical and more recent genetic studies will be considered and finally the strategies available for investigation of the molecular genetic basis of human typical absence syndromes will be outlined.

GENETIC STUDIES IN MAN

These may be divided into 'classical' and more 'recent' studies. A number of studies are likely to have included observation on patients who would now be categorised into one of the typical absence epilepsy syndromes. Lennox & Lennox (1960) undertook a large twin study, including a total of 225 twin pairs. A sub-group of these were categorised as 'without brain injury' and further sub-divided by seizure type. In the petit mal sub-group there were 20 monozygotic (MZ) pairs, of which 15 (75%) were concordant, and 14 dizygotic (DZ) pairs of which none were concordant. Similar values for concordance rates in MZ and DZ twins were observed in a further sub-group in which both tonic-clonic and typical absence seizures occurred.

Metrakos & Metrakos (1961) studied so-called 'centrencephalic' epilepsy, a term introduced by Wilder Penfield 'to identify that system within diencephalon, mesencephalon and probably rhombencephalon which has bilateral functional connections with the cerebral hemispheres'. The hallmark of this was a characteristic EEG: paroxysmal, bilaterally synchronous 3 Hz spike and wave. These patients had petit mal and/or grand mal seizures, but these terms were merely used to grade the seizures into minor and major without any other connotations. Some 211 probands with 'centrencephalic' epilepsy were studied and compared with 112 control probands. Detailed family histories and EEG studies were carried out in relatives, including parents and siblings. Only 15 of the 195 parents of the centrencephalic group had a centrencephalic type of EEG; two of 84 parents of controls had such an EEG. The interpretation of these observations is, of course, rendered difficult by the well-known age-dependent penetrance of this EEG trait which was demonstrated by sequential observations.

EEG data for 223 siblings of centrencephalic and 103 siblings of control probands were presented. A 'typical' centrencephalic EEG was observed in only 2.24% of the former, compared to none in the latter. In contrast there was a large excess of patients' siblings with an 'atypical centrencephalic' EEG (34.53% compared to 8.74%) or with an 'abnormality' of some sort (53.36% compared to 28.16%). Taking the 'typical' and 'atypical' EEGs together, it was argued that the 37% overall risk suggested a dominant gene with reduced penetrance, the low incidence observed in the parents reflecting the age-specific penetrance of the EEG trait. In retrospect, however, the criteria for a 'centrencephalic' EEG appear to have been too liberal, as an incidence of 10% in control subjects is much higher than the 2% observed in subsequent studies.

Matthes & Weber (1968) reported the EEGs of siblings of patients with petit mal absences. Of these, 9% had 3 Hz spike-waves and 3% had spike-waves of other types.

Doose et al (1973) reported an EEG study of siblings of patients with 'absence epilepsies'. Some 242 siblings of 109 index cases were examined by EEG. Unfortunately, although all index cases had 'exhibited absences with generalised 3 Hz spike-waves', they constituted a very heterogeneous group. In 46 patients grand mal attacks, some with fever, were the initial seizure type. In 61 patients petit mal was the initial seizure type, and of these 23 had 'myoclonic-astatic fits of the Lennox type'. Spike-waves were found in 8% of the siblings of index cases compared to 2% of controls. It is notable that of 105 relatives (first and second degree) who reported seizures, only 10 had absences.

'Recent' studies

Doose & Baier (1987) extended and updated their earlier studies in a report which included 400 patients with idiopathic generalised minor seizures – including absences, myoclonic and myoclonic-astatic seizures – and 4514 relatives. A distinction was drawn between seizures that manifested before (A seizures) and after (B seizures) the fifth birthday. Their Group II included 103 patients with absence seizures starting between 5 and 7 years (33 boys, 70 girls). In this group, the incidence of seizures in siblings was 10%, with siblings of girls more often affected than those of boys: 15% of 78 sisters of female probands manifested seizures, whereas there were no clinical manifestations among 25 sisters of boys. A comparable frequency was found in the parent generation. The EEG was 'abnormal' in 24 (38%) of 63 siblings investigated. Photo-sensitivity was the most frequent finding, occurring in 16 (25%), and spike-waves were observed in 11 (18%). Six of the 24 children with abnormal EEGs manifested seizures.

Degen et al (1990) recorded waking and sleep EEGs in 80 siblings of 38 patients with absence seizures. Twenty-two patients had idiopathic and 16 symptomatic absences. Fifty siblings of the idiopathic absence patients were studied. A waking EEG was recorded immediately before each sleep EEG; sleep was induced with 1 mg/kg body weight promazine-hydrocholoride given as syrup. Epileptic activity was observed in 36 (72%) of these siblings, but most of this was observed during sleep (62%); activity in the awake EEG alone was only observed in five (10%). Three siblings (3.8%) had actual absence seizures and one of these also had a febrile convulsion. In all three, generalised bilateral synchronous 3–4 Hz spike-wave discharges were noted in waking and sleep. A sibling incidence of over 50% suggests that epileptic activity on the EEG, including sleep-activated recordings, is not a valid marker for the genetic trait under study.

Beck-Mannagetta & Janz (1991) have reported results of the Berlin Pedigree Study, based on the out-patient department of the Free University of Berlin. The first degree relatives of 452 probands have been analysed in the first study to use modern syndrome categorisation for proband diagnosis. Among 671 first degree relatives of 151 probands with CAE or JAE, 33 (4.9%) were epileptic, the percentage being similar in parents, siblings and offspring. Similar numbers were observed for JME: of 600 first degree relatives of 118 probands, 35 (5.8%) were affected. A variety of epileptic syndromes was observed in these affected first degree relatives. In each group approximately one third had absence epilepsy. Of affected relatives of JME probands a further 11 (31.4%) had JME and 10 (28.6%) had epilepsy with GTCS. Of affected relatives of absence epilepsy probands, six (18.2%) had JME and 15(45.5%) had epilepsy with GTCS.

For obvious reasons, it is rather difficult to draw firm conclusions from these seven studies. They do not provide firm evidence for single-gene Mendelian inheritance of the typical absence syndromes, but do not in my view exclude segregation of a major gene of low penetrance if EEG changes are regarded as a sub-clinical marker of the epilepsy phenotype. Difficulties created by the age-specific penetrance of these syndromes render the recognition of a dominant pattern of inheritance difficult. The proportion of siblings either affected or displaying EEG changes on average tends to be above the expected population percentage but substantially below the 25% expected for an autosomal recessive disorder, ie in the range 5–10%. This is compatible with a so-called multifactorial model of inheritance.

GENETIC LINKAGE STUDIES

Juvenile myoclonic epilepsy is the sole human typical absence syndrome in which linkage studies have been undertaken and published. Greenberg et al (1988) analysed 33 families of probands with JME using classical properdin factor 8 and HLA. Analysis was carried out using various models of inheritance, penetrance and phenotype definition. A maximum lod score of 3.78 ($\theta m = f$, 0.01) was observed assuming autosomal dominant inheritance, 90% penetrance and including as affected any relatives who though asymptomatic had an abnormal EEG.

Further evidence for linkage of a locus predisposing to JME (designated EJM1) to the HLA region was obtained in a separate group of 23 families ascertained through JME probands in Berlin using serological markers (Weissbecker et al, 1991). On this occasion, the highest lod score was obtained when the 'trait' was defined to include JME or other idiopathic generalised epilepsies, but not spike-wave EEG abnormalities in asymptomatic family members. Assuming 90% penetrance and autosomal dominant inheritance, a lod score of 3.11 at $\theta m = 0.001$, $\theta f = 0.20$ was obtained. Further analysis of a sub-set of 20 of these families using HLA-DQ restriction fragment length polymorphisms gave similar results (Durner et al, 1991).

Liu et al (1991) subsequently reported a maximum total lod score of 5.5 of HLA-Bf in 24 informative families assuming autosomal dominant inheritance and 90% penetrance. The marker loci centromeric to HLA-GL01, D6S41, D6S21 were analysed and did not show evidence of linkage. These studies together provide evidence in support of a locus, EJM1, located on the short arm of chromosome 6 in the HLA region, predisposing to JME and other related idiopathic generalised epilepsies. However, the statistical significance of the lod scores observed is uncertain because so many models of inheritance were tested (Clerget-Darpoux et al, 1990; Weeks et al, 1990).

Whitehouse et al (1993) reported analysis of a third set of 25 families, including a proband with JME and at least one first degree relative with idiopathic generalised epilepsy. Eight loci spanning the HLA region on 6p were analysed. No significant evidence in favour of linkage was obtained at any of these loci. Multipoint linkage analysis generated significant exclusion data at HLA and a region of 10–30 cM telomeric to HLA. Locus heterogeneity within this epilepsy phenotype would be one explanation for these conflicting results, some families mapping to chromosome 6p and some not. The small size of the kindreds ascertained render this a difficult question to resolve, as individual pedigrees do not generate statistically significant lod scores.

STRATEGIES FOR FUTURE RESEARCH

The revolution in human molecular genetics and molecular neuroscience has provided methods which should allow the molecular genetic basis of human typical absence syndromes to be elucidated. It should be possible to identify the gene loci and their mutant alleles which predispose to these phenotypes. How can this be done? There are two principal strategies: positional cloning and candidate gene analysis. The strategies involve similar methodology and are to some extent inter-related. They are considered briefly in turn, with particular emphasis on their application to absence epilepsy.

Positional cloning: linkage analysis

In this approach, the map localisation of the locus responsible for a disease trait is first established by linkage analysis. Segregation of the trait within pedigrees is compared with that of alleles at anonymous marker loci. A linked marker will segregate with the trait, thereby revealing the location of the disease locus. The interval containing the disease gene is subsequently narrowed to a size – usually about 10^6 base-pairs – that is amenable to molecular cloning techniques and genes within that region are then identified and screened for mutations.

This strategy of positional cloning is most easily applied to Mendelian disorders, but is more difficult to apply to diseases – such as the absence epilepsies – that do not display clear evidence for segregation of a single major gene. The main difficulties arise from two uncertainties. Apparently unaffected individuals may harbour the disease-causing allele: ie, penetrance is low, either on account of other gene effects or environmental influences. Secondly, apparently identical phenotypes may be caused by mutations at different loci: ie, genetic (locus) heterogeneity is present. These difficulties can be circumvented to some extent by using non-parametric 'affecteds only' analyses. These are less powerful than conventional linkage but this loss of power is compensated for by the extraordinary resolution and informativeness of the human genome linkage maps now available (Weissenbach et al, 1992).

The age-dependent penetrance of the principal human typical absence epilepsy syndromes render 'sib-pair' analysis the optimal strategy. Contemporary rather than historical clinical data on individuals classed as affected provides secure data. Adequate power, allowing for locus heterogeneity, would be provided by between 100 and 200 sib-pairs if analysis were carried out with 300–400 highly informative micro-satellite loci spanning the genome. The small number of probands with, say, CAE who have affected siblings (5–10%) indicates that a co-ordinated effort is required to ascertain an adequate resource. The technology for marker typing has recently improved, and typing of 200 individuals at 300 loci using PCR and fluorescent primers could now be achieved within a year.

Candidate-gene analysis

In this approach, direct analysis is performed of genes which on pathophysiological grounds are possible candidates for the site of mutations causing the disease trait. Molecular neurobiology is providing an almost embarrassing number of plausible candidate genes for the epilepsies. This makes the choice of which genes to investigate difficult. Alternatively, extrapolation from animal models may be undertaken.

The pathophysiology of absence is reviewed by Berkovic et al (1987). A diffuse moderate hyper-excitability of cortical neurons causing them to respond to thalamo-cortical volleys by inducing spike-wave discharges is a reasonable supposition. Such cortical hyper-excitability could clearly arise from mutations in genes encoding proteins involved in controlling neuronal excitability such as the voltage-gated and ligand-gated ion channels. If the so-called 'microdysgenesis' which has been documented is significant (Meencke & Janz, 1984), then genes controlling this level of morphogenesis in the brain become candidates. They, of course, have yet to be identified.

An alternative approach to the identification of candidate genes lies in the study of animal models. Genetic models of absence epilepsy have been well characterised in rats and mice (Buchhalter, 1993). These allow invasive investigations of neurophysiology and neurochemistry and the application of genetic methodology to identify the genes involved. Investigations in rats have particularly implicated gamma-hydroxybutyric acid and the GABA$_B$ receptor as of primary importance (Snead et al, 1990; Bernasconi et al, 1992), but the gene for this receptor has yet to be cloned so its role in man cannot yet be investigated.

At least two mouse models of absence epilepsy exist: the tottering mouse (tg/tg) and the lethargic mouse (lh/lh) (see Ch. 4). Rapid advances in the genetic, physical and transcriptional maps of the mouse genome have rendered positional cloning of these murine genes a feasible proposition. Their identification would allow homologous genes to be investigated in man. The recent demonstration that mutations in the genes encoding the α-subunit of the glycine receptor give rise to hyperekplexia in man and the spasmodic phenotype in mice encourages the hope that murine genes causing absence epilepsy will provide useful clues to the human condition.

CONCLUSION

Human typical absence syndromes clearly have a genetic basis. Their exact mode of inheritance and molecular genetic basis remain unknown. Methods now exist which will allow the elucidation of the molecular genetics of the absence epilepsies. This will be achieved by linkage analysis, candidate gene analysis and the investigation of genetic animal models.

REFERENCES

Beck-Mannagetta G, Janz D 1991 Syndrome-related genetics in generalised epilepsy. Epilepsy Research (Suppl). 4: 105–111
Berkovic S, Andermann F, Andermann E, Gloor P 1987 Concepts of absence epilepsies: discrete syndromes or biological continuum? Neurology 37: 993–1000
Bernasconi R, Lauber J, Marescaux C et al 1992 Experimental absence seizures: potential role of gamma-hydroxybutyric acid and GABA$_B$ receptors. Journal of Neural Transmission (Suppl.) 35: 155–177
Buchhalter J 1993 Animal models of inherited epilepsy. Epilepsia 34 (Suppl. 3): 531–541
Clerget-Darpoux F, Barton M-C, Bonaiti-Pellic C 1990 Assessing the effect of multiple linkage tests in complex diseases. Genetic Epidemiology 7: 245–253
Degen R, Degen H-E, Roth C 1990 Some genetic aspects of idiopathic and symptomatic absence seizures: waking and sleep EEGs in siblings. Epilepsia 31 (6): 784–794
Doose H, Baier W 1989 Absences. In Beck-Mannagetta G, Anderson V, Doose H, Janz D (eds) Genetics of the epilepsies. Springer-Verlag, Berlin, pp34–42
Doose H, Gerkern H, Horstman T, Volzke E 1973 Genetic factors in spike-wave absences. Epilepsia 14: 57–75
Durner M, Sander T, Greenberg DA, Johnson K, Beck-Mannagetta G, Janz D 1991 Localisation of idiopathic generalised epilepsy on chromosome 6p in families of juvenile myoclonic epilepsy patients. Neurology 41 (10): 1651–1655
Greenberg DA, Delgado-Escueta AV, Widelitz H et al 1988 Juvenile myoclonic epilepsy may be linked to the BF and HLA loci on human chromosome 6. American Journal of Medical Genetics 31 (1): 185–192
Kandt R, Haines J, Smith M et al 1992 Linkage of an important gene locus for tuberous sclerosis to a chromosome 16 marker for polycystic kidney disease. Nature Genetics 2: 37–40
Lennox W, Lennox M 1960 Epilepsy and related disorders. Little, Brown, Boston
Liu AWH, Wissbecker D, Delgado-Escueta AV 1991 Centromeric markers in chromosome 6p and juvenile myoclonic epilepsy. Epilepsy 32 (Suppl. 3): 100

Matthes A, Weber H 1968 Klinische und elektroencephalographische familien untersuchungen bei pyknolepsien. Deutsche Medzin Wochenschr 10: 429–435

Meencke H, Janz D 1984 Neuropathological findings in primary generalised epilepsy: a study of eight cases. Epilepsia 25: 8–21

Metrakos K, Metrakos J 1961 Genetics of convulsive disorders II. Genetic and electroencephalographic studies in centrencephalic epilepsy. J Neurol 11: 474–483

Metrakos K, Metrakos J 1974 Genetics of epilepsy. In: Magnus O, Lorentz de Haas A (eds) Handbook of clinical neurology, Vol 15. The epilepsies. North–Holland Publishing, Amsterdam, pp429–439

Snead O, Hechler V, Vergnes M, Marescaux C, Maitre M 1990 Increased gamma-hydroxybutyric acid receptors in thalamus of a genetic animal model of petit mal epilepsy. Epilepsy Research 7 (2): 121–128

van Heyningen V 1994 One gene – four syndromes. Nature 367: 319–321

Weeks DE, Lehner T, Squires-Wheeler E, Kaufmann C, Ott J 1990 Measuring the inflation of the lod score due to its maximisation over model parameter values in human linkage analysis. Genetic Epidemiology 7 (4): 237–243

Weissbecker KA, Durner M, Janz D, Scaramelli A, Sparkes R, Spence M 1991 Confirmation of linkage between juvenile myoclonic epilepsy locus and the HLA region on chromosome 6. American Journal of Medical Genetics 38 (1): 32–36

Weissenbach J, Gyapay G, Dib C et al 1992 A second-generation linkage map of the human genome. Nature 359: 794–801

Whitehouse WP, Rees M, Curtis D et al 1993 Linkage analysis of idiopathic generalised epilepsy and marker loci on chromosome 6p in families of patients with juvenile myoclonic epilepsy: no evidence for an epilepsy locus in the HLA region. American Journal of Human Genetics 53 (3): 652–662

37. Study of concordance of symptoms in families with absence epilepsies

Amedeo Bianchi and the Italian League Against Epilepsy Collaborative Group

Strong evidence of the influence of genetic factors in idiopathic generalised epilepsies comes from studies on twins and on those with a familial risk of epilepsy (Lennox & Lennox, 1960; Anderson, 1982; Blandfort et al, 1987; Beck-Mannagetta et al, 1989; Anderson et al, 1989). Idiopathic generalised epilepsies comprise several syndromes, including childhood absence epilepsy, juvenile absence epilepsy, juvenile myoclonic epilepsy and epilepsy with generalised tonic-clonic seizures.

Moreover it is evident that there is a genetic heterogeneity of the epilepsies (Anderson et al, 1986; Bird, 1987). Animal genetic models and human diseases with clear Mendelian inheritance (autosomal dominant, autosomal recessive and X-linked recessive) with an increased seizure risk show that different genetic factors can modify the neuronal excitability threshold (Seyfried & Glaser, 1985; McKusik, 1988; Anderson et al, 1990). The first suggestions that stand out from molecular genetic research by linkage analysis are the presence of genetic heterogeneity in benign neonatal familial convulsions (Leppert et al, 1983; Ryan et al, 1991) and in juvenile myoclonic epilepsy (Greenberg et al, 1988; Durner et al, 1991; Whitehouse et al, 1993; Greenberg et al, 1993; Liu et al, 1993).

The hypothesis of a common gene for the idiopathic generalised epilepsies (Delgado-Escueta et al, 1990; Janz et al, 1992) has not been confirmed by molecular genetics which have shown evidence against a linkage between the HLA markers on chromosome 6 in families with idiopathic epilepsy and typical absences (Serratosa et al, 1993; Sander et al, 1994).

The identification of families with several cases of idiopathic generalised epilepsies has been important for molecular genetic studies, but it also allows clinical analysis of the degree of affinity existing among the several forms of idiopathic generalised epilepsy (Italian Genetic Group, 1993).

Following this strategy, the Italian League against Epilepsy has for several years collected families with more than one case of idiopathic epilepsy and saved DNA from family members (Bianchi et al, 1993; Italian Genetic Group, 1993). The aim of the present study is the analysis of the degree of concordance and of clinical affinity in families with patients affected by typical absences.

METHODS

Families with at least three affected members in one or more generation and with the proband affected by a form of idiopathic generalised epilepsy with typical absences have been collected. Twenty Italian Centers against Epilepsy have collaborated in the study.

The data bank is located in the Epilepsy Centre of Arezzo; the DNA is stored in the C Besta Institute in Milan. The diagnosis and the EEG of every case have been carefully verified by an ad hoc committee and they have been discussed in special meetings of the Italian League Against Epilepsy. Every family has been identified through a single proband. Each form has been classified according to the International Classification of Epileptic Syndromes (Commission, 1989) with the exception of relatives with epilepsy with GTCS, which was considered together with tonic-clonic seizures on awakening, idiopathic tonic-clonic seizures during sleep and random tonic-clonic seizures.

Childhood absence epilepsy and juvenile absence epilepsy have been classified according to the International Classification, while probands with eyelid myoclonia absences, juvenile myoclonic epilepsy with absences and epilepsy with photo-sensitivity, absences, myoclonia and tonic-clonic seizures are considered separately. Every identified case has had a routine EEG with activations (hyperventilation, intermittent light stimulation and sleep after sleep deprivation). As far as possible non-affected members of the families have been examined both clinically and with EEG. In the present study non-affected members with an abnormal EEG have not been considered.

RESULTS

Thirty-seven families with a total of 136 affected members have been analysed (68 males, 68 females). The mean of affected members per family is 3.7 (range 3–10) (Table 37.1). Twenty-four families have the proband affected by childhood absence epilepsy. Figure 37.1 shows the pedigrees of these families. Table 37.2 analyses the epilepsies found in affected relatives. In first degree relatives there was a high concordance (33.3%) for the same clinical form; such concordance significantly reduces in second degree relatives (10%), where there is an appreciable number of cases affected by febrile convulsions (46.7%) and by epilepsy with tonic-clonic seizures (30%). Among the 10 cases of febrile convulsions in first degree relatives, six are under 12 years of age and so may yet develop absence epilepsy. Only 7.7% of first degree relatives have juvenile myoclonic epilepsy and 2.5% have juvenile absence epilepsy.

Only five families had a clinically homogeneous form in every affected member; they had childhood absence epilepsy or childhood absence epilepsy and one member with febrile convulsions younger than 12 years (Fig. 37.2).

Table 37.1 General data

Families n = 37
Affected members (including proband) n = 136 (M=68, F=68)
Mean affected per family = 3.7 (range 3-10)

Families' characteristics

– Proband with childhood absence epilepsy	24
– Proband with juvenile absence epilepsy	3
– Proband with childhood absence epilepsy with eyelid myoclonia	4
– Proband with juvenile myoclonic epilepsy with absences	3
– Proband with epilepsy with absence, myoclonia, GTCS and photo-sensitivity	3

Table 37.2 Distribution of clinical forms in affected relatives of probands with childhood absence epilepsy

Probands 24 (M=9, F=15)	1° degree				2° degree	
	Siblings	Parents	Total	%	Relatives	%
Febrile convulsions	8	2	*10	25.7	** 14	46.7
Benign childhood epilepsy with centro-temporal spikes	0	0	0	0.0	1	3.3
Childhood absence epilepsy	8	5	13	33.3	3	10.0
Childhood absence epilepsy with eyelid myoclonia	0	0	0	0.0	0	0.0
*Epilepsy with absences, myclonia, GTCS and photo-sensitivity	0	0	0	0.0	0	0.0
Juvenile absence epilepsy	1	0	1	2.5	0	0.0
Juvenile myoclonic epilepsy	1	0	1	2.5	0	0.0
Juvenile myoclonic epilepsy with absences	1	1	2	5.2	0	0.0
*Epilepsy with GTCS	2	2	4	10.3	9	30.0
*Isolated GTCS	2	1	3	7.7	0	0.0
Generalised cryptogenic or symptomatic	0	0	0	0.0	2	6.7
Partial cryptogenic or symptomatic	0	1	1	2.5	1	3.3
Benign neonatal familial convulsions	3	1	4	10.3	0	0.0
Total	26	13	39	100.0	30	100.0

* FC<12yrs = 6 (60%)   ** FC<12yrs = 3 (21.4%)
   FC>12yrs = 4 (40%)   FC>12yrs ≡ 11 (78.6%)

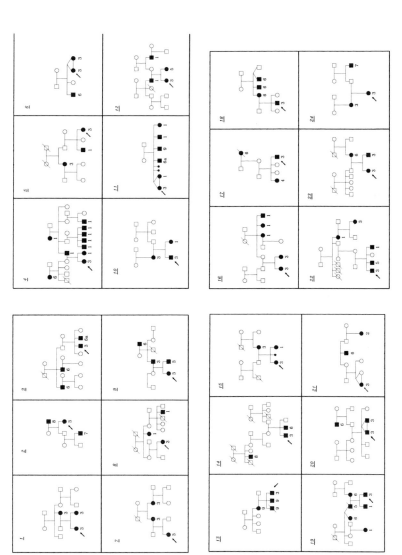

Fig. 37.1 Families with proband with childhood absence epilepsy

Proband (arrow); affected (solid squares and circles)
1. Febrile convulsions; 2. benign childhood epilepsy with centro-temporal spikes; 3. childhood absence epilepsy; 3a. childhood absence epilepsy with eyelid myoclonia; 3b. epilepsy with absences, myoclonia and photo-sensitivity; 4. juvenile absence epilepsy; 5. juvenile myoclonic epilepsy; 5a. juvenile myoclonic epilepsy with absences; 6. epilepsy with GTCS; 6a. isolated GTCS; 7. generalised cryptogenic or symptomatic; 8. partial cryptogenic or symptomatic; 9. benign neonatal familial convulsions

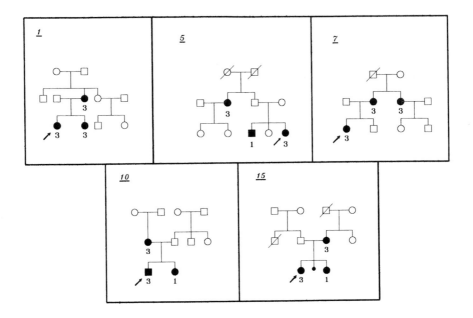

Fig. 37.2 Families with concordant form of childhood absence epilepsy in every affected member or with only another case with febrile convulsions under 12 years of age

Proband (arrow); affected (solid square and circles.
1. Febrile convulsions; 2. benign childhood epilepsy with centro-temporal spikes; 3. childhood absence epilepsy; 3a. childhood absence epilepsy with eyelid myoclonia; 3b. epilepsy with absences, myoclonia, GTCS and photo-sensitivity; 4. juvenile absence epilepsy; 5. juvenile myoclonic epilepsy; 5a. juvenile myoclonic epilepsy with absences; 6. epilepsy with GTCS; 6a. isolated GTCS; 7. generalised cryptogenic or symptomatic; 8. partial cryptogenic or symptomatic; 9. benign neonatal familial convulsions.

We found three families with a proband with juvenile absence epilepsy (Fig. 37.3). In the other members there was one case with juvenile absence, two cases with epilepsy with tonic-clonic seizures, two cases with isolated tonic-clonic seizures, two cases with generalised cryptogenic or symptomatic epilepsies but no cases with childhood absence epilepsy or juvenile myoclonic epilepsy. Four families had absence epilepsy with eyelid myoclonia (Fig. 37.4a). This is not yet an acknowledged syndrome (Jeavons, 1977; Dalla Bernardina et al, 1989; Bianchi et al, 1994a). In three families the proband had juvenile myoclonic epilepsy with absences (Fig. 37.4b) and in three families the proband was affected by absences, myoclonia, tonic-clonic seizures and photo-sensitivity (Fig. 37.4a).

Because of the relationship between myoclonia and photo-sensitivity in these three groups, we analysed the global distribution of clinical forms in the other affected relatives (Table 37.3). In first degree relatives we found juvenile myoclonic epilepsy (21.4%), epilepsy with tonic-clonic seizures (28.6%) and epilepsy with absences, myoclonia, tonic-clonic seizures and photo-sensitivity

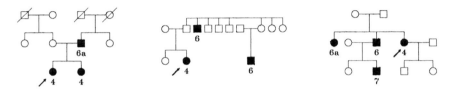

Fig. 37.3 Families with proband with juvenile absence epilepsy

Proband (arrow); affected (solid square and circles).
1. Febrile convulsions; 2. benign childhood epilepsy with centro-temporal spikes; 3. childhood absence epilepsy; 3a. childhood absence epilepsy with eyelid myoclonia; 3b. epilepsy with absences, myoclonia, GTCS and photo-sensitivity; 4. juvenile absence epilepsy; 5. juvenile myoclonic epilepsy; 5a. juvenile myoclonic epilepsy with absences; 6. epilepsy with GTCS; 6a. isolated GTCS; 7. generalised cryptogenic or symptomatic; 8. partial cryptogenic or symptomatic; 9. benign neonatal familial convulsions.

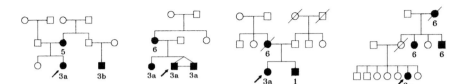

Fig. 37.4a Families with proband with childhood absence epilepsy with eyelid myoclonia

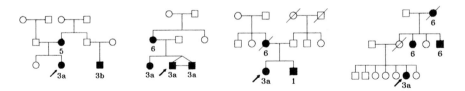

Fig. 37.4b Families with proband with juvenile myoclonic epilepsy with absences

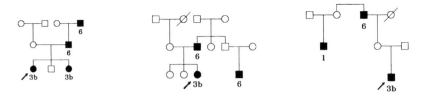

Fig. 37.4c Families with proband with epilepsy with absences, myoclonia, GTCs and photo-sensitivity

Proband (arrow); affected (solid square and circles).
1. Febrile convulsions; 2. benign childhood epilepsy with centro-temporal spikes; 3. childhood absence epilepsy; 3a. childhood absence epilepsy with eyelid myoclonia; 3b. epilepsy with absences, myoclonia, GTCS and photo-sensitivity; 4. juvenile absence epilepsy; 5. juvenile myoclonic epilepsy; 5a. juvenile myoclonic epilepsy with absences; 6. epilepsy with GTCS; 6a. isolated GTCS; 7. generalised cryptogenic or symptomatic; 8. partial cryptogenic or symptomatic; 9. benign neonatal familial convulsions.

(28.6%), while only one case presented with childhood absence epilepsy. In second degree relatives the trend to present with epilepsy with tonic-clonic seizures (70%) is confirmed. In all the 37 analysed families, benign childhood epilepsy with centro-temporal spike was very rare.

Table 37.3 Distribution of clinical forms in affected relatives of probands with childhood absence epilepsy with eyelid myoclonia, juvenile myoclonic epilepsy with absences and epilepsy with absences, myoclonia and GTCs and photo-sensitivity

Probands 10 (M=3, F=7)	1° degree				2° degree	
	Siblings	Parents	Total	%	Relatives	%
Febrile convulsions	0	0	0	0.0	2	20.0
Benign childhood epilepsy with centro-temporal spikes	0	0	0	0.0	0	0.0
Childhood absence epilepsy	1	0	1	7.1	0	0.0
Childhood absence epilepsy with eyelid myoclonia	2	0	2	14.3	0	0.0
Epilepsy with absences, myclonia, GTCS and photo-sensitivity	4	0	4	28.6	0	0.0
Juvenile absence epilepsy	0	0	0	0.0	0	0.0
Juvenile myoclonic epilepsy	1	1	2	14.3	1	10.0
Juvenile myoclonic epilepsy with absences	0	1	1	7.1	0	0.0
Epilepsy with GTCS	0	4	4	28.6	7	70.0
Isolated GTCS	0	0	0	0.0	0	0.0
Generalised cryptogenic or symptomatic	0	0	0	0.0	0	0.0
Partial cryptogenic or symptomatic	0	0	0	0.0	0	0.0
Benign neonatal familial convulsions	0	0	0	0.0	0	0.0
Total	8	6	14	100.0	10	100.0

DISCUSSION

Our selection criteria for families with at least three affected members make our case collection rather idiosyncratic and, therefore, it is not possible to draw a comparison with the literature for familial risk or for the study of transmission pattern. In the 24 families with a proband with childhood absence epilepsy we found a high concordance for the same clinical form (33.3%) in first degree relatives, while in more distant relatives febrile convulsions (46.7%) and epilepsy with tonic-clonic seizures (30%) were more common. We found that familial juvenile myoclonic epilepsy occurred rarely (7.7% of cases), in contrast with the literature (Janz et al, 1989; Delgado Escueta et al, 1990). This difference may be explained by the different family selection methods used.

Three monozygotic twins, four families with more affected cases and other sporadic cases from Bianchi et al (1994a) confirm our previous report (Bianchi et al, 1993) that epilepsy with absence seizures and eyelid myoclonia is a distinct syndrome which should be considered separately from childhood absence epilepsy. Absence epilepsy with eyelid myoclonia seems to be more similiar to juvenile myoclonic epilepsy with absences and to epilepsy with absences, myoclonia, tonic-clonic seizures and photo-sensitivity. There is a high level of concordance for juvenile myoclonic epilepsy and epilepsy with absences, myoclonia, tonic-clonic seizures and photo-sensitivity, while the association with childhood absence epilepsy seems to be very rare (one case).

These data suggest a different clinical and genetic basis to childhood absence epilepsy and juvenile myoclonic epilepsy. This may explain the first disappointing results of the molecular genetics studies in families with childhood absence epilepsy against linkage with HLA markers (Whitehouse et al, 1993; Liu et al, 1993; Sander et al, 1994). Juvenile absence epilepsy also seems to have a different syndromic characterisation, and, in particular, there is no association with childhood absence epilepsy and juvenile myoclonic epilepsy. Unfortunately, we have only three juvenile absence epilepsy families and therefore no definitive conclusions can be drawn.

Epilepsy with tonic-clonic seizures remains an open problem. This form is highly represented in families with childhood absence epilepsy, in families with juvenile absence epilepsy and in families with absences associated with myoclonia and photo-sensitivity, above all in second degree relatives. Only a critical reappraisal and a division into sub-forms will illuminate these areas. Febrile convulsions are also commonly found in relatives, and a syndromic definition is necessary here, for example, in relation to the presence of a genetic EEG pattern.

A further differentiation should be made in childhood absence epilepsy, where there is a distinction to be drawn between children having a benign course, with a rapid response to therapy, normal EEG and rare tonic-clonic seizures, and atypical cases that do not respond to therapy and have frequent tonic-clonic seizures (Bianchi et al, 1994b).

For genetic studies it is noteworthy that childhood absence epilepsy phenotype is concordant only in first degree relatives, while in more distant relatives there is a tendency toward a different phenotypic expression. Indeed, if we select among childhood absence epilepsy families only those with a homogeneous clinical form, we have again a small number (five out of 24 in our series). These families are small and nuclear, while in multi-generation families there is a tendency to a discordant clinical phenotype.

In this phase of molecular genetic research in epilepsy it could be useful to keep apart, in the analysis, the homogeneous nuclear families from the non-homogeneous multi-generation families.

CONCLUSIONS

The analysis of our series of families allows some conclusions to be formulated. Childhood absence epilepsy is distinct from juvenile myoclonic epilepsy and juvenile absence epilepsy. Childhood absence epilepsy with eyelid myoclonia is an autonomous syndrome with clinical and genetic features similar to those of juvenile myoclonic epilepsy. In childhood absence epilepsy there is a genetic familial tendency to a phenotypic concordance only in first degree relatives.

REFERENCES

Anderson VE 1982 Family study in epilepsy. In: Anderson VE, Hauser WA, Penry JK, Sing CF (eds) Genetic basis of the epilepsies. Raven Press, New York, pp103–112

Anderson VE, Hauser WA, Olafsson E, Rich SS 1990 Genetic aspects of the epilepsies. In: Sillanpaa M, Johannessen JI, Blennow G, Dam M (eds) Paediatric epilepsy. Wrightson Biomedical, pp36–56

Anderson VE, Hauser WA, Rich SS 1986 Genetic heterogeneity in the epilepsies. In: Delgado-Escueta AV, Ward Jr AA, Woodbury, Porter RJ (eds) Basic mechanisms of the epilepsies: molecular and cellular approaches. Advances in Neurology, Vol. 44. Raven Press, New York, pp59–75

Anderson VE, Wilcox KJ, Rich SS et al 1989 Twin studies in epilepsy. In: Beck-Mannagetta G, Anderson VE, Doose H, Janz D (eds) Genetics of the epilepsies. Springer-Verlag, Berlin, pp145–155

Beck-Mannagetta G, Janz D, Hoffmeister V et al 1989 Morbidity risk for seizures and epilepsy in offspring of patients with epilepsy. In: Beck-Mannagetta G, Anderson VE, Janz D (eds) Genetics of the epilepsies. Springer-Verlag, Berlin, pp119–126

Bianchi A, Tiezzi A, Buzzi G et al 1993 The characterization of clinical subforms through the study of twins with epilepsy. Epilepsia 34 (Suppl. 2): 17

Bianchi A, Avanzini G, Binelli S et al 1994: L'epilessia con assenze dell'infanzia con mioclonie palpebrali: una sottoforma sindromica. Bollettino Lega Italiana Epilessia (in press)

Bianchi A, Buzzi G, Tiezzi A, Severi S, Zolo P 1994 L'epilessia con assenze dell'infanzia: analisi della "sottoforma idiopatica benigna" o forma tipica. Bollettino Lega Italiana Epilessia (in press)

Bird TD 1987 Genetic considerations in childhood epilepsy. Epilepsia 28: S71–S81

Blandfort M, Tsuboi T, Vogel F 1987 Genetic counselling in the epilepsies. Human Genetics 76: 303–331

Commission on classification and terminology of the ILAE 1989 Proposal for revised classification of epilepsies and epileptic syndromes. Epilepsia 30: 389–399

Dalla Bernardina B, Sgrò V, Fontana E et al 1989 Eyelid myoclonias with absences. In: Beaumanoir A, Gastaut H, Naquet R (eds) Reflex seizures and reflex epilepsies. Ed Médecine et Hygiène, Geneva, pp193–200

Delgado-Escueta AV, Greenberg DA, Weissbecker KA et al 1990 Gene mapping in the idiopathic generalized epilepsies: juvenile myoclonic epilepsy, childhood absence epilepsy, epilepsy with grand mal seizures and early childhood myoclonic epilepsy. Epilepsia 31: S19–S29

Durner M, Sander T, Greenberg DA. et al 1991 Localization of idiopathic generalized epilepsy on chromosome 6p in families of juvenile myoclonic epilepsy patients. Neurology 41: 1651–1655

Greenberg DA, Delgado-Escueta AV, Widelitz H et al 1988 Juvenile myoclonic epilepsy (JME) may be linked to the Bf and HLA loci on human chromosome 6. American Journal of Medical Genetics 31: 185–192

Greenberg DA, Delgado-Escueta AV 1993 The chromosome 6p epilepsy locus: exploring mode of inheritance and heterogeneity through linkage analysis. Epilepsia 34 (Suppl. 3): S12–S18

Italian League against Epilepsy Genetic Collaborative Group 1993 Concordance of clinical forms of epilepsy in families with several affected members. Epilepsia 34 (5): 819–826

Janz D, Durner M, Beck-Mannagetta G, Pantazis G 1989 Family studies on the genetics of juvenile myoclonic epilepsy (epilepsy with impulsive petit mal). In: Beck-Mannagetta G, Anderson VE, Janz D (eds) Genetics of the epilepsies. Springer-Verlag, Berlin, pp43–66

Janz D, Beck-Mannagetta G, Sander T 1992 Do idiopathic generalized epilepsies share a common susceptibility gene? Neurology 42 (Suppl. 5): 48–55

Jeavons PM 1977 Nosological problems of myoclonic epilepsies in childhood and adolescence. Developmental Medicine and Child Neurology 19: 3–8

Lennox WG, Lennox MA (eds) 1960 Epilepsy and related disorders. Little Brown, Boston

Leppert M, Anderson VE, Quattlebaum T et al 1989 Benign familial neonatal convulsions linked to genetic markers on chromosome 20. Nature 337: 647–648

Liu WYA, Serratosa JM, Delgado-Escueta AV et al 1993 Exclusion of linkage between a large LA-Belize pedigree with juvenile myoclonic epilepsy and chromosome 6p DNA markers. Second International Workshop on Chromosome 6, Berlin

McKusick VA (ed) 1988 Mendelian inheritance in man, 8th edn. Johns Hopkins University Press, Baltimore

Ryan SG, Wiznitzer M, Hollman C, Torres MC, Szekeresova M, Scheider S 1991 Benign familial neonatal convulsions: evidence for clinical and genetic heterogeneity. Annals of Neurology 29: 469–473

Sander T, Hildmann T, Janz D et al 1994 Evidence against linkage between idiopathic generalized epilepsies and HLA-markers on chromosome 6p in families of patients with idiopathic absence epilepsy. Annals of Neurology (in press)

Seyfried TN, Glaser GH 1985 A review of mouse mutants as genetic models of epilepsy. Epilesia 26: 143–150

Serratosa JM, Delgado-Escueta AV, Liu WYA et al 1993 Exclusion of linkage between DNA markers in the juvenile myoclonic epilepsy locus of chromosome 6p and childhood absence epilepsy. Epilepsia 4 (Suppl. 2): 149

Whitehouse WP, Rees M, Curtis D et al 1993 Linkage analysis of idiopathic generalized epilepsy (IGE) and marker loci on chromosome 6p in families of patients with juvenile myoclonic epilepsy: No evidence for an epilepsy locus in the HLA region. American Journal of Human Genetics 53: 652–662

Italian League Against Epilepsy Collaborative Group

Graziano Buzzi, Alessandro Tiezzi, Sauro Severi, Paolo Zolo (organizing center)

Giuliano Avanzini, Bernardo dalla Bernardina, Raffaele Canger, Carlo A Tassinari, Federico Vigevano (LICE committee)

Antonella Antonelli, Simona Binelli, Daniela Buti, Maria P Canevini, Carlo Cianchetti, Patrizia D'Alessandro, Maria Rita De Feo, Pasquale De Marco, Stefano Di Donato, Cecilia Filati Roso, Ada Francia, Emilio Franzoni, Carlo A Galimberti, Renato Galli, Pier Gaetano Garofalo, Paola Giovanardi Rossi, Mario Manfredi, Roberto Massetani, Salvatore Mazza, Oriano Mecarelli, Antonia Parmeggiani, Andrea Pelliccia, Dario Pruna, Stefano Ricci, Raffaele Rocchi, Mariangela Rota, Amalia Saltarelli, Margherita Santucci, Giulio Sideri, Amalia Tartara, Camillo Tiacci, Giampaolo Vatti, Piernanda Vigliano (collaborative group)

Centro Epilessia, UO Neurologia, Arezzo (AB, GB, AT, SS, PZ); Istituto Neurologico 'C Besta', Milano (GA, AA, SB, SDD); Cattedra Neuropsichiatria Infantile, Verona (BDB); Centro Epilessia, Ospedale S Paolo, Milano (RC, MPC, AS); Clinica Neurologica, Ospedale Bellaria, Bologna (CAT); Divisione Neuropsichiatria Infantile, Ospedale Bambino Gesù, Roma (FV, SR); Servizio Neuropsichiatria Infantile, Ospedale Meyer, Firenze (DB, MR); Clinica Neuropsichiatria Infantile, Università Cagliari (CC, DP) Dipartimento Neuropsichiatria Infantile, Trento (PDM); Clinica Neurologica, Università Cattolica, Roma (SM); Clinica Neuropsichiatria Infantile, Roma (AP); Clinica Pediatrica, Università Bologna (EF); UO Neurofisiopatologia, Perugia (PDA, CT); I Neurofisiopatologia, Università Roma, Roma (MRDF, OM); Divisione Neurologia, Vincenza (CFG, PG); III Clinica Neurologica, Università Roma, Roma (AF, MM, GS); Istituto Neurologico 'Mondino', Pavia (CAG, AT); Cattedra Neurofisiopatologia, Pisa (RG, RM); Cattedra Neuropsichiatria Infantile, Bologna (PGR, AP, MS); Clinica Malattie Nervose e Mentali, Università Siena (RR, GV); Cattedra Neuropsichiatria Infantile, Università Torino (PV)

38. The genetics of typical absences – future research directions – consensus statement

E. Andermann

We have heard from both speakers what are the important steps that have to be taken in genetic studies. These begin with the hard work of ascertaining the probands, and extend to obtaining detailed family histories and pedigrees, as well as EEG examinations of relatives. Careful definition of the phenotypes and collection of a large number of well-defined families for each syndrome requires collaboration from dedicated researchers in many countries worldwide, in order for these studies to advance. We should not forget that in these polygenic or multifactorial conditions, the search for other markers is likely to become very important. Biochemical markers such as amino acids, and immunological markers, which have in the past been found to have associations with specific epilepsy syndromes, may now give us important clues as to which loci may be important, because many of these markers have now been mapped. This offers an alternative to make advances in the study of these diseases.

Segregation analysis is not being done as frequently at present, but it still has an important role in the study of specific syndromes where we are trying to determine the mode of inheritance more precisely.

The two main approaches which will continue to be important are linkage studies and localisation of the gene and identification of the gene product. This is also important with respect to genetic counselling; as soon as a gene is localised we may be able to bring it into genetic counselling and prenatal diagnosis. Further, the identification of the gene product will be very useful for designing rational therapies.

The type of inheritance is very important. There is a large number of single-gene disorders, tuberous sclerosis for example, in which the genes associated with epilepsy have already been mapped. However, the absence epilepsies do not seem to be associated with any single gene.

In the past a number of epilepsies were thought to be due to a single-gene disorder. The only conditions that have been found to belong to this group have been benign neonatal and benign infantile familial convulsions and the recently reported syndrome of familial frontal lobe epilepsy. We also know that most EEG traits are not single-gene disorders and many of them

338

are multifactorial. However, the 3 Hz spike-wave trait and photosensitivity may have a major gene component. Even with photo-sensitivity there may be a different genetic base as compared to the spike wave seen at rest and during hyperventilation.

There has been an evolution of the genetic concepts of generalised epilepsy: initially people talked about autosomal dominant or recessive inheritance with reduced penetrance. Then Metrakos and Metrakos talked about autosomal dominant inheritance of spike-wave EEG traits, but not of epilepsy, with age-dependent penetrance. Our own studies showed that these data on absence epilepsies fitted with the concept of multifactorial inheritance. Finally, the pendulum swung and we were back looking for single major epilepsy genes in these disorders.

By July 1992, linkage studies assigned juvenile myoclonic epilepsy to chromosome 6 and benign familial neonatal convulsions to chromosome 20. By the beginning of 1994 there were many more studies – and controversies. In September 1993 Whitehouse and colleagues excluded JME from chromosome 6 and then Delgado-Escueta found 12 families who did not map to chromosome 6. He believes that the explanation for all of this is genetic heterogeneity.

Benign familial neonatal convulsions, the first single-gene autosomal dominant idiopathic generalised epilepsy, was found to map to chromosome 20. Then a family was found who mapped to chromosome 8. It is more complex still because there are now a number of families with benign familial neonatal convulsions, even though the phenotype is identical, who do not map to either chromosome 20 or chromosome 8.

In conclusion, significant strides are being made in the molecular genetics of idiopathic generalised epilepsy, but the answers are not yet clear. Much remains to be done, with analysis of families with many affected members. As has been discussed, we also have the options of using candidate genes in the many receptors and transmitters that have now been mapped and cloned, and of using the mouse homologues in looking at these.

DISCUSSION

Berkovic: Does not locus heterogeneity complicate the analysis?

Gardiner: That is a good point but it depends on how many sib pairs there are and how much locus heterogeneity there is. If there are only two loci then one would probably see it with 100 sib pairs if the marker map were sufficiently dense. It is partly a trade-off between the number of sib pairs and the density of the marker map. A low-resolution search may never provide a marker closer than, say, 10% recombinant.

The real problem with small families is that an unlinked family and a linked family that happens to be recombinant are formally indistinguishable. If one analyses 100 sib pairs and there are two loci (so 50 are linked to one locus) and then one does a low resolution search, even though all those 50 sib pairs are at the same locus, no marker is closer than 10%. A proportion of those will appear to be recombinant; they will do nothing for the LOD score and one may not see linkage. If it is a really dense search, maybe 1000 markers instead of 300, one of the markers will be really close. All those recombinants can then be weeded out. The truly linked families will all appear as positives, and then one would see it and get a positive LOD score.

The answer to the question is that it depends on how much locus heterogeneity there really is. If there are at five different loci, so that there are never more than 20 families at one locus, then that would be a real problem without a really dense marker search.

Berkovic: What puzzles me is that if there are only two loci one would not know which 50 are at the locus.

Gardiner: One would do the linkage and get all the individual family results and look for heterogeneity. There is a computer analysis called HOMOG which would show whether it is a reasonable proposition that a sub-set of families are really linked. HOMOG knows that with a lot of nuclear families there will be a few positives and a few negatives and this is why I am so worried about some of the approaches to the JME families where there has been a tendency to say that one family has a positive score so it is linked and another family has got a negative score so it is not. That is not true for small nuclear families. It is all right if there are enough meioses to push it to <-2 or $+3$ in one family, but with small nuclear families one can only look at a lot of them. With a dense marker map and a close marker only 20 or 30 sib pairs would be needed to see the linkage.

Wolf: Surely it would be useful to try and locate the photo-sensitivity gene? It seems that this is definitely a separate trait with its own inheritance (if we are lucky with one gene, perhaps with several), and it goes across all the syndromes of idiopathic generalised epilepsy and blurs the picture. It might be that some of the problems we encounter with JME are due to this because the trait is very frequent there, but by no means omnipresent.

Gardiner: I would agree entirely. I suspect that the problem there is discovering enough families in which a high-quality assessment has been done. But the European concerted action group is working on this.

Janz: In the light of the findings of Dr Bianchi that juvenile myoclonic epilepsies and absence epilepsies are not only clinically but genetically different, I should like to ask whether we should restrict our investigations only to concordant forms? Would that perhaps improve the possibility of positive results?

Gardiner: I certainly agree that the most cautious and safest approach is to study families in which there is a stringent definition of the phenotype and to deal with those separately.

I think JME sib pairs and CAE sib pairs would be the most appropriate families to investigate in the first instance. If there is linkage one can then examine the other families to see what the situation is.

Janz: We may not have enough sib pairs for JME and CAE, but concordant families in which multi-generational concordance is present may be easier to find.

Gardiner: Yes, one can do that and still use the affected individual approach. The only reason why I was emphasising sib pairs is that I feel that if the affected individuals are contemporary with the whole of the data available now, it is a generally superior. I agree, in a group like Bianchi's with very good documentation of a parental or grandparental generation then it might be safe. But usually, if these families must be acquired by way of neurologists, the quality of the clinical data on the parental or the grand-parental generation is likely to be poor. However, with a couple of siblings who are right there, one can be a bit more sure.

Panayiotopoulos: How many of the results will be made more difficult by contaminated disease? If for example, eyelid myoclonia with absences is classified as childhood absence epilepsy and vice versa?

Gardiner: We do not know whether inclusion of these variant types is nec-essarily a bad thing in the sense that they do not correspond to the same phenotype. I would agree entirely that, having recognised them, the cau-tious thing would be to exclude them.

One of the real problems is that the families we would really like are those that clinicians are not interested in. The families we really like are the barn door families, not all these subtle variations. I suppose the question is whether we can be sure that such a family really is a CAE, as narrowly defined, without having all the videos. In practical terms, if we start demanding that it may become an impossible project.

I do not think one should be too worried. As long as, for example, there is a description of the seizures I do not think one should be too worried about the phenotype or one might end up with no families at all.

Hirsch: I want to raise the relationship between absence epilepsy and benign rolandic epilepsy. These two entities can be compared because they have approximately the same age of onset, around the age of 6–12 years. Can the geneticists confirm that these conditions are not related (which from the statistics given by Bianchi seems to be the case)? In the literature it has been stated that people with rolandic epilepsy have had siblings with gener-alised spike and wave, and that people with absences might have rolandic spikes. It has recently been demonstrated that this was not the case and this point needs to be finally clarified.

Marescaux: Is it fair to say that this form of absence with eyelid myoclonia and with photo-sensitive seizures in the older generation is essentially photo-sensitive absence?

Bianchi: Yes. We have three families with absences, photo-sensitivity and myoclonia, but have no clearly defined sub-types of this.

Marescaux: I think there is something like a consensus on absences induced either by eye closure or by photic stimulation. According to the data obtained in Italy this form is the dominant one. I wonder whether this form is the best one to begin the genetic study.

Tassinari: The Italian group have identified two types of photo-sensitivity but they are different. One is eyelid myoclonia, which is facilitated by eye closure. The second is the multiple spike and wave induced by intermittent light stimulation which is not the same thing. They are different inasmuch as we do not get the same response in different patients. We have not succeeded in transforming one response to the other. They are different and the EEG patterns are also different. One is a multiple spike and wave discharge frontal and the other is more of a posterior discharge, which eventually spreads from the back and moves forward.

Panayiotopoulos: There is not the slightest possibility of inducing eyelid myoclonia with absences in patients who have absences on photic stimulations. They are two entirely different electro-clinical phenomena.

Wolf: In his childhood absence group, Dr Bianchi had quite a few relatives with benign familial neonatal convulsions. Do they all belong to one family?

Bianchi: One family, and in this family we found only one child with childhood absence epilepsy and other cases in the three generations with benign neonatal familial convulsions.

F Andermann: It is very clear that the level of co-operation in Italy is extraordinarily good. What are the chances of getting this kind of co-operation between the other 200-odd million people in Europe? How does this approach compare with looking for a transmitter abnormality or using other approaches which might give an answer about the mechanism of idiopathic generalised epilepsy?

Gardiner: Putting together collaboration is extraordinarily difficult. The problem is persuading people that they cannot do it on their own with a small number of families and then persuade them that if they chip their families in they will not then be quietly ignored by the people to whom they have contributed themselves. I must admit I oscillate between the linkage and the candidate gene approaches. I think they are evenly balanced and that which approach is best depends on what the underlying mechanism of inheritance is, and we do not know what it is.

Duncan: Can we bring in the basic scientists, for their best guesses for the candidate genes that should be addressed.

Noebels: The potassium channel genes have a very high probability of being defective in an excitability disorder.

Gardiner: One of the best hopes is the mouse genes. There are so many mouse/man homologies, murine genes that cause exactly the same disease in man, and the mouse genes are so much easier to get at, that in some ways perhaps the focus should be on those first. For example, with the potassium channels there is a whole group on chromosome 6 in the mouse and chromosome 12 in man, and there are several mouse phenotypes that are in that locality. There is one called Deof waddler and another called Opisthotonos in which there are seizures, so it may well be there are human phenotypes caused by mutations in those K-channels but they do not happen to occur in JME or CAE.

Coulter: The problem with epilepsy is we are modulating excitability but we cannot get one of the major players and knock it out and hope just to modulate excitability. I talked about the T-current a couple of days ago. My feeling is if the properties of the T-current get changed excessively, the oscillator will not work correctly. Understanding the mechanisms of ictogenesis is essential. I do not think that abnormalities of any of the major players are involved. It is something that is modulating that process and I think K-channels are a good place to begin.

Mirsky: What would Professor Gardiner think of the use of behavioural markers to include in their genetic analysis? There is a parallel in the genetic analysis of schizophrenia. Patients with schizophrenia and first-degree relatives show anomalous smooth pursuit eye movements. The relationship to the other symptoms is not clear, but on the basis of adding that marker to some familial studies the power of the analysis may be increased.

In the case of absence epilepsy, inability in sustained attention tasks is a very characteristic trait, and it may or may not be found in association with spike-wave discharges. What would be the value of adding this kind of marker?

Gardiner: Potentially it could be of considerable value. Anything that allows a more precise definition of the trait is potentially valuable. The parallel to something like smooth eye movements in schizophrenia would be to include EEG traits in the definition. It is very plausible that alterations on the EEG are a component of the trait. For example, in CAE I am sure one could boost the number of possible pairs by doing EEGs on them all and finding those with the characteristic EEG trait. A behavioural trait would be comparable.

The real difficulty would be that this would require time and expertise and be very expensive.

39. Impact on life: psychological, social and occupational aspects of absence seizures

Ann Jacoby   Gus A. Baker

The social and psychological consequences of epilepsy in adults are well documented. Adults with epilepsy are prone to have poorer self-esteem and higher levels of anxiety and depression than people without epilepsy (Collings, 1990). They are more likely to be un- or under-employed; and lower rates of marriage and greater social isolation have been noted in adults with epilepsy (Dodrill et al, 1984; Arntson et al, 1986). People with epilepsy sometimes feel stigmatised by their condition (Jacoby, 1993).

In children with epilepsy there is evidence of increased emotional and behavioural morbidity compared with other conditions (Rutter et al, 1970; Austin et al, 1994). In addition, it has been shown that parents fear that their children with epilepsy will suffer intellectual deterioration and personality disorder, and that adverse drug effects will alter their emotions and behaviour (Austin & Dunn, 1993).

Although much is known about the effects of epilepsy per se, there is little evidence in the literature of the psycho-social consequences of different seizure types. In this chapter we review the evidence of social and psychological correlates of absence seizures and present evidence from a recent community study. We address the important question whether there are any differences between patients with absence seizures and those with other seizure types in relation to their social and psychological sequelae.

What little evidence is available about absence seizures suggests that around a third of patients with typical absence seizures experience social maladjustment problems (Loiseau et al, 1983). These authors reported that patients with absence seizures often had psychiatric problems; their social adaptability was poor compared with patients experiencing other seizure types. In a recent study of 58 young adult patients with absence seizures persisting since childhood (Olsson & Campenhausen, 1993) the authors reported a number of cognitive and psycho-social difficulties. Of 50 patients still receiving anti-epileptic drug treatment, 62% reported side-effects of their medication, including drowsiness, difficulties with concentration and memory problems. Some 74% believed their epilepsy had an impact upon schooling, occupational and leisure activities, relations with friends, daily routine and housing (this was independent of whether or not they had achieved seizure control).

In this chapter we present evidence about the psychological, social and occupational aspects of absence seizures using data from a recently completed study of an unselected population of adults and children with epilepsy of varying aetiology, duration and severity (Jacoby, 1993).

METHODS

The aim of the study was to examine the quality of life and medical care of a population of individuals with active epilepsy (defined as a history of seizures in the last two years or currently taking anti-epileptic drugs and with a previous history of seizures). The study was undertaken in one health region of the UK, the Mersey region (population just under 2.5 million). We identified 1347 patients with active epilepsy through the morbidity and repeat prescription records of a random sample of 31 general practices. Information was collected both from general practice medical records and through postal questionnaires to adults aged 16 years and over and to the parents of children aged 5–15 years.

The questionnaire covered a number of areas, including: seizure type and frequency; injuries associated with seizures; anti-epileptic drug side-effects (Baker et al, in preparation); the perceived impact of epilepsy (Jacoby et al, 1993); feelings of stigma because of the diagnosis of epilepsy (Jacoby, 1994); and extent of worry over epilepsy, anxiety and depression (Zigmond & Snaith, 1983); life fulfilment (Baker et al, 1994); and overall perception of quality of life (Andrews & Withey, 1976). In the parents' questionnaire, information was collected using the Rutter Behavioural Checklist (Rutter et al, 1970), an impact of epilepsy scale, a seizure severity scale and an adverse drug effects profile (Baker et al, in preparation).

General practitioners were asked to provide information from the records about the diagnosis of epilepsy, including the classification of seizure type. The diagnosis had been made by a consultant or other hospital doctor in 78% of cases and by the general practitioner in 8%. In the remaining 14% information about who had made the diagnosis was missing from the notes. Of the 1347 patients identified, 4% were classified as having absence seizures only, a further 9% as having absence and other seizure types. A total of 54% were classified as having other seizure types only, and 33% were unclassifiable from the notes.

Not all identified patients were eligible to receive a psycho-social questionnaire. Those with known learning disability, or those considered by the general practitioner too ill or infirm, were excluded. In all, questionnaires were sent to 1185 patients and returned by 789, of whom 696 were adults.

RESULTS

Adults

Clinical status

Twenty-seven adults identified from the medical records as having absence seizures only returned a psychosocial questionnaire, as did 65 identified as having absence seizures and other seizure types, and 400 of those having other seizure types only. The mean age of the adults in the study was 46, with no differences between the groups. In the absence only group, 41% were men, as were 45% of those in the group having absences and other seizure types, and 53% of the group having only other seizure types.

The mean duration of epilepsy in each of the groups was 19, 18, and 14 years. Of the 27 adults in the absence group, 78% reported epilepsy of more than two years' duration, compared with 83% of those who had both absence and other seizure types and 75% of those who had only other seizure types.

In relation to frequency of seizures, 44% of the absence only group reported no seizures in the last year, 19% less than one seizure a month and 37% one or more per month. Of those having absence seizures plus other seizure types, 38% reported none in the last year, 26% less than one per month, and 31% one or more per month. For the remaining 5%, information about seizure frequency was missing. Of those having only other types of seizures, 52% reported none in the last year, 23% less than one per month, 24% one or more per month; information was missing for the remaining 1%.

Eleven per cent of the absence only group were not on any anti-epileptic (AED) medication, compared with 2% of the absence and other seizure types group and 6% of the other seizure types only group. Among those on AED, rates for monotherapy were 67%, 63%, and 73% respectively.

Social and occupational status

There was no difference in the marital status of adults with absence seizures only, absence and other seizures and other seizures only (Table 39.1). There were no statistically significant differences in the age at which full-time education was completed or in the level of qualifications obtained, although there was a suggestion from the data that those with absence seizures only were more likely than the rest to have gained some formal qualifications.

Adults who had absence seizures only were more likely than the rest to be in full-time employment, and this difference was statistically significant when those with absence seizures only were compared to those with other seizure types only (Table 39.1). Fifty per cent of all adults were currently employed in non-manual occupations (based on OPCS Standard Classification of Occupations, 1990), a proportion similar to that in the general population (Central Statistical Office, 1994). Although it was not statistically significant, there was a trend in the data: among those currently employed, individuals with absence seizures only were most likely to be working in non-manual occupations (64%); and those with other seizure types only were least likely to be doing so (51%).

Table 39.1 Comparison of psycho-social status of adults with different seizure types

| | Seizure type: | | | |
| | Absence only | Absence + other types | Other types only | All adults[+] |
	(n=24*)	(n=60*)	(n=379*)	(n=655*)
Marital status:				
Single	27%	29%	27%	27%
Married	62%	57%	59%	58%
Divorced/separated	–	12%	8%	8%
Widowed	11%	2%	6%	8%
Age at which full–time education completed:				
16 and under	71%	75%	81%	80%
Educational qualifications obtained:				
No qualifications	39%	44%	52%	52%
CSE/GCSE/O level	27%	29%	25%	24%
A level	11%	8%	3%	4%
College/univ. degree	4%	6%	8%	7%
Other	19%	13%	12%	13%
Current employment status:				
Employed full-time	46%	32%	28%	28%
Employed part-time	–	5%	8%	7%
Unemployed	12%	8%	11%	10%
Retired	19%	8%	20%	20%
Permanent sick	12%	17%	15%	15%
Housewife	11%	25%	13%	15%
Other	–	5%	5%	5%

*   Bases on which percentages were calculated excluding adults for whom this information was missing. Quoted 'n' is the lowest number on which percentages were calculated.
[+]   Includes some adults for whom seizure type could not be classified from the notes.

Psychological status

Based on their scores on the Hospital Anxiety and Depression Scale, 30% of adults in the absence only group were classified as anxious, and a further 11% as borderline. In those with both absence and other seizures, 20% were classified as anxious, and a further 12% as borderline; the figures for those having other seizure types only were 25% and 13% respectively. Seven per cent of individuals in the absence only group were classified as depressed, 15% as borderline. In the other two groups, these figures were 7% and 12%, and 10% and 16% respectively.

Feelings of stigma were measured using a three-item scale, developed originally to measure patient perceptions of the stigma of another neurological condition, stroke, and reworded for epilepsy. Respondents were asked to say whether, because of their epilepsy, they felt that other people were uncomfortable with them, treated them as inferior, and preferred to avoid them. They scored one for each item with which they agreed and their overall score was the sum of their positive responses. Sixty-two per cent of adults in the study did not feel stigmatised by their epilepsy, independent of their seizure type. Of those who reported feeling stigmatised, there were no differences in their scores according to seizure type.

Adults' perceptions of the impact of epilepsy

Subjects were asked to what extent they thought their epilepsy affected various aspects of everyday living (Table 39.2). The percentage of individuals with absence seizures only who reported a significant impact on their relationships with partners, other close family members and friends did not differ significantly from the other two groups. Those with absence seizures only were least likely to report that epilepsy significantly affected their social life and activities, though the differences between the groups were not statistically significant. There was no difference between the groups in the percentages reporting that epilepsy affected their ability to undertake paid employment. Around a third of adults in each group reported that epilepsy had a significant impact on their health overall. Those with absence seizures only were less likely to report that epilepsy affected the way they felt about themselves, and their plans for the future (though the differences were not statistically significant). There were no differences between the groups in the percentages reporting an impact of epilepsy on their standard of living.

When asked how they felt about their life as a whole, 89% of the adults with absence seizures only described themselves as happy and the rest as unhappy. Among those with both absence and other seizures, 73% described themselves as happy, 21% as neutral and 6% as unhappy. Figures for individuals with other seizure types only were 73%, 13% and 13% respectively.

Children

Clinical status

There were 93 children identified from the medical records for whom parents completed a psycho-social questionnaire. Of these, nine had absence seizures only, 11 had absence seizures and other seizure types and 53 had other seizure types only. In the remaining 20 children, seizure type was not classifiable from the notes. Since the numbers are so small, it is not possible to look at children with absences only as a separate group. We have combined them with children who had other seizure types also, and compared this group with those having only other seizure types.

Table 39.2 Perceived impact of epilepsy on adult's daily functioning

	Seizure type:			
	Absence only (n=21*)	Absence + other (n=48*)	Other only (n=279*)	All adults[+] (n=456*,+)
Felt epilepsy affected a lot/some:				
Relationship with partner	14%	16%	23%	21%
Relationship with other family members	26%	25%	23%	23%
Social life and activities	22%	28%	34%	31%
Ability to work in paid employment	23%	29%	29%	28%
Overall health	30%	31%	36%	37%
Relationships with friends	19%	19%	22%	21%
Feelings about self	22%	38%	38%	37%
Plans and ambitions for the future	22%	41%	34%	33%
Standard of living	22%	31%	30%	29%

*   Bases on which percentages were calculated excluding adults for whom this information
      was missing. Quoted 'n' is the lowest number on which percentages were calculated.
[+]   Includes some adults for whom seizure type could not be classified from the notes.

The mean age of children in the study was 11 years. There were equal numbers of boys and girls in each of the groups. Mean age of onset was seven years; the mean duration of epilepsy was five years. Age of onset was lower in the absence group than in the rest (four years compared with nine years). There was no significant difference between children with absence seizures and the rest for duration of epilepsy. Overall, 29% of children had been seizure-free in the last 12 months, 31% had had less than one seizure a month and the remaining 40% had had at least one a month. There was no difference in seizure frequency between children with absences and the rest. Fourteen per cent of children were not taking any AED medication, 67% were on one AED only and 19% were taking two or more AEDs. There was no difference between groups in the percentage on no, one, or two or more AEDs.

Psychosocial status

A high proportion of children in the study (38%) were in receipt of special education for learning difficulties. A further 12% required remedial help, although in mainstream schooling. There were no differences between groups in the percentages receiving special education or remedial help.

The prevalence of behavioural problems was assessed using the Rutter Behavioural Checklist (Rutter et al, 1970). Taking all children together, 54% were perceived by their parents as having behavioural problems. The percentages for children with absences and those with other seizure types only were 40% and 58% respectively (not statistically significant).

Parents were asked to say to what extent epilepsy affected a number of different aspects of their child's daily life (Table 39.3). The differences in parents' perceptions of the impact of epilepsy on daily functioning were small and not statistically significant between the group with absence seizures and those with other seizure types only. When all the children were considered as a single group, the percentages of parents who felt that epilepsy affected 'a lot' or 'some' the various aspects of their daily life, with the exception of schooling, feelings about self, and plans and ambitions for the future were small. For these three areas, around a third of parents felt that epilepsy had a significant impact.

Table 39.3 Impact of epilepsy on children's daily lives by seizure type

	Seizure type:		
	Absence +/– others (n=18*)	Other only (n=47*)	All children[+] (n=79*)
Parent felt epilepsy affected a lot/some their child's:			
Relationship with responding parent	20%	15%	16%
Relationship with respondent's partner	(17%)	13%	13%
Relationship with siblings	20%	17%	16%
Relationship with friends	25%	15%	18%
Interests and hobbies	20%	20%	18%
Schooling	35%	36%	32%
Health overall	10%	21%	18%
Feelings about self	25%	32%	28%
Plans and ambitions for the future	35%	44%	37%

*   Bases on which percentages were calculated excluding children for whom this information was missing. Quoted 'n' is the lowest number on which percentages were calculated.
( )   Percentages in brackets are those where the base was less than 20.
[+]   Includes some children for whom seizure type could not be classified from the notes.

DISCUSSION

It is clear from these results that the secondary psycho-social consequences of epilepsy are not confined to any one seizure type; nor does having a potentially less stigmatising seizure disorder necessarily protect individuals against them. Among adults in the study, there were no significant differences between the three groups in marital or employment status, level of educational qualifications or social class. Between 20 and 30% of adults, independent of seizure type, were classified as anxious, a result similar to findings from a recent hospital-based study (Baker et al, 1993). Rates of depression were similar between the three groups and slightly lower than reported in previous studies. There was no difference between the three groups in the level of reported stigma, and there were few significant differences between the groups in their perceptions of how epilepsy affected their daily lives.

Overall, only a relatively small percentage of adults reported a significant impact on their relationship with partners, though a quarter of the population reported a significant impact on their relationship with other close family members. Adults with absence seizures only reported less of an impact on their social life than those with other seizure types, but there was no significant difference between the groups in their perceived ability to work in paid employment. Approximately a third of all adults reported an effect of epilepsy on their health and this was not different by seizure type; approximately a fifth reported an impact on their relationships with friends. Adults with absence seizures only reported a significantly lower impact of epilepsy on the way they felt about themselves and their plans for the future.

Comparing the results with those from a long-term follow-up study of 58 adults with absence seizures (Olsson & Campenhausen, 1993), adults in this study reported significantly less impact of their absence seizures on various aspects of daily life. Olsson & Campenhausen (1993) reported that 74% of their patients believed that their epilepsy had exerted an impact on their lives in a number of areas, including schooling, occupation, daily living, leisure activities, relations with friends and housing. This was not the experience of our population.

The small number of children in the study having absence seizures only means that it is not possible for us to draw clear conclusions about the impact of this particular seizure type on psycho-social status. However, the data suggest that there is no direct relationship between seizure type and psycho-social outcome.

In the Anti-epileptic Drug Withdrawal Study (Jacoby et al, 1992), in which a significant proportion of patients had been seizure-free for some time, many reported a good quality of life, suggesting that whether or not patients attain remission from seizures is more important than seizure type in determining the psycho-social consequences of their condition.

Acknowledgements

We would like to thank Professor David Chadwick for his support and encouragement with our work in an ongoing programme of research into the quality of life of people with epilepsy. We also thank the Wellcome Trust for funding this research and the patients and parents for taking time to complete the questionnaires.

REFERENCES

Andrews FM, Withey SB 1976 Social indicators of well-being. Plenum Press, New York
Arntson P, Droge D, Norton R, Murray E 1986 The perceived psychosocial consequences of
  having epilepsy. In: Whitman S, Hermann B (eds) Psychopathology in epilepsy: social
  dimensions. Oxford University Press, New York, p143
Austin JK, Dunn DW 1993 Children with newly diagnosed epilepsy: impact on quality of life.
  In: Chadwick DW, Baker GA, Jacoby A (eds) Quality of life and quality of care in epilepsy:
  Update 1993. Royal Society of Medicine, Round Table Series 31, London, p14
Austin JK, Smith MS, Risinger MW, McNelis AM 1994 Childhood epilepsy and asthma:
  comparisons of quality of life. Epilepsia 35: 608–615
Baker GA, Smith DF, Dewey M, Jacoby A, Chadwick DW 1993 The initial development of a
  health-related quality of life model as an outcome measure in epilepsy. Epilepsy Research 16:
  65–81
Baker GA, Jacoby A, Smith DF, Dewey M, Chadwick DW 1994 The development of a novel
  scale to assess life fulfilment as part of the further refinement of a quality of life model for
  epilepsy. Epilepsia 35: 597–607
Central Statistical Office 1994 Social trends 24. HMSO, London
Collings J 1990 Psychosocial well-being and epilepsy: an empirical study. Epilepsia 31:
  418–426
Dodrill CB, Batzel L, Queisser HR, Temkin NR 1984 An objective method for the assessment
  of psychological and social problems in epileptics. Epilepsia 25: 176–183
Jacoby A, Johnson AL, Chadwick DW 1992 Psychosocial outcomes of antiepileptic drug
  discontinuation. Epilepsia 33: 1123–1131
Jacoby A 1993 Quality of life and care in epilepsy. In: Chadwick DW, Baker GA, Jacoby A
  (eds) Quality of life and quality of care in epilepsy: Update 1993. Royal Society of Medicine
  Round Table Series No 31, London, p66
Jacoby A 1994 Felt versus enacted stigma: a concept revisited. Social Science and Medicine 38:
  269–274
Jacoby A, Baker GA, Smith DF, Dewey M, Chadwick DW 1993 Measuring the impact of
  epilepsy: the development of a novel scale. Epilepsy Research 16: 65–81
Loiseau P, Pestre M, Dartigues JF, Commenges D, Barberger-Gateau C, Cohadon S 1983
  Long-term prognosis in two forms of childhood epilepsy. Annals of Neurology 13: 642–8
Olsson I, Campenhausen G 1993 Social adjustment in young adults with absence epilepsy.
  Epilepsia 34 (5): 846–851
OPCS 1990 Standard occupational classification. HMSO, London
Rutter M, Graham P, Yule W A 1970 A neuropsychiatric study in childhood. Spastics
  International Medical Publications, London
Zigmond AS, Snaith RP 1980 The hospital anxiety and depression scale. Acta Psychiatrica 67:
  361–370

DISCUSSION

Brodie: This is interesting and it puts paid to the suggestion that absences are a benign form of epilepsy. We found that many children with absences are having behavioural problems at school and at home. I wonder whether they are having many more absences than we appreciate.

Duncan: In contrast, anecdotally I see a fair number of children with the benign form of CAE and I have been struck by how normal they are in terms of being very bright and getting on well at school. I was quite surprised by Dr. Jacoby's finding.

Robinson: One thought occurs to me about the lack of difference between the groups. If people are more psycho-socially disadvantaged are they more or less likely to return the questionnaires?

Jacoby: That is a good question. It is very difficult to know what we have lost in our non-responders. All I can do is to look at the clinical information that I have for them all and see if the people who did not send back questionnaires are different.

Something I did do in the MRC drug withdrawal study was to go back and compare responders' and non responders' clinical data and I did not find any difference there, so I felt reasonably confident about the conclusions that I drew from that data. I shall do the same with this study.

Gloor: I suspect that because the candidates were selected from GP populations there must be a high contamination of the absence group by patients with temporal lobe epilepsy, especially the adults (in whom it is a frequent form of epilepsy). That would upset the apple cart completely as we know they have a high incidence of problems.

I would not want to conclude from this study that patients with absence seizures have the same range of problems as the others. A much more carefully selected population is needed to come to that conclusion.

Jacoby: We have got the information about who made the diagnosis and this was usually in hospital.

Duncan: To what extent do you think the findings of your study are determined by the methodology? Would a structured interview have elicited far more problems than a questionnaire?

Jacoby: In my experience the difference when using interviews is not that more things come out but they yield more information. I have not compared interviews and questionnaires in studies in epilepsy but I have in another area, about maternity services and women's views of that. We found that we did not pick up new facts from the interviews but people were far more expansive about what they were saying.

E Andermann: I was wondering whether one of the reasons for your findings would be that on the whole the GPs would have the milder cases and the very severe cases would tend to be followed by neurologists.

Jacoby: That is certainly what happens in many of the studies of psychosocial outcome and quality of life, but in fact these patients were chosen on a community basis by sifting through all the notes. They may be being treated at the hospital but the GP will still hold notes about their epilepsy. A community-based study is very important if selection bias is to be avoided.

Mirsky: I am very pleased to hear the results, particularly with the children. We who do laboratory studies often get criticised that our work has nothing to do with real life. Clearly the kinds of deficits that we describe in patients with absence seizures are reflected in real life, and 50% of these children are having difficulty at school.

40. Treatment strategies for typical absences and related epileptic syndromes

John S. Duncan

This chapter draws together some of the principles and points made in other chapters and is intended to give an overview of the treatment of the patient with typical absences and idiopathic generalised epilepsy.

INITIATION OF DRUG TREATMENT

Diagnosis of seizures and syndrome

Before starting anti-epileptic drug treatment it is clearly necessary to be certain that the diagnosis of typical absences is correct and that the patient does not have blank spells that are atypical absences or complex partial seizures, or even are non-epileptic in basis. As emphasised in Section 2 (see Chs 17–35), diagnostic certainty is essential and the history, examination and routine EEG may, in difficult cases, be usefully supplemented by prolonged video-EEG telemetry, including sleep and hyperventilation.

A diagnosis of the patient's epilepsy syndrome should also be made, although this may be difficult at the outset of the condition when the patient has only had a few absences and other features of a typical syndrome phenotype have not yet emerged. In a patient with juvenile myoclonic epilepsy, for example, typical absences may antedate the occurrence of myoclonic and tonic-clonic seizures by several years. An accurate syndromic diagnosis aids choice of initial drug therapy, decisions regarding subsequent treatment options and is necessary if the patient is to be given a realistic prognosis and appropriate advice about the risks of relapse should medication be withdrawn after 2–3 years of seizure control.

Avoidance of precipitating stimuli

In some patients it is evident that seizures are precipitated by certain stimuli, particularly sleep deprivation and flickering light in predisposed individuals. There is non-uniformity of the incidence of photo-sensitivity between the syndromes of idiopathic generalised epilepsy; 20% of patients with childhood absence epilepsy are photo-sensitive, as are 10–20% of patients with juvenile absence epilepsy and 50% of patients with juvenile myoclonic epilepsy. Susceptible individuals should be counselled to avoid these stimuli so far as possible by ensuring that they get adequate sleep and avoid sitting close up to television screens and monitors, particularly when playing video games. Some photo-sensitive patients, particularly children, appear to derive pleasure from inducing serial absences by gazing at sunlight and passing their fingers rapidly before their eyes. This should be discouraged by counselling and explanation. There have been reports of fenfluramine being useful in this situation (Aicardi & Gastaut, 1985), but experience is limited and the treatment is not without risk for a condition that is usually benign and self-limiting. In patients who have eyelid myoclonia with typical absences, absences are often brought on by bright light, even if this is not flickering; avoidance and the wearing of coloured lenses may be helpful.

Anti-epileptic drug treatment

The commencement of prophylactic anti-epileptic drug treatment should not be a reflex action in a patient who presents with typical absences. This should be considered if absences are continuing despite the avoidance of precipitating stimuli and if absences are adversely affecting learning, cognitive function (see Ch. 14) and quality of life (see Ch. 39). In some patients the case for regular prophylactic anti-epileptic drug treatment is overwhelming – for example, the child with childhood absence epilepsy who is having hundreds of absences a day or the adolescent with juvenile myoclonic epilepsy who also has myoclonic and generalised tonic-clonic seizures. At the other extreme, some patients having only occasional absences which do not concern them prefer not to take regular anti-epileptic drugs, particularly if these are associated with any adverse effects.

As with the treatment of other forms of epilepsy the goal is to achieve complete seizure control without adverse effects from anti-epileptic drugs. Patients and their relatives need to be counselled on the aims, expectations, limitations and adverse effects of drug treatment and that drug therapy is long term and needs to be taken regularly and reliably if it is to be effective.

THE INTENSITY OF TREATMENT

Once medication has been commenced doses are best titrated according to clinical response and the development of any adverse effects. While the goal of the patient becoming totally seizure-free is laudable, this should not be regarded as a holy grail that must be pursued relentlessly whatever the costs in terms of drug side-effects. For many patients whose absences do not respond well it is preferable to have some absences continue and have no adverse effects from medication rather than have no absences and to be sedated by the drugs taken. In general, the two most important issues in older adolescents and adults are driving and pregnancy. If they wish to obtain a driving licence patients will tend to want to take higher doses of medication, to suppress all absences. In contrast, if they are planning a conception they are likely to prefer to take the minimum dose of a single agent that gives reasonable control of their absences so that the teratogenic risk is minimised.

If a patient with absences who is receiving appropriate drug treatment complains of poor concentration it may be difficult to be certain whether this is the consequence of frequent absences or the medication itself. A useful way of resolving this difficulty is to undertake a prolonged video-EEG recording and to perform a neuropsychological assessment during the period of monitoring. This approach allows quantification of the absences and also whether any neuropsychological impairments are the direct consequence of absences.

WHICH DRUG FOR WHICH PATIENT

The typical absences found in some forms of idiopathic generalised epilepsy, eg childhood absence epilepsy, respond equally well to ethosuximide and valproate given as monotherapy (Bourgeois, 1989) and for the majority of patients a single agent controls the absences. A point in favour of ethosuximide is the concern about severe valproate-related hepatic reactions (see Ch. 41). It is important to consider the epilepsy syndrome and not just the seizure type. An advantage of valproate is that it is also effective against tonic-clonic and myoclonic seizures, which may also affect the patient. Of patients with juvenile myoclonic epilepsy, 30% have absences as their first seizure type, subsequently developing myoclonic jerks and then tonic-clonic seizures (Grunewald et al, 1992). Overall, 30–40% of children presenting with typical absences will subsequently develop tonic-clonic and/or myoclonic seizures. If valproate or ethosuximide do not provide adequate control of absences it is appropriate to try the other, and then the two agents in combination, as in some individuals the combination of these two drugs appears to be significantly more effective than each agent given in isolation (Sato et al, 1982; Rowan et al, 1983). Some sub-types of idiopathic generalised epilepsy (for example, eyelid myoclonia with typical absences) appear to respond poorly to valproate or ethosuximide in isolation, but well to the combination.

Second-line drugs

Second-line medications for intractable absences include: clonazepam, acetazolamide and lamotrigine. There are no controlled clinical studies of the effect of these drugs on absences. The use of the first two is often complicated by the development of tolerance and clonazepam use is frequently limited by drowsiness. There is anecdotal experience of lamotrigine benefiting otherwise intractable absences, especially when given with valproate (Timmings & Richens, 1992; Panayiotopoulos et al, 1993a).

TREATMENT OF COMMON SYNDROMES WITH TYPICAL ABSENCES

Childhood absence epilepsy

Ethosuximide and sodium valproate are equally effective in treating the absences of childhood absence epilepsy, achieving a total suppression in over 70% of patients. If one of these drugs does not give adequate control, it is appropriate to change to the other, and if that is not successful to prescribe the two in combination (Sato et al, 1982; Rowan et al, 1983). In about 40% of patients with childhood absence epilepsy, tonic-clonic and/or myoclonic seizures also occur. In these cases sodium valproate is generally the drug of choice, as there is the possibility of control of all seizure types with a single anti-epileptic drug and there is an argument for initiating therapy with sodium valproate.

The reservation about commencing valproate therapy in young children is concern about hepatotoxicity (see Ch. 41). If control is difficult, it is generally best to avoid adverse effects of high doses of medication and to accept the continuation of some absences. If the patient, parents and teachers complain of a child's poor concentration, and it is not apparent whether this is due to frequent absences or adverse effects of anti-epileptic drugs, it is helpful to obtain a 24 h ambulatory EEG to determine if frequent absences are occurring and to check the serum concentrations of the anti-epileptic drugs. If absences remain intractable, lamotrigine and clonazepam are worth considering. If remission occurs it is usually long-lasting and the risk of relapse on tapering anti-epileptic drugs after seizure control for 2–3 years is small, probably between 10–15%.

Juvenile absence epilepsy

The principles are similar to those for childhood absence epilepsy. Sodium valproate and ethosuximide appear to be equally effective against absences. The former is the drug of choice if generalised tonic-clonic and/or myoclonic seizures also occur. As with childhood absence epilepsy, about 80% of patients with juvenile absence epilepsy become seizure-free with medication. Both absences and generalised tonic-clonic seizures may, however, persist into adulthood. The risk of relapse on subsequent withdrawal of medication is not clearly defined. The clinical and EEG features of juvenile absence epilepsy place it between childhood absence epilepsy and juvenile myoclonic epilepsy if one accepts the hypothesis of a biological continuum of the various idiopathic generalised epilepsy syndromes. In this case the risk of relapse after two to three years' freedom from seizures, on medication, is probably between the 10–15% of childhood absence epilepsy and the 80–90% of juvenile myoclonic epilepsy should medication be withdrawn.

Juvenile myoclonic epilepsy

Patients should be counselled to avoid precipitating factors, such as excessive alcohol, sleep deprivation and, if they are photo-sensitive, flashing lights. Sodium valproate is the drug of first choice and is effective in 80% of cases. There are anecdotal reports of lamotrigine being a useful addition to valproate if seizures are continuing. To date, however, there have not been any controlled studies to evaluate this issue.

Up to 90% of patients with juvenile myoclonic epilepsy become seizure-free with optimal medication. There is, however, a very high relapse rate if medication is subsequently withdrawn, even if the patient has been seizure-free for several years. The prognosis for a relapse in patients in their forties, however, has not been studied in detail and is uncertain at the present time (Grünewald & Panayiotopoulos, 1993).

Eyelid myoclonia with typical absences

Eyelid myoclonia with typical absences does not usually respond to treatment with sodium valproate or ethosuximide given alone, but is often well controlled by giving these medications in combination (Jeavons, 1977; Appleton et al, 1993). It should be recognised at the outset that the prognosis for seizure control is less good than in other idiopathic generalised epilepsy syndromes and patients who have eyelid myoclonia with typical absences often continue to have some seizures, even if medication is effective at reducing the frequency of attacks. The condition does not appear to remit in adolescence, but there have not been sufficient long-term studies to allow predictions of the prognosis through adulthood.

Perioral myoclonia with absences

Perioral myoclonia with absences has been described recently (Panayiotopoulos et al, 1993b) and is not yet recognised by the International League against Epilepsy. Perioral myoclonus consisting of rhythmic lip protrusion occurs at the time of absences. The small number of patients described with this feature appear to be resistant to anti-epileptic drug treatment.

PREGNANCY

If the epilepsy is still active most women will wish to continue through pregnancy with anti-epileptic drug treatment that gives optimal seizure control. It is appropriate to try to treat with monotherapy from before conception if at all possible. The risk of fetal malformation is increased from a background of 3% to 7% if one anti-epileptic drug is taken and to about 12% if two drugs are taken through pregnancy (Nakane et al, 1980). The risk of malformation is also dose-related, so attempts should be made to establish the patient on the minimum effective dose. Higher daily doses of valproate (>1000 mg per day) probably carry greater risk than lower doses (Lindhout et al, 1992) and there is some evidence that high peak serum concentrations of valproate may be associated with increased risk, with the consequence that some risk reduction may be achieved by fractionating the dose of valproate into three or even four daily doses, or by using slow-release valproate. As yet, however, there is no proof that this is a useful manoeuvre.

If a woman with typical absences has been seizure-free on medication for 2–3 years it is appropriate to consider the respective merits of discontinuing therapy prior to conception or continuing through the pregnancy. The key factors to consider are the syndrome, previous seizure types and hence the risk of relapse should medication be withdrawn, and the impact of such a relapse on the patient. The major effect on such patients' lives is usually driving, particularly in countries such as the United Kingdom in which the recurrence of a single absence would result in suspension of a driving licence for one year.

It is now widely agreed that all women with epilepsy who are taking anti-epileptic drugs and are planning a pregnancy should take folic acid to minimise the risk of neural tube defects (Medical Research Council Vitamin Study Research Group, 1991; Czeizel & Dudas, 1992; Rosenberg, 1992), particularly if valproate is being taken. The risk of neural tube defects is probably reduced by about 75% by folic acid supplementation. The dose of folic acid that was shown to be effective in clinical trials was 4 mg per day. This is almost certainly more than is needed, but does not appear to be associated with any adverse effects. The role of measuring red blood cell folate concentrations to determine whether folic acid supplementation is adequate to achieve a maximal protective effect has not yet been established.

REFERENCES

Aicardi J, Gastaut H 1985 Treatment of self-induced photosensitive epilepsy with fenfluramine. New England Journal of Medicine 313: 1419

Appleton R, Panayiotopoulos CP, Acomb AB et al 1993 Eyelid myoclonia with absences: An epilepsy syndrome. Journal of Neurology Neurosurgery and Psychiatry 56: 1312–1316

Bourgeois BFD 1989 Valproate; clinical use. In: Levy RH, Mattson RH, Meldrum BS, Penry JK, Dreifuss FE (eds) Antiepileptic drugs, 3rd edn. Raven Press, New York, pp633–642

Czeizel AE, Dudas I 1992 Prevention of the first occurrence of neural-tube defects by periconceptional vitamin supplementation. New England Journal of Medicine 327: 1832–1835

Grunewald RA, Panayiotopoulos CP 1993 Juvenile myoclonic epilepsy. A review. Archives of Neurology 50: 594–598

Grunewald RA, Chroni E, Panayiotopoulos CP 1992 Delayed diagnosis of juvenile myoclonic epilepsy. Journal of Neurology, Neurosurgery and Psychiatry 55: 497–99

Jeavons PM 1977 Nosological problems of myoclonic epilepsies in childhood and adolescence. Developmental Medicine and Child Neurology 19: 3–8

Lindhout D, Omtzigt JGC, Cornel MC 1992 Spectrum of neural-tube defects in 34 infants prenatally exposed to antiepileptic drugs. Neurology 42 (Suppl. 5): 111–118

Medical Research Council Vitamin Study Research Group 1991 Prevention of neural-tube defects: results of the Medical Research Council Vitamin Study. Lancet 338: 131–137

Nakane Y, Okuma T, Takahishi R et al 1980 Multi-institutional study on the teratogenicity and fetal toxicity of anticonvulsants: a report of a collaborative study group in Japan. Epilepsia 21: 663–680

Panayiotopoulos CP, Ferrie CD, Knott C, Robinson RO 1993a Interaction of lamotrigine with sodium valproate. Lancet 341: 445

Panayiotopoulos CP, Chroni E, Daskopoulos C, Baker A, Rowlinson S, Walsh P 1993b Typical absence seizures in adults: clinical, EEG, video-EEG findings and diagnostic/syndromic considerations. Journal of Neurology, Neurosurgery and Psychiatry 55: 1002–1008

Rosenberg IH 1992 Folic acid and neural-tube defects – time for action? New England Journal of Medicine 327: 1875–1876

Rowan AJ, Meijer JW, de Beer-Pawlikowski N, van der Geest P, Meinardi H 1983 Valproate-ethosuximide combination therapy for refractory absence seizures. Archives of Neurology 40: 797–802

Sato S, White BG, Penry JK, Dreifuss FE, Sackellares JC, Kupferberg HJ 1982 Valproic acid versus ethosuximide in the treatment of absence seizures. Neurology 32: 157–63

Timmings PL, Richens A 1992 Lamotrigine in primary generalized epilepsy. Lancet 339: 1300

41. Ethosuximide and valproate

Alan Richens

Prior to the discovery of the succinimide drugs, there was no specific treatment for absence seizures. Ethosuximide was the first to be developed, in the Parke-Davis laboratories in the early 1950s, and the first report of its efficacy in absences appeared in 1958 (Zimmerman & Burgmeister, 1958). This drug soon established itself as a highly effective treatment but it became clear that it was ineffective in tonic clonic seizures and therefore it had to be used in combination with a drug active in the latter type of seizure when both seizure types co-existed. A second major development occurred in the early 1960s with the discovery of the anti-epileptic activity of valproic acid in France (Meunier et al, 1963). Subsequent clinical trials indicated that it was active in all seizure types and could therefore be given as sole therapy when absences were accompanied by other seizure types. This chapter will review briefly the evidence for efficacy of these two drugs and their relative merits in absence seizures.

ETHOSUXIMIDE

The succinimide drugs were developed at a time when the classification of seizures and epilepsy syndromes was less satisfactory than at present. Therefore, the criteria for admission of patients to clinical trials were less clearly defined and often incompletely explained in publications. As a result it is often not possible to determine the proportion of patients who had typical absences compared with those who had absences of another type, or associated with syndromes other than childhood absence epilepsy. In some instances it is clear that some had partial seizures and were often on a variety of other anti-epileptic drugs.

Furthermore, the discipline of the controlled clinical trial was in its infancy at that time and therefore most studies were non-comparative and some were retrospective in nature. These qualities, together with the recognised difficulty of quantifying absence seizure activity by clinical observation, severely limits the interpretation of such studies.

In Table 41.1 a number of open, non-comparative studies are summarised. In most of these trials, ethosuximide was added to existing therapy. The overall response rate, namely 52% of patients experiencing complete control of seizures, is probably an under-estimate for the reasons given above.

Table 41.1 Ethosuximide in absence seizures: open, non-comparative trials

Authors	n	Seizure-free	% Seizure-free
Zimmerman & Burgmeister (1958)	18	11	61
Heathfield & Jewesbury (1961)	50	27	54
Gordon (1961)	14	6	43
Goldensohn et al (1962)	62	29	47
Mann & Habenicht (1962)	24	15	63
Livingston et al (1962)	62	8	38
Guinena et al (1963)	18	13	72
O'Donohoe (1964)	23	11	48
Weinstein & Allen (1966)	67	33	49
Blomquist & Zetterlund (1974)	11	8	73
Total	349	161	Mean 46

One comparative study has been published in which a placebo control was used under single blind conditions (Browne et al, 1975); but treatments were not randomised, the one-week placebo treatment always preceding the eight-week ethosuximide treatment. Thirty-seven patients aged 5-15 years were included, none of whom had been treated previously with drugs. All had absence seizures which were defined clinically, but 14 had other seizure types, including partial, akinetic, myoclonic and tonic-clonic seizures. It is unclear whether all the patients had 3 Hz spike and wave activity in their EEG. Complete control of absences was obtained in only seven of the patients (Table 41.2) but most had a seizure reduction of 50% or greater with doses of 6.5-36.7mg/kg/day. Plasma ethosuximide concentrations were significantly correlated with dose but not with seizure control.

Table 41.2 Ethosuximide in absence seizures: placebo-controlled single-blind trial (Browne et al, 1975)*

Patient		Control n (%)		
n	age (yrs)	100%	90-100%	50-100%
37	5-15	7(19)	18(49)	35(85)

*   Patients were previously untreated and were assessed by observation by professional staff and parents and by video-EEG recording.

It is difficult to ascertain from these studies what proportion of previously untreated patients with typical absences will respond to ethosuximide. The inclusion of many patients with atypical absences probably biased the results against ethosuximide.

VALPROATE

When valproate was introduced into clinical practice, ethosuximide had become the established treatment for absence seizures. Some of the early reports assessed valproate in patients whose absences had failed to respond to ethosuximide. However, several trials involved valproate monotherapy given either to patients who had received other drugs previously or to newly diagnosed patients without prior treatment (Table 41.3); 92% had their absences completely controlled by valproate.

Table 41.3 Valproate in absence seizures: open, non-comparative trials of valproate monotherapy

Authors	n	Seizure-free	% Seizure-free
Convanis et al (1982)	12	11	92
Dulac et al (1982)	23	21	91
Feuerstein (1983)	17	16	94
Henriksen & Johannessen (1982)	16	14	88
Bourgeois et al (1987)	21	20	95
Total	89	82	92

A wider spectrum of non-comparative trials in children were analysed by Davis et al (1994), including patients on combination therapy as well as monotherapy: 90% showed a 75% or greater reduction in absence seizure frequency, and this was better than the response with myoclonic seizures (69%) or tonic-clonic seizures (68%).

Two placebo-controlled trials of valproate have been reported (Table 41. 4). Both of these were single blind sequential trials. Villareal et al (1978) recruited adult patients with absences, usually in association with other seizure types, including partial seizures. Most patients were receiving other anti-epileptic drugs during the study. A placebo preparation was added on for two weeks, followed by 10 weeks' valproate therapy. Assessment was based on spike and wave EEG discharges. Forty-six per cent showed a 75% or greater reduction in the number of spike and wave EEG discharges but there was no correlation with the plasma level of valproic acid. Erenberg et al (1982) studied children with mainly refractory absences associated with other seizure types, again giving 10 weeks' valproate therapy after two weeks of placebo. Eighty-two per cent of the children had a 75% or greater reduction in absence seizures but there was no correlation between the response and plasma valproic acid level.

Table 41.4 Valproate in absence seizures: placebo-controlled trials

Authors	Patients		Valproic acid dose mg/kg/day	Control (≥75% reduction) n(%)
	n	age (yrs)		
Villareal et al (1978)*	24	14–39	18–62	11(46)
Erenberg et al (1982)†	17	5–16	20–66	14(82)

* Assessment based on spike and wave EEG discharges before and after 10 weeks' valproic acid therapy.
† Assessment based on clinical absences before and after 10 weeks' valproic acid therapy.

COMPARATIVE STUDIES OF ETHOSUXIMIDE AND VALPROATE

In order to assess the relative efficacy of the two drugs, comparative trials are particularly helpful. In an add-on comparative study of valproate and ethosuximide in 35 children who had principally absence seizures Suzuki et al (1972) found no difference in the efficacy of the two drugs, about 70% experiencing a 75% or greater reduction in seizure frequency. Three subsequent randomised comparative studies are summarised in Table 41.5. The double-blind study of Sato et al (1982) involved two groups of patients: one who had not previously received drug therapy and a second group with absences refractory to maximally tolerated doses of ethosuximide. The primary measures of efficacy were the frequency and duration of 3 Hz spike and wave activity in the 12-h telemetered EEG. A cross-over design was used in which only those who failed to achieve 100% control (previously untreated patients) or 80% control (refractory patients) were allowed to receive the second treatment. It can be seen that the refractory patients responded less well to either drug than the previously untreated patients.

Table 4.5 Comparative trials of ethosuximide and valproate

Authors	Patients		Maximum doses (mg/day)		Responders n(%)	
	n	age (yrs)	ESM	VPA	ESM	VPA
Sato et al (1982)*	16	4–18	1500	30‡	6/11(54)	9/12(75)
Callaghan et al (1982)†	28	4–15	1500	2400	8/14(57)	6/14(43)
Martinovic (1983)†	20	5–8	500	450	8/10(80)	7/10(70)
Sato et al (1982)††	29	7–18	1500	60‡	9/26(35)	5/25(20)

Responder= complete control of absence seizures ESM = ethosuximide VPA = Valproate

* Randomised double-blind response-conditional cross-over trial in previously untreated patients; assessment based on telemetered EEG
† Randomised non-blind study; assessment based on clinical seizures.
†† As in * but in patients with refractory absences
‡ mg/kg/day

The trials of Callaghan et al (1982) and Martinovic (1983) were randomised but non-blind studies in which seizure frequency was assessed by parents or other carers in newly-diagnosed children with typical absence seizures. Callaghan et al (1982) included patients with typical absences only, whereas Martinovic (1983) recruited some children with other seizure types. Despite this, and the lower doses used by the latter author, the responses to both drugs were greater than those found by Callaghan et al (1982). None of the studies revealed a significant difference in efficacy between the two drugs, but the numbers of patients included were sufficient only to detect a large difference.

ETHOSUXIMIDE-VALPROATE COMBINATION THERAPY

It has been generally accepted that a combination of valproate and ethosuximide may be effective in absence seizures which have failed to respond to one drug alone. No randomised controlled study has been undertaken to support this view, but Rowan et al (1983) reported five patients who responded well to the combination when they had failed to do so to valproate or both drugs given alone. All had 3 Hz spike and wave EEG activity but also had focal abnormalities, three with obvious secondary generalisation. All five showed a marked therapeutic response judged by the EEG and, clinically, they became seizure-free.

Although this combination probably works by additive pharmacodynamic effects (ie, pharmacological actions on the brain), the possibility of a pharmacokinetic interaction needs to be considered. Mattson & Cramer (1980) showed that the addition of valproate to ethosuximide increased the plasma concentration of ethosuximide in four of five patients studied. The concentration increased by a mean of 53% from 73 to 112 mg/l. This observation has been confirmed by Pisani et al (1984) and accords with knowledge that valproate inhibits the metabolism of other drugs – for example, lamotrigine and phenobarbitone. There are no reports of ethosuximide affecting valproic concentrations. It is likely, therefore, that a pharmacokinetic interaction might explain, at least in part, the good effect of combination therapy.

PLASMA DRUG CONCENTRATIONS

Plasma ethosuximide and valproic concentrations were measured in a number of the studies discussed above. The ranges of concentrations measured in patients whose seizures were completely controlled in four studies are given in Table 41.6. It should be noted, however, that none of these studies was designed to define the therapeutic range of plasma concentrations by titrating the level against therapeutic effect. Furthermore, there was usually a poor correlation or none at all between the concentration and effect, suggesting that some patients whose seizures are sensitive to the drug in question respond at a low concentration whereas others with more resistant seizures do not respond to much higher concentrations (Browne et al, 1975; Villareal et al, 1978). On the other hand a good correlation between dose and plasma concentration has been demonstrated for both drugs (Browne et al, 1975; Chadwick, 1985). These two sets of observations do not support the usefulness of drug level monitoring in absence seizures because one pre-requisite is that plasma levels should correlate better with efficacy than the dose. This does not appear to be so with either drug. Furthermore, the EEG is an accurate method of assessing the frequency of absence seizures because of the good relationship between 3 Hz spike and wave activity and clinical absence seizures. However, notwithstanding these comments, Sherwin et al (1973) reported that monitoring plasma ethosuximide concentrations in a prospective study in 70 patients with absence seizures resulted in a significant improvement in clinical control.

Table 41.6 Plasma ethosuximide and valproate concentrations in patients with complete control of typical absences

Authors	Concentrations	(mg/l)
	Ethosuximide	Valproate
Callaghan et al (1982)	26–88	47–121
Sato et al (1982)	63–97	49–115
Martinovic (1983)	51–114	68–131
Blomquist & Zetterlund (1985)	25–139	–
Range	25–139	32–131

CONCLUSION

This chapter has concentrated on the efficacy of ethosuximide and valproate in typical absences. No clear difference emerges but comparative studies are few and the power to detect a difference was low. Either drug can therefore be chosen, but valproate has a clear advantage in that it is effective against other seizure types when they occur concurrently. There is no clear benefit in measuring plasma drug levels. Adverse drug reactions have not been considered here. Little comparative data is available and therefore each prescriber will be influenced by his own perspective.

REFERENCES

Blomquist HK, Zetterlund B 1985 Evaluation of treatment in typical absence seizures. The role of long-term EEG monitoring and ethosuximide. Acta Paediatrica Scandinavica 74: 409–415
Blomquist HK, Zetterlund B 1974 Evaluation of treatment in typical absence seizures. Acta Paediatrica Scandinavica 985: 409–415
Bourgeois B, Beaumanoir A, Blajev B et al 1987 Monotherapy with valproate in primary generalized epilepsies. Epilepsia 28 (Suppl. 2): S8–S11

Browne TR, Dreifuss FE, Dyken PR et al 1975 Ethosuximide in the treatment of absence (petit mal) seizures. Neurology 25: 515–524

Callaghan N, O'Hara J, O'Driscoll D, O'Neill B, Daly M 1982 Comparative study of ethosuximide and sodium valproate in the treatment of typical absence seizures (petit mal). Developmental Medicine and Child Neurology 24: 830–836

Chadwick DW 1985 Concentration – effect relationships of valproic acid. Clinical Pharmacokinetics 10: 155–163

Covanis A, Gupta AK, Jeavons PM 1982 Sodium valproate: monotherapy and polytherapy. Epilepsia 23: 693–720

Davis R, Peters DH, McTavish D 1994 Valproic acid. A reappraisal of its pharmacological properties and clinical efficacy in epilepsy. Drugs 47: 332–372

Dulac O, Stern D, Rey E, Perret A, Arthuis M 1982 Monotherapie par le valproate de sodium dans les epilepsies de l'enfant. Archives Francais Pediatriques 39: 347–352

Erenberg G, Rothner AD, Henry CE, Cruse RP 1982 Valproic acid in the treatment of intractable absence seizures in children. American Journal of Diseases of Children 136: 526–529

Feuerstein J 1983 A long term study of monotherapy with sodium valproate in primary generalized epilepsy. British Journal of Clinical Practice (Suppl. 27): 17–25

Goldensohn ES, Hardie J, Borea ED 1962 Ethosuximide in the treatment of epilepsy. Journal of the American Medical Association 180: 840–842

Gordon N 1961 Treatment of epilepsy with alpha-ethyl-alpha-methylsuccinimide (PM671). Neurology 11: 266–268

Guinena YH, Taker Y, Elwan O, Amin N 1963 Zarontin therepy in petit mal. European Journal of Neurology Psychiatry and Neurosurgery 4: 51–55

Heathfield KWG, Jewesbury ECO 1961 Treatment of petit mal with ethosuximide. British Medical Journal 3: 565–567

Henriksen O, Johannessen SI 1982 Clinical and pharmacokinetic observations on sodium valproate – a 5 year follow-up study in 100 children with epilepsy. Acta Neurologica Scandinavica 56: 504–523

Livingston S, Pauli L, Najmabadi A 1962 Ethosuximide in the treatment of epilepsy. Journal of the American Medical Association 180: 822–825

Mann LB, Habenicht HA 1962 The use of ethosuximide (Zarontin) in petit mal epilepsy. Bulletin of the Los Angeles Neurological Society 27: 155–159

Martinovic Z 1983 Comparison of ethosuximide with sodium valproate. In: Parsonage M, Grant RHE, Craig AG, Ward AA (eds) Advances in Epileptology XIVth Epilepsy International Symposium. Raven Press, New York, pp301–305

Mattson RH, Cramer JA 1980 Valproic acid and ethosuximide interaction. Annals of Neurology 7: 583–584

Meunier H, Carraz G, Menrier Y, Eymard P, Aimard M 1963 Propriétés pharmacodynamiques de l'acide n-dipropylacetique. Therapie 18: 435–438

O'Donohoe NV 1964 Treatment of petit mal with ethosuximide. Developmental Medicine and Child Neurology 6: 498–501

Pisani F, Narbone MC, Trunfio C, Fazio A, La Rossa G, Oteri G, Di Perri R 1984 Valproic acid-ethosuximide interaction. A pharmacokinetic study. Epilepsia 25: 229–233

Rowan AJ, Meijer JWA, de Beer-Pawlikowski N, van der Geest P 1983 Valproate ethosuximide combination therapy for refractory absence seizures. Archives of Neurology 40: 797–802

Sato S, White BG, Penry JK, Dreifuss FE, Sackellares JC, Kupferberg HJ 1982 Valproic acid versus ethosuximide in the treatment of absence seizures. Neurology 32: 157–163

Sherwin AL, Robb JP, Lechter M 1973 Improved control of epilepsy by monitoring plasma ethosuximide. Archives of Neurology 28: 178–181

Suzuki M, Maruyama H, Ishibashi Y et al 1972 A double-blind comparative trial of sodium dipropylacetate and ethosuximide in epilepsy in children with special emphasis on pure petit mal seizures. Medical Progress (Japan) 82: 470–488

Villareal HJ, Wilder BJ, Willmore LJ, Bauman AW, Hammond EJ, Bruni J 1978 Effect of valproic acid on spike and wave discharges in patients with absence seizures. Neurology 28: 886–891

Weinstein AW, Allen RJ 1966 Ethosuximide treatment in petit mal seizures. American Journal of Diseases in Children 3: 63–67

Zimmerman FT, Burgmeister BB 1958 A new drug for petit mal epilepsy. Neurology 8: 769–775

42. Acetazolamide, benzodiazepines and lamotrigine

Lennart Gram

ACETAZOLAMIDE

Acetazolamide (AZM) was introduced for the treatment of epilepsy by Bergstrøm et al (1952). Holowach & Thurston (1958) have summarised the results of the early trials with AZM, which indicate that the drug may be effective in various forms of epilepsies/seizure types. With regard to typical absences a number of studies have shown that AZM may be very effective against this seizure type. In a study of 178 patients proving refractory to a number of other drugs (Chiao & Plumb, 1961), 14 suffered from absences with 3 Hz spike-wave activity on the EEG. Treatment duration with AZM varied from six months to three years. Ten of the 14 patients with absences obtained 80–100% seizure control, which was actually the seizure type demonstrating the best result in this study. However, nothing was said about development of tolerance.

Lombroso & Forsythe (1960) investigated 91 patients with absences as their only seizure type. Although the study mentions nothing in particular about EEG, since 80 of these patients were less than 12 years old it is conceivable that the majority may have suffered from typical absences. They had all experienced treatment failure on at least one conventional antiepileptic drug before receiving AZM. Forty-eight were treated with AZM monotherapy, the group in which the effect of AZM against absences can be most clearly documented. After three months' treatment nine patients (40%) had experienced at least a 99% reduction in seizure frequency, while 23 (48%) had at least a 90% reduction. After one year 17 (35%) were 99% absence free and eight (17%) had at least a 90% reduction. After two years' AZM treatment the figures were 10 (21%) 99% seizure-free and four (8%) 90% controlled; by three years this had changed to eight (17%) 99% controlled and two (4%) 90% seizure-free. In the group of 43 patients receiving AZM as add-on treatment the results were identical to those in the monotherapy treatment group.

The results of this study demonstrate one of the major drawbacks of AZM, the development of tolerance observed in other studies (Ansell & Clark, 1956; Lombroso et al, 1956). This problem seriously limits the efficacy of AZM in the treatment of epilepsy. It has been claimed that the frequency of tolerance development may be diminished if AZM is used as add-on treatment (Forsythe et al, 1981). However, apart from problems with toxicity, the development of tolerance is probably the main reason for the infrequent use of AZM in the treatment of epilepsy.

BENZODIAZEPINES

The first report of successful treatment of epilepsy with a benzodiazepine was by Naquet et al (1965), who treated status epilepticus with intravenous diazepam. Since then a number of benzodiazepines have been applied in the treatment of epilepsy. Several reviews of their use in epilepsy have appeared (Browne & Penry, 1983; Robertson, 1986). With regard to treatment of typical absences, clonazepam (CZP) is by far the most extensively investigated benzodiazepine, including several controlled trials. Mikkelsen et al (1976) compared CZP and placebo in a single-blind cross-over trial, with two 4-week treatment periods, comprising 10 patients with therapy-resistant absences. CZP proved to be significantly better than placebo in that eight out of 10 patients became completely free of seizures, while one experienced more than a 75% reduction. However, nine out of 10 patients experienced side-effects during CZP treatment, mainly in the form of varying degrees of sedation. It should be noted that the duration of this trial was too short to evaluate the problem of development of tolerance to clonazepam.

Seventy-nine children with absences featured in a double-blind comparative trial of CZP and ethosuximide. The duration of treatment was 17 weeks. Unfortunately, the results of this study have only been published in abstract form (Sato et al, 1977), while an early phase of the study has been published in full (Dreifuss et al, 1975). A difference in completing the study was observed, since 91.7% of patients on ethosuximide and only 69.8% of patients on CZP completed the study. The main reason for withdrawal from CZP was behavioural changes in the form of hyper-activity. No further data concerning the results of this trial have been provided. However, the conclusion of the abstract seems to indicate that development of tolerance was observed during treatment with CZP.

In most other studies which have been performed with CZP it has been used as add-on treatment in cases with refractory epilepsy. In one of these studies combined treatment with CZP and valproate was investigated, also in patients with typical absences (Mireles & Leppik, 1985). The study comprised six patients with this seizure type, one experiencing a 75–100% reduction in seizures, four obtaining a 50–74% seizure reduction and one exhibiting unchanged seizure frequency during combined treatment with CZP, valproate and possible other concomitant drugs. Consequently, the investigators could not confirm the risk of developing absence status caused by combined treatment with CZP and valproate, which had been pointed out by others (Jeavons et al, 1977).

In order to try to improve the situation with regard to toxicity as well as tolerance development a 1,5-benzodiazepine has been synthesised, clobazam (CLB), which is used in the treatment of epilepsy. A number of controlled and open studies have confirmed the effect of CLB in various seizure types. Apparently with regard to toxicity this drug represents progress compared to CZP, while with regard to tolerance development CLB represents no improvement. Except one, the studies of CLB did not include patients with typical absences. The study of the Canadian Clobazam Cooperative Group (1991) comprised 53 patients with typical absences, but unfortunately the results are reported in such a way that it is impossible to interpret the specific effect of CLB on this particular seizure type.

LAMOTRIGINE

Lamotrigine (LTG) was recently introduced in the treatment of epilepsy. Several reviews of the drug have already appeared (Miller et al, 1986; Gram, 1989; Yuen, 1991; Goa et al, 1993). Like all other anti-epileptic drugs the initial controlled clinical testing of LTG has been performed in therapy-resistant patients with partial epilepsies and a number of placebo-controlled studies have confirmed the efficacy of LTG compared to placebo. However, reports have appeared which seem to suggest that LTG may be more effective in the treatment of generalised rather than partial epilepsies. Stewart et al (1992) reported on their treatment of 72 drug-resistant patients, four of whom had idiopathic generalised epilepsy, with LTG. While 30% of patients with partial seizures had a 50% reduction in seizures during treatment with LTG, two of the four with generalised epilepsy became seizure-free (for several years), while the other two patients experienced reductions in seizure frequency of more than 75%.

Timmings & Richens (1992) reported on treatment with LTG of 82 persons on a named patient basis. Of the patients with partial seizures, 48% obtained at least a 50% reduction in seizure frequency, while 79% of patients with idiopathic generalised epilepsy obtained this seizure reduction. Consequently, these data could point towards an effect of LTG in the treatment of typical absences. However, so far no formal studies addressing specifically this seizure type have been performed.

Richens & Yuen (1991) compiled the results, according to different seizure types, of 27 open studies of LTG, comparing the effect in the 12-week treatment period with a retrospective 12-week baseline. Of 24 patients with typical absences 46% obtained at least a 50% reduction. The only seizure types with better results were tonic-clonic and atypical absences, the latter seizure type being consistent with findings of another study (Gibbs et al, 1992). A number of studies which have so far only been reported in abstract form also seem to indicate that LTG is effective in the treatment of typical absences. Sander et al (1991) reported on treatment of 23 patients with refractory generalised seizures with multiple seizure types, of whom 19 had absences. This seizure type responded most favourably to LTG and one patient became seizure-free. Exactly the same result was obtained by Schlumberger et al (1992) in 58 children with uncontrolled epilepsy. Yuen & Rafter (1992) summarised the results of five paediatric studies of LTG totalling 323 children with refractory epilepsy. Although no details were provided in the abstract typical absences were one of the seizure types responding well to treatment with LTG.

A single report on the efficacy of combined treatment with LTG and valproate of intractable typical absences has appeared (Panayiotopoulos et al, 1993). Two patients, not responding to either valproate alone or combined with ethosuximide, became seizure-free on a combination of LTG and valproate. That the effect was not simply due to the well-known pharmacokinetic interaction between the drugs was demonstrated in that withdrawal of valproate resulted in seizure relapse, despite tripling the dose of LTG. At the same time, however, the authors report on two additional patients with the same seizure type who did not respond to combined treatment with LTG and valproate.

A recent paper reports on the effect of LTG in the treatment of myoclonic absences, a rare syndrome first identified by Tassinari et al (1969) (see also Ch. 23). This syndrome has distinct characteristics which allow its separation from typical childhood absences in that resistance to conventional treatment is an almost constant feature and it is often accompagnied by intellectual impairment. Manonmani & Wallace (1994) investigated eight patients with this syndrome, two of whom obtained at least a 75% reduction (defined as response) in myoclonic absences either on valproate alone or combined with ethosuximide. Of the six patients treated with LTG, three obtained a response when it was combined with valproate and ethosuximide, one on a combination of LTG and valproate and one on combined LTG, valproate and CZP, while one patient did not respond at all. The authors suggest further studies of the effect of LTG in this syndrome.

CONCLUSION

Acetazolamide may be a useful therapy for typical absences that have not responded to first-line drugs, although tolerance may be a problem. Benzodiazepines may be helpful, but tolerance is a common problem, and clonazepam in particular has been associated with behavioural disturbance. Anecdotal and uncontrolled data suggest that lamotrigine may be effective against typical absences. Controlled studies are required.

REFERENCES

Ansell B, Clark E 1956 Acetazolamide in the treatment of epilepsy. British Medical Journal 1: 650–661

Bergstrøm WH, Garzoli RF, Lombroso C et al 1952 Observations on metabolism and clinical effect of carbonic anhydrase inhibitors in epileptics. American Journal of Diseases of Children 84: 71–74

Browne TR, Penry JK 1983 Benzodiazepines in the treatment of epilepsy. A review. Epilepsia 14: 277–310

Canadian Clobazam Cooperative Group 1991 Clobazam in treatment of refractory epilepsy: the Canadian experience. A retrospective study. Epilepsia 32: 407–416

Chiao DH, Plumb RL 1961 Diamox in epilepsy. A review of 178 cases. Journal of Pediatrics 58: 211–218

Dreifuss FE, Penry JK, Rose SW et al 1975 Serum clonazepam concentrations in children with absence seizures. Neurology 25: 255–258

Forsythe WI, Owens JR, Tothill C 1981 Effectiveness of acetazolamide in the treatment of carbamazepine-resistant epilepsy in children. Developmental Medicine and Child Neurology 23: 761–769

Gibbs J, Appleton RE, Rosenbloom L et al 1992 Lamotrigine for intractable childhood epilepsy. A preliminary communication. Developmental Medicine and Child Neurology 34: 368–371

Goa KL, Ross SR, Chrisp P 1993 Lamotrigine. A review of its pharmacological and clinical efficacy in epilepsy. Drugs 46: 152–176

Gram L 1989 Potential new antiepileptic drugs: Lamotrigine. In: Levy RH, Mattson R, Meldrum BS et al (eds) Antiepileptic Drugs, 3rd edn. Raven Press, New York, pp947–953

Holowach J, Thurston DL 1958 A clinical evaluation of acetazolamide (Diamox) in the treatment of epilepsy in children. Journal of Pediatrics 53: 160–171

Jeavons PM, Clark JE, Maheshwari MC 1977 Treatment of generalized epilepsies of childhood and adolescence with valproate ("Epilim"). Developmental Medicine and Child Neurology 19: 9–25

Lombroso CT, Forsythe I 1969 Long-term follow-up of acetazolamide (diamox) in the treatment of epilepsy. Epilepsia 1: 493–500

Lombroso CT, Davidson DT, Grossi-Bianchi ML 1956 Further evaluation of acetazolamide (diamox) in the treatment of epilepsy. Epilepsia 1: 493–500

Manonmani V, Wallace SJ 1994 Epilepsy with myoclonic absences. Archives of Diseases in Childhood 70: 288–290

Mikkelsen B, Birket-Smith E, Brandt S et al 1976 Clonazepam in the treatment of epilepsy. Archives of Neurology 33: 322–325

Miller AA, Sawyer DA, Roth B et al 1986 Lamotrigine. In: Meldrum BS, Porter RJ (eds) New anticonvulsant drugs. John Libbey, London, pp165–177

Mireles R, Leppik IE 1985 Valproate and clonazepam comedication in patients with intractable epilepsy. Epilepsia 26: 122–126

Naquet R, Soulayrol R, Keogh HJ et al 1965 First attempt at treatment of experimental status epilepticus in animals and spontaneous status epilepticus in man with diazepam (valium). Electroencephalography and Clinical Neurophysiology 18: 427

Panayiotopoulos CP, Ferrie CD, Knott C, Robinson RO 1993 Interaction of lamotrigine with sodium valproate. Lancet 341: 445

Richens A, Yuen AWC 1991 Overview of the clinical efficacy of lamotrigine. Epilepsia 32 (Suppl. 2): S13–S16

Robertson MM 1986 Current status of the 1,4- and 1,5-benzodiazepines in the treatment of epilepsy. The place of clonazepam. Epilepsia 27 (Suppl. 1): S27–S41

Sander JWAS, Hart YM, Patsalos PN et al 1991 Lamotrigine in generalised seizures. Epilepsia 32 (Suppl. 1): 59

Sato S, Penry JK, Dreifuss FE et al 1977 Clonazepam in the treatment of absence seizures: a double-blind clinical trial. Neurology 27: 371

Schlumberger E, Chavew F, Dulac O 1992 Open study with lamotrigine (LTG) in child epilepsy. Seizure (Suppl. 1A) pp9–21

Stewart J, Hughes E, Reynolds EH 1992 Lamotrigine for generalised epilepsy. Lancet 340: 1223

Tassinari CA, Lyagoubi S, Santos V et al 1969 Etude des décharges de pointes ondes chez l'homme. II – Les aspects cliniques et électroencéphalographiques des absences myocloniques. Revue Neurologique 121: 379–383
Timmings PL, Richens A 1992 Lamotrigine in primary generalised epilepsy. Lancet 339: 1300
Yuen AWC 1991 Lamotrigine. In: Pisani F, Perucca E, Avanzini G et al (eds) New antiepileptic drugs. Epilepsy Research (Suppl. 3) Elsevier, Amsterdam.
Yuen AWC, Rafter JEW 1992 Lamotrigine (Lamictal) as add-on therapy in pediatric patients with treatment-resistant epilepsy: an overview. Epilepsia 33 (Suppl. 3): 82–83

DISCUSSION

Brodie: Is there anything more about lamotrigine and valproate that has not been said by Dr Gram?

Panayiotopoulos: We have found that eight of 14 patients with absences became seizure-free after the addition of lamotrigine to sodium valproate.

Marescaux: In a few children we got the same surprising effect, seeing their seizures disappear after adding a small dose of lamotrigine to valproate. In rats we found that lamotrigine potentiates the effect of valproic acid, but only to a very small extent. I think it is something completely different to what we see in humans. We find a tendency to potentiation but nothing comparable to what we see in humans.

Stephenson: We used to use ethosuximide as the first choice for typical absences. One reason was that supposedly we would be able to see if somebody got other seizure types, tonic-clonic and myoclonic, which we might not do with certain other drugs. I have been concerned about the side-effects of ethosuximide, which might be more than any serious toxicity with valproate, such as lupus erythematosus and agranulocytosis.

E Andermann: I should like to comment on the question of teratogenicity. We have all heard that polytherapy is bad for teratogenic effects, but with valproic acid this does not seem to be generally the case, unlike most other drugs. There have been a number of studies that have shown this, the first being by Lindhout and Schmidt which clearly showed that with valproate monotherapy the risk of neural tube defects was 2.5% versus 1% in polytherapy. The reason for this is probably because when valproate is used in polytherapy, especially with phenytoin and also with the barbiturates and carbamazepine, the valproate levels are much lower. We have recently been able to show that there is a significant correlation between the plasma level of valproate and teratogenicity.

However, there are a number of other factors to be considered. One is the pharmacogenetic susceptibility to these malformations. We have had several patients who have had neural tube defects repeatedly picked up on ultrasound in their pregnancies who have been on very low levels of valproate (e.g., 750 mg per day). I believe that these patients have some kind of genetic abnormality in the way that they metabolise valproate, as this has been shown for phenytoin. It is much more difficult to demonstrate with valproate because of the more complex ways that valproate can be metabolised.

The vast majority of pregnancies on valproate result in normal children and those that are abnormal can be picked up quite early now with high-definition ultrasound for the neural tube defects and fetal echocardiogram for the cardiac defects.

Finally, pre-pregnancy and periconceptional folate definitely reduces the risk significantly not only of neural tube defects but of other malformations, by about two-thirds.

Sanofi Winthrop: Sanofi Winthrop are collaborating with Wellcome in a study of idiopathic generalised epilepsy, a comparative study of valproate versus lamotrigine. I was interested to hear Dr Andermann's comments about teratogenicity and plasma concentration. I find it surprising that there was a reduced incidence of teratogenicity with polytherapy. I do not think it can be ascribed solely to the reduced concentrations of valproate but I would be very interested to see the data on plasma concentrations.

Marescaux: Professor Richens says that he believes that typical absences which do not react to valproic acid must be considered as a separate group, as something not as typical as classical typical absences. Is the pharmacological reaction some new way of thinking about classification of absences, or should we believe that it may be only a metabolic point of view, that these are people who are unable to tolerate adequate doses of valproic acid?

Does anybody know if the potentiation that Dr Panayiotopoulos described with the combination of valproic acid and lamotrigine is also seen for negative effects? Is there an increased risk for teratogenicity in patients using lamotrigine simultaneously with valproic acid?

Duncan: We described three patients in the Lancet in 1993 who had significant side-effects with the combination of valproate and lamotrigine. Their seizures got better; they did not have typical absences. The concentrations of valproate and lamotrigine were not that high, but they all had incapacitating tremor such that they could not walk, could not feed themselves, had gross nystagmus and ataxia. We have no data, however, with regard to teratogenicity.

Richens: There was a question to my pharmacological classification of the absences. I think the answer is no. All I was hinting at was that in the literature there is the fairly strong suggestion that typical absences respond better to valproate or to ethosuximide than do other types of absences. I was not suggesting that we could classify them in pharmacological terms.

F Andermann: First a comment about driving and some of these problems. In Canada myoclonus is not a bar to driving.

Second, adult patients who have occasional absences are not uncommon.

These represent a particular problem because they do not want to take medication, they say that they have occasional absences, but they may have more, and they vigorously resist all attempts to have them take medication, and in fact it may not be reasonable to insist on this. I do not know what we can do about this. Theoretically they are not allowed to drive, but these people represent a definite sub-group who are not dealt with specifically.

Thirdly, in Canada a driving licence is restored after one full year seizure-free, including absence. But if the doctor reduces the medication and they have any recurrence it is three months suspension after the dose is increased again.

Finally, lamotrigine is probably a useful anti-absence agent and it is pleasing that it is now to be formally evaluated in idiopathic generalised epilepsy.

Gram: A major problem with valproate is weight gain and if we have a new compound which is as effective as valproate and does not have this side-effect this could be a very welcome competitor.

43. Gabapentin and felbamate

David Chadwick

The quality and quantity of published information on the therapeutic effects of any anti-epileptic drugs in typical absence is poor. There are, to the author's knowledge, no randomised placebo-controlled studies of established anti-epileptic drugs against absence seizures and only three studies have compared the efficacy of sodium valproate and ethosuximide (Suzuki et al, 1972; Callaghan et al, 1982; Sato et al, 1982).

There are a number of obvious reasons for this deficit. Absence seizures are uncommon outside childhood and, until recently, there have been considerable ethical reservations about including children in randomised controlled trials of anti-epileptic drugs. Furthermore, typical absences are readily suppressed by existing drugs such as ethosuximide and valproate; thus, there is no major incentive to test agents in this seizure type. The relative rarity of absence epilepsy syndromes and the satisfactory drug response means that it is extremely difficult to collect sufficient numbers of newly diagnosed (incident) cases or drug-resistant (prevalent) cases to mount statistical trials with sufficient power to determine effects.

The measurement of outcome presents further difficulties. Typical absence seizures are brief and can be frequent and are therefore extremely difficult to count and to document adequately. Certainly, clinical seizure frequency counts are likely to be somewhat unreliable and the only alternative would be some form of ambulatory or video-telemetry monitoring with quantification of spike-wave activity in the EEG. This has been pursued by Sato et al (1982).

It is, nevertheless, important to consider the potential effectiveness or otherwise of new anti-epileptic drugs in those syndromes of idiopathic generalised epilepsy that include typical absence seizures. Once anti-epileptic drugs are licensed and introduced to the market they may be given to patients with such seizure types before there is satisfactory definition of the spectrum of activity of the anti-epileptic drug. This on the one hand could be potentially harmful in that some drugs anecdotally seem capable of exacerbating absence seizures (which has been the author's experience with vigabatrin).

GABAPENTIN

Gabapentin was originally designed as a GABA analogue but it cannot be shown to have significant GABA-ergic activity (Chadwick, 1994). The drug has been licensed in a number of countries consequent on studies showing efficacy against partial seizures with or without secondary generalisation. Early open studies, however, suggested that some patients with frequent absence seizures experienced some improvement (Bauer et al, 1989). Because of this a large randomised parallel group study of gabapentin 1200 mg per day compared with placebo as add-on treatment was commenced in patients with refractory generalised epilepsies, at the same time as the UK Gabapentin Study Group commenced a similarly designed study in partial epilepsy (UK Gabapentin UK Study Group, 1990).

The study in generalised epilepsies has not yet been reported but preliminary analyses have been undertaken. In all, 129 patients were randomised, 71 to placebo and 58 to gabapentin. Fifty-seven patients in the placebo group were reported to have absence seizures and 42 in the gabapentin group. The primary outcome variable in this study was the number of primary generalised tonic-clonic seizures but counting of absence and myoclonic seizures was also undertaken. For tonic-clonic seizures 17.5% of patients receiving placebo showed a 50% or greater reduction following randomisation compared to 27.5% of patients randomised to gabapentin. These differences just failed to reach statistical significance. For absence seizures there was a small reduction following randomisation in both the placebo and gabapentin groups. When this was expressed as an RR ratio, mean RR ratio for placebo was -0.078 compared to -0.117 on gabapentin. The response ratio is a normally distributed function of the change from baseline (B) to treatment (T) seizure frequency such that the response ratio RR $= T-B/T+B$. It can be seen that the differences are small and certainly of no clinical significance. This is, to the author's knowledge, the only satisfactory data from a randomised controlled trial in absence seizures.

There is a further unpublished study which compared 15–20 mg/kg/day gabapentin with placebo in a parallel group study in 33 children with EEG quantification of bursts of 3 Hz spike-wave in excess of 1 s in a 24-h EEG and a diagnosis of previously untreated absence seizures. Both gabapentin and placebo were associated with a small reduction in the amount of spike-wave in the EEG but there were no statistically significant differences.

FELBAMATE

Felbamate is a dicarbamate whose precise mode of action remains unclear. The pharmacokinetics and potential interactions with this drug are considerable and greatly complicate assessment of its efficacy. Plasma concentrations of felbamate are increased during co-administration of valproic acid and decreased with phenytoin and carbamazepine. Plasma concentrations of phenytoin and valproic acid are increased by felbamate, while those of carbamazepine are decreased. At the same time those of the carbamazepine-epoxide metabolite are increased (Patsalos & Duncan, 1994).

Felbamate has been licensed on the basis of a number of clinical trials in partial epilepsies. Some of these are of very novel designs which include periods of monotherapy in patients with relatively refractory partial epilepsy (Gram & Schmidt, 1993). The author is unaware of any randomised studies against typical absences but one study has been undertaken in the Lennox–Gastaut syndrome (Ritter et al, 1993). In this latter study children and adults diagnosed as having Lennox–Gastaut syndrome were randomised to add-on therapy with either felbamate or placebo. Doses of valproate and phenytoin were reduced prior to the commencement of the baseline phase. The primary outcome variables were close-circuit monitoring and EEG for restricted periods of time during the baseline and treatment phases and parents or guardians counting atonic seizures. Felbamate was associated with a mean 34% reduction of atonic seizures, compared with a 9% reduction on placebo. It is clear that patients in the study probably had atypical absences but there is no reporting of any effects on atypical absences and no clear reporting of potential pharmacokinetic interactions in this study. There have been no studies reported of efficacy against typical absences.

CONCLUSION

On the basis of current evidence it is not possible to recommend either gabapentin or felbamate for the treatment of the small numbers of children and adults with typical absences refractory to either ethosuximide or valproate.

EDITORS' NOTE

Felbamate has since been withdrawn in Europe and has a restricted licence in the USA because of an incidence of aplastic anaemia of approximately 1 in 10 000 and reports of cases of liver failure.

REFERENCES

Suzuki M, Maruyama H, Ishibashi Y et al 1972 A double-blind comparative trial of sodium dipropylacetate and ethosuximide in epilepsy in children with special emphasis on pure petit mal seizures. Medical Progress 82:470–488 (in Japanese)
Callaghan N, O'Hare J, O'Driscoll D et al 1982 Comparative study of ethosuximide and sodium valproate in the treatment of typical absence seizures (petit mal). Developmental Medicine and Child Neurology 24: 830–836
Sato S, White BG, Penry JK et al 1982 Valproic acid versus ethosuximide in the treatment of absence seizures. Neurology 32:157–163
Chadwick D 1994 Gabapentin. Lancet 343:89–91
Bauer G, Bechinger D, Castell M, Deisenhammer E et al 1989 Clinical studies with gabapentin. Advances in Epileptology 17: 219–220
Gram L, Schmidt D 1993 Innovative designs of controlled clinical trials in epilepsy. Epilepsia 34 (Suppl. 7): S1–S6

UK Gabapentin Study Group (Andrews J, Chadwick D, Bates D et al) 1990 Gabapentin in partial epilepsy. Lancet i: 1114–1117

Patsalos PN, Duncan JS 1994 New antiepileptic drugs. A review of their current status and clinical potential. CNS Drugs 2: 40–77

Ritter FJ, Leppik IE, Dreifuss FE et al 1993 Efficacy of felbamate in childhood epileptic encephalopathy (Lennox–Gastaut syndrome). New England Journal of Medicine 1993; 328:29–33

DISCUSSION

Berkovic: The dose of gabapentin in that study was 1200 mg. May higher doses be beneficial in absences?

Duncan: I do not know the answer to that question. Certainly in the partial seizures one sees a dose response relationship and 2400 mg/day is better than 1200 mg/day. I do not know of any study or anecdotal experience where larger doses have been used for typical absences and I do not think the data is available.

Member of audience: We did a study in newly diagnosed typical absence with up to 1800 mg and it really was no better.

Berkovic: Vigabatrin is a good drug for partial seizures but does not work too well in generalised seizures. Is it your opinion that it is not worth trying in patients with refractory absences?

Duncan: It has been my experience that it can be positively dangerous. I have had more than one patient in whom I have made a wrong syndromic diagnosis; I thought they had partial and secondary generalised seizures and not absences and GTCS. They were on carbamazepine and valproate and I switched the valproate to vigabatrin and they developed status myoclonicus and absence status.

F Andermann: A question arises about the compliance of subjects. There are drugs that patients do not like to take because they make them uncomfortable. The question is, how much of the variability between drugs may be due to differential compliance and how do we evaluate that?

Brodie: Compliance is something we keep under the carpet. We are all aware that compliance in patients with seizure disorders is very variable and sometimes we get very unpleasant surprises. But it is very difficult to know what to do about it.

Duncan: Certainly in controlled trials one needs to do as rigorous a compliance check as one can, with tablet counts, counselling and surprise drug levels. In open studies it is even more of a problem.

Brodie: What sort of experience do our American colleagues have with felbamate in typical absences?

Dreifuss: I can only give you anecdotal information because there have not been any randomised studies to date on absence seizures. The effects are quite variable. Some people have reported it works very well and others have not found any significant effect.

In my own experience we have had some remarkably effective experiences with patients who have had absence seizures for years, uncontrolled by standard medications, who suddenly stopped having them after the introduction of felbamate. As far as the atypical absences are concerned, certainly in the ones with Lennox–Gastaut syndrome, they are so variable from day to day in their natural history that the patient may have 50 or 60 one day and none the next. We found them extremely difficult to estimate with any kind of statistical validity and therefore preferred not to assign any particular percentage improvement, although there was some tendency toward improvement while on the medication.

Marescaux: Listening to these presentations, it occurs to me that there is a tremendous difference between the average child with good intelligence and easily controlled typical absences, and what have been called people with uncontrollable absence. They are a very special group of individuals and there are several questions about background activity, about their intelligence, about their various risk factors. With these people it is hard to know whether it is post hoc or what but they are really quite a different group of patients compared with the majority of people who have typical absences, and yet nobody has ever looked at this critically that I know of.

Panayiotopoulos: Certain drugs not only are not helpful, but they exaggerate absences. For instance, the animal experiments with carbamazepine and phenytoin. I wonder if we can address what these drugs do in clinical practice.

The problem in clinical trials with absences is that clinically one cannot count them. Recently we evaluated the Monolog device which can count spike and slow-wave activity through 24 h. It is not accurate for numbers of events, but it is very good on the duration of the spike and slow-wave activity and we found it highly accurate.

Brodie: I agree that we become fixated on the patients who have responded well to medication and we are missing out a great deal of information on those who get worse. We should perhaps concentrate also on these patients – not just specifically on their seizure types, but on what it is telling us about the modes of action of the drugs and the pathophysiology of the seizures. This is an area that has a lot to teach us if we are prepared to look at it and gather data in a more consistent fashion.

44. The treatment of typical absences and related epileptic syndromes – consensus statement

Martin J. Brodie

The aim of management in all patients with typical absences and related epileptic syndromes should be complete seizure control without drug-related adverse effects. The treatment of choice is sodium valproate since it is not possible to predict at presentation whether the patient will go on to develop myoclonic jerks or generalised tonic-clonic seizures. These seizure types can be expected to complicate the clinical picture in 30–40% of cases. A small minority of participants favoured initial therapy with ethosuximide in patients with uncomplicated typical absences, particularly girls, to avoid the possibility of excessive weight-gain and later teratogenesis. This approach may also be appropriate for children under three years of age, in whom there is a small risk of microvesicular steatosis with valproate. Sodium valproate would be substituted if the patient experienced another seizure type.

An occasional patient reporting very few typical absences may not require pharmacotherapy at all. Everyone agreed also that carbamazepine and phenytoin might exacerbate typical absences and should be discontinued whenever possible. Avoidance of precipitating stimuli, such as sleep deprivation and photo-sensitisation, seems a sensible precaution for those few patients in whom such a trigger can be identified. Patients with eyelid myoclonia may benefit from wearing coloured lenses. Counselling the patient and family on the aims of therapy and the importance of total compliance with medication was regarded as an essential part of routine management.

OTHER STRATEGIES

If valproate is not well tolerated by a patient with only typical absences, ethosuximide should be substituted. If ethosuximide itself is not tolerated, methsuximide could be a useful alternative in those countries in which it is licensed. If valproate is not wholly effective but is well tolerated, combining the two drugs is regarded as a logical next step. This is likely to be necessary for the treatment of eyelid myoclonia with typical absences, which does not usually respond fully to monotherapy with either valproate or ethosuximide. If the seizure disorder remains refractory, a combination of valproate and lamotrigine may be tried. Preliminary anecdotal reports have suggested that these drugs may be synergistic for this clinical indication. If these strategies are unsuccessful, other possible options include prescribing sodium valproate together with clobazam or triple therapy with valproate, ethosuximide and lamotrigine. Some people also recommend the use of acetazolamide and lorazepam as alternative adjunctive therapy in refractory cases.

It is agreed that all drugs should be introduced at low dosage and titrated slowly according to clinical response and the emergence of side-effects. Potential side-effects should be discussed at an early stage with the patient and his or her family to anticipate later problems, and to allow for the development of tolerance, particularly to somnolence. If seizures persist despite all the pharmacological measures previously discussed, it is important to consider quality of life. In some patients optimal management means as few seizures as possible, without the intolerable burden of drug toxicity.

MONITORING

If a child or adolescent is seizure-free according to his or her own testimony and that of the parents and teacher, then little more needs to be done. Most participants would also arrange a routine surface EEG at this stage to ensure that the trace is free of 3 Hz per s spike-wave activity. If there is uncertainty as to the quality of seizure control, some participants would ask the patient to count his or her breaths while hyperventilating for three minutes to try to trigger a typical absence; others would undertake 24 h EEG telemetry. All would measure anti-epileptic drug concentrations to ensure good compliance with medication. In children, evidence from school is also considered essential. Behaviour, vigilance, attention, academic performance and social skills all need to be discussed with teachers.

DISCONTINUING TREATMENT

In pure childhood absence epilepsy drug therapy can be withdrawn in a seizure-free patient after 2–3 years. Around 10–15% of such patients can be expected to relapse. If the patient has a myoclonic syndrome, withdrawal of medication should not be contemplated until he or she has been free from all epileptic events for at least five years, as the prognosis is known to be less good.

There was some discussion about the time over which a drug should be discontinued. Opinions range from six weeks to six months. The lower figure is acceptable for patients with just typical absences, while a longer timescale should be employed in patients with other syndromes. If myoclonic seizures are a feature, drug withdrawal should be slower and with smaller dosage reductions. Therapy should be returned rapidly to the status quo if the patient develops myoclonic jerks. In all patients, one drug should be withdrawn at a time.

FURTHER RESEARCH

Sodium valproate (tremor, weight-gain, hair-loss, teratogenesis, hepatotoxicity, thrombocytopenia, pancreatitis) and ethosuximide (gastro-intestinal intolerance, headache, drowsiness, psychosis, rashes, lupus-like syndrome, blood dyscrasias) have many side-effects and are not effective in all patients. Lamotrigine (headache, nausea and vomiting, dizziness, rash) is not yet licensed for absence syndromes as no controlled clinical trials have been undertaken for these seizure types. Clobazam is sedative and tolerance develops in some patients. All participants agreed that sodium valproate and, in certain circumstances, ethosuximide are currently the treatment of choice, but new anti-epileptic drugs for the treatment of typical absences and related epileptic syndromes are awaited with interest. Ideally, these should have a broad spectrum, to cover (and also to be effective against) concomitant myoclonic and tonic-clonic seizures.

Index